Optical Diagnostics and Imaging

Optical Diagnostics and Imaging

Editor: Macie Holloway

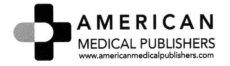

AMERICAN
MEDICAL PUBLISHERS
www.americanmedicalpublishers.com

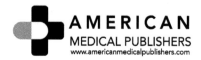

AMERICAN
MEDICAL PUBLISHERS
www.americanmedicalpublishers.com

Cataloging-in-Publication Data

Optical diagnostics and imaging / edited by Macie Holloway.
   p. cm.
Includes bibliographical references and index.
ISBN 978-1-63927-769-8
1. Optical fiber detectors--Diagnostic use. 2. Lasers--Diagnostic use. 3. Lasers--Therapeutic use.
4. Diagnostic imaging. 5. Optical fibers in medicine. 6. Lasers in medicine. 7. Imaging systems in medicine.
I. Holloway, Macie.
R857.O6 O68 2023
616.075 4--dc23

American Medical Publishers,
41 Flatbush Avenue,
1st Floor, New York,
NY 11217, USA

ISBN 978-1-63927-769-8 (Hardback)

Contents

Preface

Over the recent decade, advancements and applications have progressed exponentially. This has led to the increased interest in this field and projects are being conducted to enhance knowledge. The main objective of this book is to present some of the critical challenges and provide insights into possible solutions. This book will answer the varied questions that arise in the field and also provide an increased scope for furthering studies.

Light-based technologies help diagnose an array of pathological disorders of biological tissues. Innovation and progress in the field of medical science and technologies has enabled medical practitioners to identify various diseases in a non-invasive manner in the initial stages. The optical technologies use laser radiation to capture light-tissue interaction, which helps in obtaining information with respect to the morphological structure and biochemical state of the body area that has been examined. In optical diagnostics, light is passed through the tissues of particular organs of a patient under investigation using optical radiation and the results are recorded. Several imaging and spectroscopic techniques are used in optical non-invasive diagnostics such as laser speckle contrast imaging, optical coherence tomography, optoacoustic tomography, near infrared spectrophotometry, confocal spectroscopy, and fluorescence spectroscopy and imaging. The book aims to shed light on some of the unexplored aspects of optical diagnostics and imaging, and the recent researches in this field. Those with an interest in this field would find this book helpful.

I hope that this book, with its visionary approach, will be a valuable addition and will promote interest among readers. Each of the authors has provided their extraordinary competence in their specific fields by providing different perspectives as they come from diverse nations and regions. I thank them for their contributions.

Editor

Optical Density Optimization of Malaria Pan Rapid Diagnostic Test Strips for Improved Test Zone Band Intensity

Prince Manta [1][ID], Rupak Nagraik [2], Avinash Sharma [2], Akshay Kumar [3], Pritt Verma [4], Shravan Kumar Paswan [4], Dmitry O. Bokov [5], Juber Dastagir Shaikh [6], Roopvir Kaur [7], Ana Francesca Vommaro Leite [8][ID], Silas Jose Braz Filho [8], Nimisha Shiwalkar [9][ID], Purnadeo Persaud [10] and Deepak N. Kapoor [1],*

[1] School of Pharmaceutical Sciences, Shoolini University of Biotechnology and Management Sciences, Solan 173212, India; princemanta@gmail.com

[2] School of Bioengineering and Food Technology, Shoolini University of Biotechnology and Management Sciences, Solan 173212, India; rupak.nagraik@gmail.com (R.N.); avinashsubms@gmail.com (A.S.)

[3] Department of Surgery, Medanta Hospital, Gurugram 122001, India; drakshay82@gmail.com

[4] Departments of Pharmacology, CSIR-National Botanical Research Institute, Lucknow 226001, India; preetverma06@gmail.com (P.V.); paswanshravan@gmail.com (S.K.P.)

[5] Institute of Pharmacy, Sechenov First Moscow State Medical University,8 Trubetskaya St., Moscow 119991, Russia; bokov_d_o@staff.sechenov.ru

[6] Department of Neurology, MGM Newbombay Hospital, Vashi, Navi Mumbai 400703, India; jubershaikh703@yahoo.com

[7] Department of Anesthesiology, Government Medical College, Amritsar 143001, India; roopvirsaini@gmail.com

[8] Department of Medicine, University of Minas Gerais, Passos 37902-313, Brazil; francescavommaroleite@gmail.com (A.F.V.L.); silasbrazf@gmail.com (S.J.B.F.)

[9] Department of Anesthesiology, MGM Hospital, Navi Mumbai 410209, India; dr.nimisha4u@gmail.com

[10] Department of Medicine, Kansas City University, Kansas City, MO 64106, USA; narpaulpersaud@hotmail.com

* Correspondence: deepakpharmatech@gmail.com

Abstract: For the last few decades, the immunochromatographic assay has been used for the rapid detection of biological markers in infectious diseases in humans and animals The assay, also known as lateral flow assay, is utilized for the detection of antigen or antibody in human infectious diseases. There are a series of steps involved in the development of these immuno-chromatographic test kits, from gold nano colloids preparation to nitrocellulose membrane coating (NCM). These tests are mostly used for qualitative assays by a visual interpretation of results. For the interpretation of the results, the color intensity of the test zone is therefore very significant. Herein, the study was performed on a malaria antigen test kit. Several studies have reported the use of gold nanoparticles (AuNPs) with varying diameters and its binding with various concentrations of protein in order to optimize tests. However, none of these studies have reported how to fix (improve) test zone band intensity (color), if different sized AuNPs were synthesized during a reaction and when conjugated equally with same amount of protein. Herein, different AuNPs with average diameter ranging from 10 nm to 50 nm were prepared and conjugated equally with protein concentration of 150 µg/mL with $K_D = 1.0 \times 10^{-3}$. Afterwards, the developed kits' test zone band intensity for all different sizes AuNPs was fixed to the same band level (high) by utilization of an ultraviolet-visible spectrophotometer. The study found that the same optical density (OD) has the same test zone band intensity irrespective of AuNP size. This study also illustrates the use of absorption maxima (λ max) techniques to characterize AuNPs and to prevent wastage of protein while developing immunochromatographic test kits.

Keywords: lateral flow assay; immuno-chromatographic; gold nanoparticles sensor; UV/Vis spectrophotometer; malaria pan rapid diagnostic strip; point-of-care

1. Introduction

Malaria is caused by parasites that are transmitted to humans via the bites of the infected female Anopheles mosquito. While preventable and curable, it still remains a paramount cause of morbidity and mortality in developing countries. Malaria is estimated to kill between 1.5 to 2.7 million people annually [1]. Malaria morbidity is estimated at about 300–500 million annually, and malaria clinical diagnosis is most effective at 50%. Malaria immunoassays use the inherent sensitivity, specificity and binding affinity of antibodies to respective antigens for the detection of antigens in a sample. In immunoassays, the sample tested includes whole blood, urine, saliva, serum, etc. [2]. In the Malaria Pan Antigen rapid test kit, the sample used is Red Blood cells containing specific antigens of *P. vivex* and *P. malariae/P. ovale* [3]. The red blood cells get lysed by a buffer solution to allow antigen–antibody binding at the test site. Immunoassay signals emanate from the gold-labeled antibody set for the antigen on a substratum at the binding site (Test line). Typical antibody labels include fluorescent molecules, nano- or microparticles, or enzymes. Gold nanoparticles (NPs) are the most widely used label [4]. Such immunoassays can be used in industry, clinical or laboratory settings, doctor's offices, or as over-the-counter tests [2]. At the test line, the naked eye will see a gold-labelled marker as a pink/red line [5]. In most countries, the diagnosis of malaria challenges multiple laboratories [3]. The laboratories require longer than one hour to analyze the findings, leading to less consistency in the analysis of the results.

1.1. Components of Immuno-Chromatographic Test Kits

The Immuno-Chromatographic kit is composed of components shown in Figure 1. The parts of the kits are attached on an inert polyvinyl chloride (PVC) backing material and further packed in a plastic cassette with a specimen port and reaction window displaying the capture and control zones [2]. The Immunochromatographic Test Kit has a sample pad, conventionally composed of glass fibres. The sample pad is selected to have zero cross-reactivity with the specimen. The sample pad is pretreated with a buffer for specimen pH adjustment and extraction of unspecific antigen form specimens [6]. One of the vital parts of the strip is nitrocellulose membrane (NCM). In this, the interaction between antigen and antibody takes place. Typically, a hydrophobic nitrocellulose membrane is used on which anti-target analyte antibodies are immobilized in a line that crosses the membrane to act as a capture zone on the test line [2]. The NCM membrane should be chosen based upon pore size [7]. Other parts of test strips are glass fibres or non-woven fibres based conjugate pads which can be pre-treated to avoid any cross-reactivity [8]. Conclusively, the conjugate pad is prepared by dipping the glass fibers into a colloidal solution of gold protein and then used after drying. In addition, an absorbent pad is present in the kit, which is designed to collect extra specimen samples passing the reaction membrane [9].

1.2. The Protein

In the Malaria Pan immunoassay, antibody protein is used for AuNP conjugation. Plasmodium lactate dehydrogenase (pLDH) and goat anti-mouse (GAM) protein are used for binding at test and control lines, respectively. An ultraviolet-visible spectrophotometer optimization technique was demonstrated in this work by formulating an immuno-chromatographic detection kit for Malaria Pan using AuNPs as an indicator. Various research works attempted to optimize the AuNP size [10–13], and the AuNPs of about 30–40 nm were reported to be optimal [11,12]. Khlebtsov and Byzova et al. also tried to determine the optimum concentration of protein required for AuNP conjugation [14,15].

In present research, gold nanoparticles (AuNPs) were utilized as labels, and the concentration of AuNPs with conjugate antibodies was tailored to a fine-tuned optical density (OD). The gold nanoparticles of various sizes (10 nm to 50 nm) were prepared, by quantifying λ max (absorption maxima) and dynamic light scattering (DLS). The relationship of AuNP diameters with a concentration of target protein was monitored to develop a better test kit. Finally, the developed immuno-chromatographic test kit test zone band intensity was tested using RGB and HSV color models. The reason to select a malaria test kit for the study is to create a more cost-effective rapid diagnostic test kits because malaria cases are found in countries where cost-effectiveness is significant. The study aim to improve test band intensity irrespective of AuNP size using a fixed quantity of protein while optimizing the optical density.

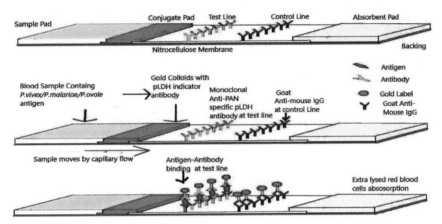

Figure 1. Presentation of lateral flow strip that works on sandwich assay. Blood sample lysed with buffer solution is added to the sample pad. *P. vivex/P. malariae/P. ovale* malaria antigens attach to antibodies in the red colored gold conjugate pad and the complex formed attaches to test line monoclonal anti-PAN specific pLDH antibodies. The excess labeled antibodies bind with Goat anti-mouse IgG antibodies in the control line. The extra lysed red blood cells get absorbed in the absorbent pad.

2. Materials and Methods

2.1. Reagents, Instruments and Other Support Materials

For the fabrication of immunochromatographic strip assay, sodium hydrogen phosphate, sucrose, disodium hydrogen phosphate, sodium chloride and bovine serum albumin (BSA) were purchased from Merck, Darmstadt, Germany. The gold chloride used for the synthesis of gold nanoparticles was purchased from Sigma-Aldrich, Tokyo, Japan. The Plasmodium lactate dehydrogenase (pLDH) antibodies' molecules and control line Goat anti-mouse protein were purchased from Fapon Biotech, Shenzhen, China. All the other chemicals and reagents used in the present study were of analytical grade reagents. The Delsa™ Nano Submicron Particle Size Zeta Potential instrument of Beckman Coulter, Brea, CA, USA was used for analyzing AuNP diameters. An ultraviolet-visible spectrophotometer 1900i of Shimadzu, Kyoto, Japan was used to measure optical density and absorbance maxima. The nitro cellulose membrane was coated with XYXYZ3210™ dispense platform of Bio-dot, Irvine, CA, USA. The centrifuge of Remi RM-12C, Mumbai, India was utilized for AuNP–protein conjugate centrifugation, and the magnetic stirrer of Remi, Mumbai, India was also used in the study. The nitrocellulose membrane was purchased form Nupore System Pvt. Ltd., Ghaziabad, India and Glass fibre sample pad and conjugate pad were purchased from Advanced Micro Devices, Ambala, India.

2.2. Experimental

2.2.1. Preparation of Gold Nanoparticles (AuNPs)

The gold nanoparticles were prepared by classical classical Turkevich and Fern methods by citrate reduction. In general, the Turkevich and Fern process reaction leads to formation of AuNPs of size range 10 nm to 100 nm [16,17]. Utilizing raw gold chloride (AuHCl$_4$) [18], the 1% light yellowish color solution was prepared by dissolving 1 gm of gold chloride in 100 mL of ultra-mili-Q water. The aforementioned 1% gold solution was furthermore dissolved into ultra-milli-Q water in order to obtain the optical density between 0.7 and 0.9 at λ max (absorption maxima) by taking a solution spectrum scan at wavelength between 700 nm and 400 nm. Now, the final gold solution had been refluxed for 30 min at 100 °C. The above-diluted gold solution was reduced by adding 1% (1 g of sodium citrate in 100 mL of water) sodium citrate solution of pH 7.80 ± 0.5 with refluxing until bright red color develops. Initially, the addition of a 1% solution of sodium citrate turns the color of the solution black. The color change from mildly yellowish to brick red confirms the synthesis of nanoparticles. The change in colour solution is due to the surface plasmon resonance effect (SPR) in which electrons excited to its higher state and produces a colour change. During the reduction mechanism, metal salts get converted into their ionic form when it combines with water. Different chemical functional groups of reducing agents combine with metal ions whether they are bivalent or monovalent and reduce it into a zerovalent state of small size [19].

The color transforms from red to pink to blue as the reaction proceeds. As the solution color turns pink, the reaction was stopped by decreasing the temperature to room temperature in the ice bath. Particle size distribution of synthesized nanoparticles was analysed by dynamic light scattering.

The five gold nanoparticles of the sizes 10 nm, 20 nm, 30 nm, 40 nm and 50 nm were chosen for protein conjugation after AuNP characterisation. The prepared pink-colored gold solution was characterized by spectrophotometric absorbance maxima (λ max) by scanning in a visible wavelength range of 700 nm to 400 nm.

2.2.2. Protein Conjugation with Gold NPs

For all the above-prepared AuNPs of size 10 nm to 50 nm, pH was adjusted separately to 7.00 ± 0.1 with 0.2 M Potassium Carbonate solution of pH 12.00 ± 0.5. The pH adjustment is predicated on the protein's isoelectric point, which varies from protein to protein. The pH was measured with the help of pH paper. The antibody pLDH (Plasmodium lactate dehydrogenase) reagents have been diluted to 150 µg/mL from the stock solution with 10 mM of Sodium Dihydrogen Phosphate buffer of pH 8.50 ± 0.1. Afterwards, the protein pLDH of 150 µg/mL concentration was conjugated to all five AuNPs (10 nm to 50 nm). Conjugation of the AuNPs and protein was achieved by stirring the solution to 10 ± 2 min. Following this, 1% BSA (Bovine Serum Albumin) was added into the gold conjugate solution and stirred for 30 ± 2 min for stabilisation and abstraction of unbound protein. For all five sizes of AuNPs, the single tuned protein concentration was used to detect the effect of gold nanoparticle size on the band intensity of developed kits.

2.2.3. Centrifugation

The above five separately prepared AuNP–protein conjugate solutions were centrifuged. The centrifugation was performed with a Relative Centrifugal Force (RCF) of 7000× g for 45 min at 4 °C to 8 °C temperature. The centrifugation of an AuNPs–protein conjugate solution at a force higher than 7000× g RCF can sometimes shows aggregation while centrifugation at a force slower than 7000× g RCF may give less residue with a dark supernatant. Centrifugation at 7000× g RCF gives a stable and good yield of the residue or pellet. The supernatant's aspiration was performed in a different beaker, and gold pellets were resuspended in the phosphate-buffered saline (PBS) buffer. The absorbance of the supernatant was measured at a 520 nm wavelength. If the OD was greater than 0.05, then the supernatant's re-centrifugation is performed one more time. The supernatant was discarded if the OD was less than 0.05. This will enable conjugate recovery and prevent wastage. The supernatant aspiration is performed in a separate beaker, accumulating the AnNP–protein pellets. Carefully, the supernatant aspiration and the residue re-suspension was accomplished in a re-suspension buffer. Figure 2 represents the protein conjugation and centrifugation procedure.

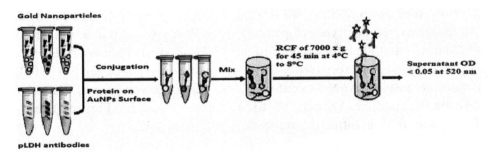

Figure 2. The diagrammatical representation of the protein conjugation and centrifugation methodology.

2.2.4. Conjugate Pad Prepration

All five separately re-suspended AuNPs—protein conjugate above solutions were diluted (ultra-pure mili-Q water) to a constant OD of 3.00 at 520 nm wavelength.

Following the dilution, five conjugate pads were prepared by dipping the glass fibre pad into the conjugate solution. In comparison, the other changes through the entire development of the kit was held constant, e.g., test line concentration and control line protein.

2.2.5. Membrane Coating

The five nitrocellulose membranes were coated at the test (Pan) and control line (C). The test and control line coating on the nitrocellulose membrane (NCM) was achieved with the use of a Bio-dot dispensing machine. First of all, the bio-dot machine stripping system (tubing and jets) was flushed with de-ionized water over ten cycles. The control and test solutions were then coated on NCMs. For drying, membrane sheets were kept in the oven at 30 °C for 30 min after coating. The concentrations of test and control line reagents were as follows:

2.2.6. Test Line Reagents Concentration

To obtain the final test solution, the pLDH (Plasmodium lactate dehydrogenase) antibody was diluted from the stock solution to 50 µg/mL with 1% sucrose solution in the PBS buffer. The antibody protein mixing in PBS buffer was performed with a magnetic stirrer, and a 0.22-micron filter was used to eliminate the suspended particles.

2.2.7. Control Line Reagents Concentration

To obtain the final control line solution, Goat Anti Mouse IgG was diluted from stock solution to 400 µg/mL with a 0.5 percent sucrose in the PBS buffer. To extract the suspended particles, mixing and filtration were achieved using a 0.22-micron filter.

3. Results and Discussion

3.1. Gold NP Characterization

Firstly, we prepared the most stable AuNPs of an average of of 10 nm to 50 nm in diameter. The AuNPs with absorbance maxima (λ max) ranging between 520 to 570 wavelengths were considered for the development of the Malaria Pan Antigen detection test kit. In this range of λ max, the AuNP size ranges from 10 nm to 50 nm as determined by the particle sizer. Figure 3A–E represent the AuNP size measured in dynamic light scattering (DLS). AuNPs of this range were selected due to their smaller particle size and lower polydispersity index (PDI). It has been observed that smaller sized nanoparticles have better conjugation with the protein [10–12,20]. The size of gold NPs depends on the sodium citrate content used [18]. The concentration of sodium citrate in gold solution affects the size of AuNPs, which can be controlled by measuring absorbance maxima (λ max). The sodium citrate of viz 0.2, 0.4, 0.6, 0.75 and 0.90 mg/mL in gold solutions produces nanoparticles (NPs) with average diameters of 10 nm (size distribution of 8 to 12 nm), 20 nm (size distribution of 17 to 23 nm),

30 nm (size distribution of 26 to 35 nm), 40 nm (size distribution of 32 to 50 nm) and 50 nm (size distribution of 36 to 80 nm), respectively (Figure 3). AuNPs shows λ max at varying wavelengths of 520 (10 nm), 530 (20 nm), 540 (30 nm), 560 (40 nm) and 570 (60 nm). Figure 4A–E represent the λ max of AuNPs. The optical density of prepared AuNPs at λ max ranges between 8.0 to 9.0. When sodium citrate concentration increases in AuNP solution, AuNP size does too. When the size of the gold NPs increases, the absorbance maxima (λ max) shift to higher wavelengths (Figure 5), and the color of the solution turns from pink to blue, reflecting nanoparticles' instability.

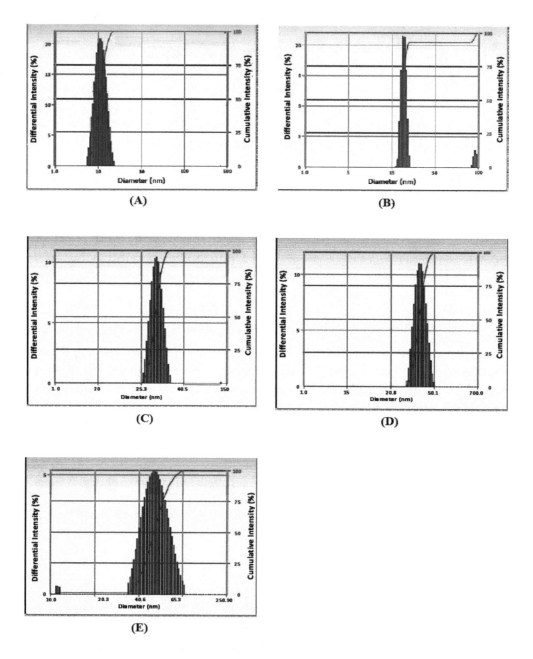

Figure 3. Synthesized gold nanoparticles' size distribution measured by the Zeta Seizer. The sodium citrate solutions of 0.2, 0.4, 0.6, 0.75 and 0.90 mg/mL in gold solutions' produced nanoparticles (NPs) with average diameters of **(A)** 10 nm (size distribution of 8 to 12 nm); **(B)** 20 nm (size distribution of 17 to 23 nm); **(C)** 30 nm (size distribution of 26 to 35 nm); **(D)** 40 nm (size distribution of 32 to 50 nm); and **(E)** 50 nm (size distribution of 36 to 80 nm).

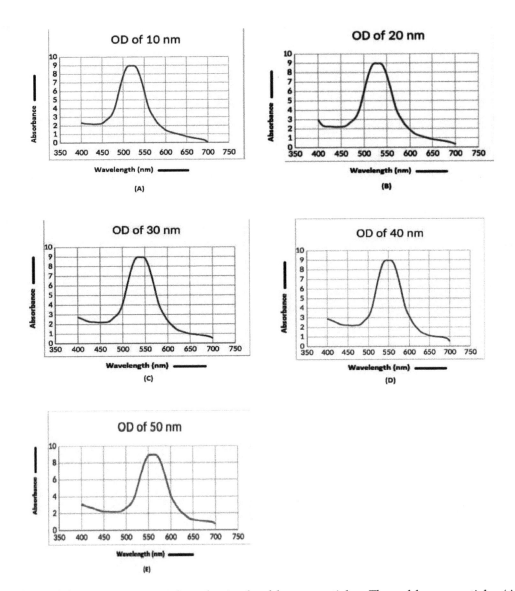

Figure 4. Optical density spectrum of synthesized gold nanoparticles. The gold nanoparticles (AUNPs) show different λ max (absorbance maxima) at different sizes; i.e., **(A)** λ max 520 nm at diameter of 10 nm; **(B)** λ max 530 nm at diameter of 20 nm; **(C)** λ max 540 nm at diameter of 30 nm; **(D)** λ max 560 nm at diameter of 40 nm; **(E)** λ max 570 nm at diameter of 50 nm.

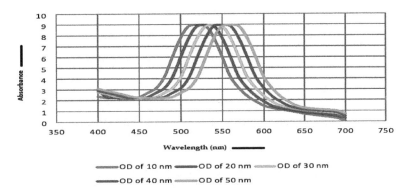

Figure 5. The graph shows a correlation of synthesized gold nanoparticles (10 nm, 20 nm, 30 nm, 40 nm and 50 nm) λ max (absorbance maxima) and Optical Density. With an increase in the size of the gold NPs, the absorbance maxima (λ max) shifts to higher wavelengths (520 nm to 570 nm), reflecting nanoparticle instability.

As the average diameters increase, the nanoparticles' size distribution increases, which causes the instability of AuNPs (Figure 3). This technique is widely used for the determination of particle size in colloidal solution, which, in turn, used to measure the thickness of capping or stabilizing agent along with its actual size of metallic core. These studies also determined the hydrodynamic diameter of the synthesized nanoparticles. These results also suggested that there is an absence of large aggregates when these nanoparticles were dispersed in aqueous medium [21].

3.2. Monitoring the Protein Loss

After centrifigation of AuNP–protein conjugate, a small portion of re-suspended solution was diluted (1 in 100) into ultra-pure mili-Q water to facilitate OD measurement at 520 nm. The OD values obtained are shown in Table 1.

Table 1. Optical density (OD) measurement results of synthesized gold nanoparticles–protein centrifuged re-suspension conjugate solution when diluted in 1–100.

S. No.	Gold Nanoparticles (AuNP) Size	Optical Density (OD) Observation
1	10 nm	0.301
2	20 nm	0.354
3	30 nm	0.368
4	40 nm	0.426
5	50 nm	0.385

Figure 6 and Table 1 indicate that 40 nm AuNPs have high OD, and thus AuNPs have maximum protein binding with AuNPs of 40 nm size. In contrast, the other AuNPs had less binding. This indicates that the supernatant lost extra unbound protein. This means that the additional unbound protein was lost in the supernatant. The protein depletion can also be checked with the use of UV/Vis spectrophotometer OD analysis.

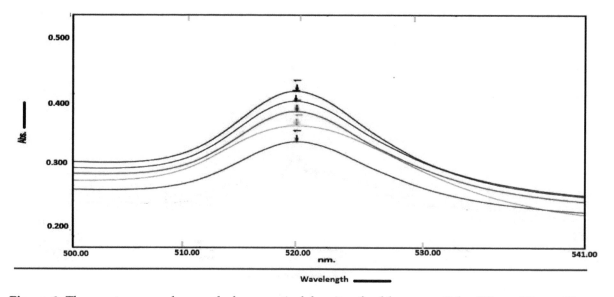

Figure 6. The spectrum overlay graph shows optical density of gold nanoparticles (10 nm, 20 nm, 30 nm, 40 nm and 50 nm) and protein conjugate solution (1–100 mL) measured at 520 nm of wavelength. The gold nanoparticles of average diameter of 40 nm have maximum optical density (0.426), which reflects the maximum protein binding.

3.3. Test Line Intensity Analysis

The developed kits were tested to find out the kit test zone band intensity (results) when equivalent protein ratios are conjugated with different AuNP sizes. The five immunochromatographic rapid test kits were formulated using a conjugate pad (10 nm to 50 nm) prepared above. Then, all five of the immunechromatographic test kits were assembled. Now, the five developed test kits were tested for band intensity using 5 μL of malaria (*P. vivax*) positive blood specimens of concentration 150 parasites/μL. The three specifications were given to test line viz. high test line intensity was ranked as +3, medium test line intensity was ranked as +2, and weak test line intensity was ranked as +1. Upon testing all kits with the same specimen samples, all kits showed an equal band intensity of +3 (high) as shown in Table 2. In this analysis, it was noticed that, if the final OD is tuned to one point, there will be no effects of AuNPs sizes on kit results (test zone intensity). OD-adjustment will refine the final test zone band intensity. Figure 7 is the systematic representation of the results. All five test kits developed after OD tuning to 3.0 were additionally verified for their specificity with 5 μL of Malaria Pf (Falciparum) antigen blood specimens of concentration 40 parasites/μL to find out test kit susceptibility for *P. Falciparum*. The specificity results of developed kits (Table 3) were found without any false positive indication (no Pan line appears), and the the control band intensity was high (+3).

Table 2. Test line intensity results of five Malaria Pan Ag immunochromatographic rapid test kits formulated using different diameter AuNPs. The kit final OD is tuned to one point (3.00) after conjugation with protein. Kit's test line intensity was tested using *P. vivax* positive blood specimen of a concentration of 150 parasites/μL. The band intensity for test (Pan) and control (C) line is ranked as: high test (+3), medium (+2) and weak (+1). Upon testing, all developed kits showed an equal sensitivity of +3 (high).

Test Zone Intensity of Kit Developed by 10 nm of AuNPs	Test Zone Intensity of Kit Developed by 20 nm of AuNPs	Test Zone Intensity of Kit Developed by 30 nm of AuNPs	Test Zone Intensity of Kit Developed by 40 nm of AuNPs	Test Zone Intensity of Kit Developed by 50 nm of AuNPs

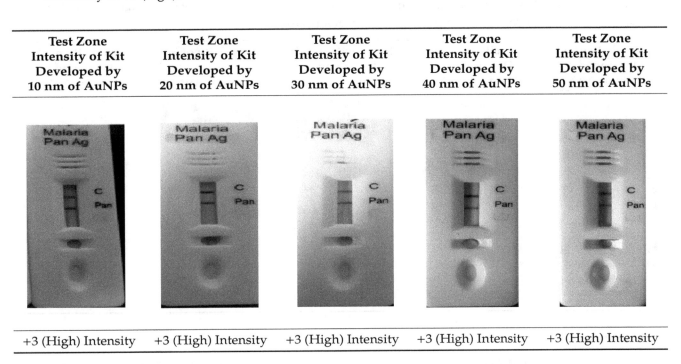

| +3 (High) Intensity | +3 (High) Intensity | +3 (High) Intensity | +3 (High) Intensity | +3 (High) Intensity |

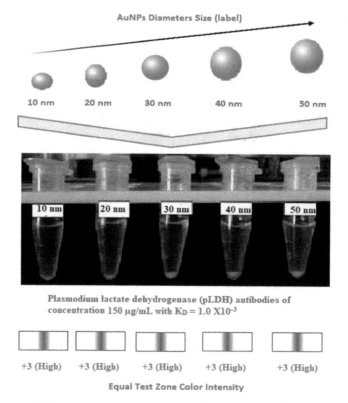

Figure 7. The diagram systematically represented the results.

Table 3. Specificity results of five Malaria Pan Ag immunochromatographic rapid test kits formulated using different sizes AuNPs. Kit's specificity was tested using *P. Falciparum* positive blood specimens of concentration 40 parasites/µL. The color band intensity for control (C) line was +3 (high) and no line appears on the test zone (Pan) indicating absence of any cross reactivity.

Specificity of Kit Developed by 10 nm of AuNPs	Specificity of Kit Developed by 20 nm of AuNPs	Specificity of Kit Developed by 30 nm of AuNPs	Specificity of Kit Developed by 40 nm of AuNPs	Specificity of Kit Developed by 50 nm of AuNPs

4. Conclusions

It can be concluded from the above study that the particle size of AuNPs has no effect on the test zone band intensity of Malaria Pan rapid diagnostic test kits if optical density of AuNP–protein conjugate is adjusted at 520 nm. The test zone band intensity was also observed to be maximum at 520 nm and optical density 3.0. It was found from the study that any quantity of protein can be utilized for AuNP conjugation, if the final optical density (OD) is adjusted correctly. It can also be concluded that, by optimizing the optical density, an enhanced test zone band intensity can be obtained while reducing the total number of trial and wastage of reagents.

Author Contributions: Conceptualization: P.M. and D.N.K.; Methodology: R.N and A.S.; Validation: A.K., J.D.S. and R.K.; Formal Analysis: A.F.V.L.; Investigation: S.J.B.F.; Data Curation: N.S.; Writing—Original Draft Preparation: P.M., R.N. and A.S.; Writing—Review and Editing: A.K.; Visualization: P.P.; Funding acquisition: D.O.B., S.K.P. and P.V.; Supervision: D.N.K. All authors have read and agreed to the published version of the manuscript.

References

1. Mishra, M.N.; Misra, R.N. Immunochromatographic methods in malaria diagnosis. *Med. J. Armed Forces India* **2007**, *63*, 127–129. [CrossRef]
2. Manta, P.; Agarwal, S.; Singh, G.; Bhamrah, S.S. Formulation, development and sensitivity, specificity comparison of gold, platinum and silver nano particle based HIV $\frac{1}{2}$ and hCG IVD rapid test kit (Immune chromatoghraphic test device). *World J. Pharm. Sci.* **2015**, *4*, 1870–1905.
3. Maltha, J.; Gillet, P.; Jacobs, J. Malaria rapid diagnostic tests in endemic settings. *Clin. Microbes Infect.* **2013**, *19*, 399–407. [CrossRef] [PubMed]
4. Koczula, K.M.; Gallotta, A. Lateral flow assays. *Essays Biochem.* **2016**, *60*, 111–120. [CrossRef] [PubMed]
5. Gronowski, A.M. *Handbook of Clinical Laboratory Testing during Pregnancy*; Springer Science & Business Media: Berlin, Germany, 2004. [CrossRef]
6. Benjamin, G.Y.; Bartholomew, B.; Abdullahi, J.; Labaran, L.M. Prevalence of Plasmodium falciparum and Haemoglobin Genotype Distribution among Malaria Patients in Zaria, Kaduna State, Nigeria. *South Asian J. Parasitol.* **2019**, *23*, 1–7. [CrossRef]
7. Ramachandran, S.; Singhal, M.; McKenzie, K.G.; Osborn, J.L.; Arjyal, A.; Dongol, S.; Baker, S.G.; Basnyat, B.; Farrar, J.; Dolecek, C.; et al. A rapid, multiplexed, high-throughput flow-through membrane immunoassay: A convenient alternative to ELISA. *Diagnosis* **2013**, *3*, 244–260. [CrossRef] [PubMed]
8. Tsai, T.T.; Huang, T.H.; Chen, C.A.; Ho, N.Y.; Chou, Y.J.; Chen, C.F. Development a stacking pad design for enhancing the sensitivity of lateral flow immunoassay. *Sci. Rep.* **2018**, *8*, 1–10. [CrossRef] [PubMed]
9. Wong, R.; Tse, H. *Lateral Flow Immunoassay*; Springer Science & Business Media: Berlin, Germany, 2008. [CrossRef]
10. Lou, S.; Ye, J.Y.; Li, K.Q.; Wu, A. A gold nanoparticle-based immunochromatographic assay: The influence of nanoparticulate size. *Analyst* **2012**, *137*, 1174–1181. [CrossRef] [PubMed]
11. Kim, D.S.; Kim, Y.T.; Hong, S.B.; Kim, J.; Heo, N.S.; Lee, M.K.; Lee, S.J.; Kim, B.I.; Kim, I.S.; Huh, Y.S.; et al. Development of lateral flow assay based on size-controlled gold nanoparticles for detection of hepatitis B surface antigen. *Sensors* **2016**, *16*, 2154. [CrossRef] [PubMed]
12. Fang, C.; Chen, Z.; Li, L.; Xia, J. Barcode lateral flow immunochromatographic strip for prostate acid phosphatase determination. *J. Pharm. Biomed. Anal.* **2011**, *56*, 1035–1040. [CrossRef] [PubMed]
13. Safenkova, I.; Zherdev, A.; Dzantiev, B. Factors influencing the detection limit of the lateral-flow sandwich immunoassay: A case study with potato virus X. *Anal. Bioanal. Chem.* **2012**, *403*, 1595–1605. [CrossRef] [PubMed]
14. Banerjee, S.; Gautam, R.K.; Jaiswal, A.; Chattopadhyaya, M.C.; Sharma, Y.C. Rapid scavenging of methylene blue dye from a liquid phase by adsorption on alumina nanoparticles. *RSC Adv.* **2015**, *5*, 14425–14440. [CrossRef]
15. Kaur, K.; Forrest, J.A. Influence of particle size on the binding activity of proteins adsorbed onto gold nanoparticles. *Langmuir* **2012**, *28*, 2736–2744. [CrossRef]
16. Turkevich, J.; Stevenson, P.C.; Hillier, J. A Study of the nucleation and growth processes in the synthesis of colloidal gold. Discuss. *Faraday Soc.* **1951**, *11*, 55–75. [CrossRef]
17. Frens, G. Controlled Nucleation for the Regulation of the Particle Size in Monodisperse Gold Suspensions. *Nat. Phys. Sci.* **1973**, *241*, 20–22. [CrossRef]
18. Khlebtsov, B.N.; Tumskiy, R.S.; Burov, A.M.; Pylaev, T.E. Quantifying the Numbers of Gold Nanoparticles in the Test Zone of Lateral Flow Immunoassay Strips. *ACS Appl. Nano Mater.* **2019**, *2*, 5020–5028. [CrossRef]

19. Byzova, N.A.; Safenkova, I.V.; Slutskaya, E.S.; Zherdev, A.V.; Dzantiev, B.B. Less is more: A comparison of antibody–gold nanoparticle conjugates of different ratios. *Bioconjugate Chem.* **2017**, *28*, 2737–2746. [CrossRef] [PubMed]

20. Larm, N.E.; Essner, J.B.; Pokpas, K.; Canon, J.A.; Jahed, N.; Iwuoha, E.I.; Baker, G.A. Room-temperature turkevich method: Formation of gold nanoparticles at the speed of mixing using cyclic oxocarbon reducing agents. *J. Phys. Chem. C* **2018**, *122*, 5105–5118. [CrossRef]

21. Sujitha, M.V.; Kannan, S. Green synthesis of gold nanoparticles using Citrus fruits (Citrus limon, Citrus reticulata and Citrus sinensis) aqueous extract and its characterization. *Spectrochim. Acta Part A Mol. Biomol. Spectrosc.* **2013**, *102*, 15–23. [CrossRef]

2

In Vivo Endoscopic Optical Coherence Tomography of the Healthy Human Oral Mucosa: Qualitative and Quantitative Image Analysis

Marius Albrecht [1], Christian Schnabel [1,2], Juliane Mueller [2], Jonas Golde [2], Edmund Koch [2] and Julia Walther [1,*]

1   Department of Medical Physics and Biomedical Engineering, Technische Universitaet Dresden, Carl Gustav Carus Faculty of Medicine, Fetscherstraße 74, 01307 Dresden, Germany; marius.albrecht@mailbox.tu-dresden.de (M.A.); christian.schnabel@tu-dresden.de (C.S.)
2   Department of Anesthesiology and Intensive Care Medicine, Technische Universität Dresden, Clinical Sensoring and Monitoring, Carl Gustav Carus Faculty of Medicine, Fetscherstraße 74, 01307 Dresden, Germany; juliane.mueller3@tu-dresden.de (J.M.); jonas.golde@tu-dresden.de (J.G.); edmund.koch@tu-dresden.de (E.K.)
*   Correspondence: julia.walther@tu-dresden.de

Abstract: To date, there is still a lack of reliable imaging modalities to improve the quality of consultation, diagnostic and medical examinations of the oral mucosa in dentistry. Even though, optical technologies have become an important element for the detection and treatment of different diseases of soft tissue, for the case of oral screenings the evidence of the benefit in comparison to conventional histopathology is mostly still pending. One promising optical technology for oral diagnostics is optical coherence tomography (OCT). To prove the potential of OCT, even the amount of freely accessible OCT data is not sufficient to describe the variance of healthy human oral soft tissue in vivo. In order to remedy this deficiency, the present study provides in vivo OCT cross sections of the human oral mucosa of the anterior and posterior oral cavity as well as the oropharynx of 47 adult volunteers. A collection of representative OCT cross sections forms the basis for a randomized blinded image analysis by means of seven criteria to assess the main features of the superficial layers of the human oral mucosa and to determine its correlation to regional features known from hematoxylin and eosin (HE) stained histology.

Keywords: optical coherence tomography; endoscopy; noninvasive; healthy human oral mucosa; epithelial thickness; adults, histology

1. Introduction

According to the results of the global burden of disease study, diagnosis and treatment of oral cancer is still challenging because of at least >350,000 new cases and >170,000 deaths every year [1]. The most common type of oral cancer is the squamous cell carcinoma (SCC) (90% of all oral malignancies [2]) developing within the few ten microns thin epithelium, which is replaced by a neoplastic tissue associated with a progressive dysplasia [2,3]. The highest incidence is found between the ages of 55 and 75 years corresponding to a mean age of onset of about 63 years for male and 66 years for female patients [4]. With regard to demographic aging, the global incidence of oral cancer is predicted to increase of almost two thirds in 2035 [4]. Even though, treatment methods have been improved over the last decades and leading risk factors like smoking, excessive consumption of alcohol and HPV infection are well-known, the overall 5 year survival remains low of about 63% being significantly decreased in advanced stages [2–6]. The reason for this lies primarily in the high number of initial diagnoses at a late stage underlining the necessity for an improved early diagnosis [4].

With regard to the routine diagnostic process, the general anamnesis is complemented by a visual examination and a subsequent endoscopy for difficult-to-access regions of the posterior oral cavity as well as oropharynx [7]. Depending on the reported symptoms, that may include oral bleeding, persisting pain or progressive swelling, as well as existing visually suspect lesions, the indication for an invasive biopsy with histopathological evaluation is set by means of the medical opinion [7,8]. Although, incisional and excisional biopsies represent the current gold standard of an accurate and complete diagnosis [7–9], the procedure is painful and requires a surgical intervention leading to a reduced compliance of the patient [9,10]. Especially for the case of extensive and/or numerous lesions, the decision on the location and size of the tissue sample for a representative biopsy is challenging [9,10]. Moreover, missing out on recurrences and relapses (second primary cancer) or redundant biopsies is problematic [11].

In this context, the implementation of optical techniques provides the opportunity to examine the oral mucosa in a non-invasive and non-ionising way before the decision of starting the tissue extraction [12]. Optical coherence tomography (OCT) is such an emerging optical technology enabling cross-sectional sub-surface in vivo imaging of biological tissues with a common spatial resolution of about 5–20 μm [13,14]. By the implementation of adapted rigid or fiber optics, endoscopic OCT can be used for the non-invasive examination of human oral soft tissue [15,16]. As tissue elements of the mucosal sublayers result in various scattering behaviour, information about the appearance and geometry of the epithelium and the underlying lamina propria becomes accessible [14,17]. Ongoing research has occasionally proposed perspective measurement parameters, such as the mean epithelial thickness, the occurrence of a keratinized layer and the course of the basement membrane, for the detection of (pre-)malignant changes of the oral epithelium by means of OCT [14,17]. Furthermore, OCT image scoring was performed using hamster cheek pouches, concentrating on the presence of irregular epithelial stratification in combination with broadened rete pegs and basal hyperplasia [18]. Beyond that, diagnostic scoring was done on human oral soft tissue in the context of preliminary studies [19]. Moreover, several ex vivo studies as well as an increasing amount of in vivo investigations have described key features of suspicious lesions and oral squamous cell carcinoma, such as the increase in epithelial thickness as well as the loss of the basement membrane during the progress of malignant transformation [17,20]. Regarding oral lesions alongside the upper aerodigestive tract, measurement of epithelial thickness provided large differences resulting in a moderate sensitivity and specificity in order to distinguish noninvasive from invasive proliferation [21]. Along with the process of epithelial thickening, changes in the standard deviation of the OCT signal have been reported offering the possibility to differentiate between the stages of oral dysplasia in a more reliably way [22–24]. However, the correct identification of early dysplasia by means of intensity-based OCT was stated to be difficult because of a similar appearance compared to benign lesions [20].

As requirement for the accurate evaluation of pathological changes of the human oral mucosa, healthy oral soft tissue was investigated by only a few studies mostly realized with small numbers of volunteers [25–27]. The majority of OCT images were obtained from examinations within the anterior parts of the oral cavity, like the labial, buccal and sublingual mucosa, whereas OCT cross sections of the posterior areas, such as the oropharynx and the palatine tonsils, likewise typical sites of oral cancer, have only been presented rarely. Ridgway et al. [26] showed a collection of OCT cross sections depicting the normal oral mucosa of fifteen different locations as well as a combination of benign and malign lesions. Image material was gained from measurements with a flexible handheld OCT probe including a total of forty-one patients. Within the examples, epithelium was described as hyporeflective layer followed by the basement membrane and the hyperreflective lamina propria consisting of connective tissue, minor salivary glands and blood vessels [26]. Prestin et al. [25] intended to determine reference values for the mean epithelial thickness by investigating 143 healthy test persons. A commercial fiber-based OCT device was used to conduct in vivo measurements at seven points, among them the buccal mucosa, the mouth floor, the palatine arch, the uvula and the hard palate. Further results were published by Stasio et al. [27] involving 28 healthy adult volunteers and six defined areas of the oral soft tissue, the labial mucosa, the buccal mucosa, the gingiva, the mouth floor as well as the ventral and dorsal tongue. Measurements were done by means of a commercial swept-source OCT system with a grip type probe.

Against this background, the demand for a comprehensive study with the aim of assessing the variance of appearance of the healthy oral mucosa, in dependence of the localization within the oral cavity, and with this the ground truth arises [17,26]. Moreover, systematic reviews suggest that the visual interpretation of OCT data sets is often strongly user-dependent due to a lack of established standards for the image analysis [17], which leads to the aim of defining qualitative and quantitative criteria for an improved optical biopsy by OCT. On the other hand, there are several studies dealing with an automatic evaluation of OCT images of oral pathologies [28,29]. Here, changes in the speckle pattern of the epithelium as well as in the signal intensity within the single A-scans offer the possibility to serve as indicators for the development of oral malignancy [28]. Besides, the measurement of the epithelial thickness and the determination of the basement membrane can be done by means of an automatic segmentation algorithm [29]. For this purpose, corresponding histopathological images are used to confirm the findings in the OCT cross sections reaching a solid base for software training in regards to the detection of malign lesions. However, in order to improve the current state of knowledge concerning healthy oral soft tissue, the aim of the presented study is the detection and analysis of in vivo OCT data sets representing characteristic and cancer-relevant parts of normal mucosa alongside the whole oral cavity, which forms the fundamental basis for further developments in functional and endoscopic OCT [26,27,30–33] as well as subsequent clinical research.

2. Materials and Methods

2.1. Study Population

Forty-seven healthy adult volunteers participated in the presented in vivo study. Before starting the measurement, volunteers were screened visually by an experienced physician for exclusion criteria including suspicious oral lesions (i.e., erythroplakia, leukoplakia and ulcers), chronic or recently occurred disorders (i.e., mucous membrane and connective tissue diseases) as well as alcohol- and smoking-induced tissue damage. In addition, common oral symptoms (i.e., dry mouth, recurrent pain, gingival bleeding, increased sensitivity) were registered within anamnesis. Reactive changes in the mucosa related to alcohol and tobacco were considered by quantifying alcohol intake (g/day) and smoking habits (cigarettes per day; pack years). According to a systematic review of Burger et al. [34], mucosa was classified as healthy, if the mean consumption did not exceed the tolerable upper alcohol intake level (TUAL; 10–12 g/day for healthy adult women; 20–24 g/day for healthy adult men). Concerning the use of tobacco, the tolerance level corresponds to a frequency of less than 10 cigarettes per day and a total amount of less than 10 pack years leading to a similar likelihood ratio for oral cancer compared to never smokers [35]. Finally, sex and age were noted and used to categorize groups (male/female; <25 years, 25–45 years and >45 years). All participants have declared their informed consent before the examination. The study was approved by the ethics commission of the Faculty of Medicine of the Technische Universitaet Dresden (EK 96032018; 2018-11-16).

2.2. Endoscopic OCT System

Acquisition of OCT image series was realized by the use of a customized optical probe (lateral resolution: 17.4 µm, working distance: 7.5 mm) based on a commercial rigid endoscope (8711 AGA, Karl Storz GmbH & Co. KG, length: 200 mm, insertion diameter: 10 mm, angle of view: 0°) [36] in combination with a self-built spectrometer-based OCT system using a fiber-coupled superluminescent diode (SLD-371-HP1, Superlumdiodes Ltd., center wavelength: $\lambda = 840$ nm, FWHM: $\Delta\lambda = 45$ nm) and a customized spectrometer [37], providing an axial resolution in air of 11.6 µm. Cross-sectional OCT images (64 B-scans) consisting of 480 A-scans were detected with increments of $\delta x = 5\ \mu m$ (fast scanning axis) and $\delta y = 10\ \mu m$ (slow scanning axis) to cover a scanning field of 2.4 mm × 0.6 mm in about 2.5 s ($f_{A\text{-scan}} = 11.88$ kHz). The whole endoscopic OCT system was in accordance with the requirements for a positive ethics committee vote concerning the aspect of disinfection and sterilization.

2.3. Measurement Protocol

Endoscopic OCT image series were detected at 16 measurement points within seven regions of the oral cavity in accordance to the measurement plan in Figure 1. Corresponding zones that are expected to be characterized by comparable structure and ratio of the mucosal layers are presented in the same color. The sequence of measurements was set from outer to inner oral cavity with additional points alongside the buccal and sublingual region enabling the comparison of anterior and posterior regions. Within the oral vestibule, measurement points were situated alongside the upper and lower part of the labial and alveolar mucosa. In this context the term "alveolar mucosa" defined the oral soft tissue that is located between the attached gingiva and the adjacent labial mucosa. In this study, lining oral mucosa was mainly recorded since deeper structures of the masticatory and specialized oral mucosa, such as strongly keratinized attached gingiva and dorsal tongue, are unreliably detected because of the limited penetration depth as a result of increased backscattering of the probing light. Thus, with the exception of the masticatory mucosa of the hard palate, the presented study particularly considers the measurement of the lining mucosa of the oral cavity and the oro-pharyngeal isthmus with respect to common sites of oral cancer.

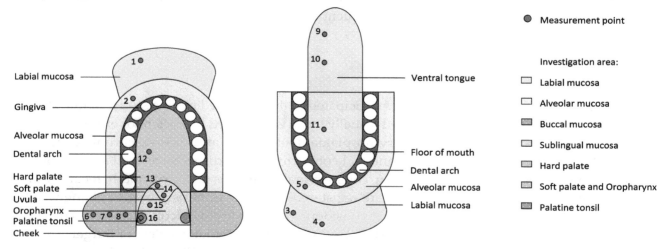

Figure 1. Schematic illustration of the human oral cavity with seven investigation areas (colored zones) and selected measurement points (red dots) in consideration of common sites of oral cancer.

The examination with the rigid handheld OCT endoscope was supported by a chin and head rest that ensures the reduction of patient movement and consequently motion artefacts. The entire examination was performed in sitting position whereby measurement points were scanned without direct contact to the local mucosa as well as unilateral on the subject's right side to minimize measurement time. Recording two stacks of 64 B-scans in each case results in a total examination time of approximately 20 min. To reach all of the points to be investigated, common tools (i.e., tongue depressor, cotton cloth) were used including the minor active involvement of the volunteer (e.g., participants were instructed to turn down their lips for imaging the labial region).

The image processing contained the visual selection of a series of five B-scans for each measurement position being used for the subsequent image analysis. By means of defined criteria (see Section 2.4), each cross section was examined by a prospective physician well-versed in OCT in agreement with a skilled histologist. Quantitative and qualitative evaluation of the selected OCT cross sections has been done with ImageJ [38]. A random choice of 200 images served as training set before the analysis. Finally, a characterization of the anatomical regions by means of OCT was created, summarizing the results of corresponding measurement points and regions.

2.4. OCT Image Analysis

As illustrated in Table 1, the OCT image analysis was manually performed using a set of criteria concerning the epithelium (EP) and the adjacent lamina propria (LP) (Figure 2). Within this section, evaluation is methodically explained and exemplified by five sample images.

Table 1. Criteria of the OCT image analysis.

Criterion	Evaluation
Surface integrity	intact/with alterations
Surface profile	even/uneven
Epithelial homogeneity	homogeneous/inhomogeneous
Epithelial thickness	mean value of 25 measurements (µm)
Basement membrane	intact/unsharp/not assessable
Tissue vascularization	low (<0.10)/moderate (0.10–0.30)/high (>0.30)
Additional components	Description of regional features within the lamina propria

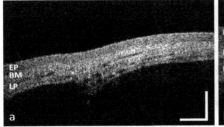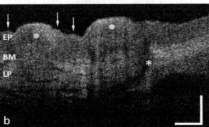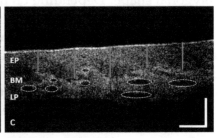

Figure 2. Representative OCT images of the sublingual mucosa (**a**), the hard palate (**b**) and the labial mucosa (**c**) demonstrating the principle of the visual image analysis. EP: epithelium, BM: basement membrane, LP: lamina propria; Arrows in (**b**): epithelial surface alteration, Yellow dots: palatal ridges (uneven surface profile), Asterisk: salivary gland opening; Vertical lines in (**c**): epithelial thickness measurement, Ellipsoidal shapes: marked regions of vascularization. Scale bar: 200 µm.

First of all, the integrity of the epithelial surface is assessed by searching for lesions. The surface is called "intact", if the number of single lesions does not exceed one; otherwise the term "with alterations" is used. The sublingual mucosa depicted in Figure 2a shows an intact surface, whereas the mucosa of the hard palate in Figure 2b contains numerous epithelial surface alterations (arrows). Moreover, the surface profile is evaluated by differentiating between "even" and "uneven" course. The term "even" underlined that the epithelial surface is free from crypts (concave) and ridges (convex) larger than 200 µm in diameter (cp. Figure 2a). Therefore, epithelium with an uneven surface is exemplarily presented by means of the plicae ridges of the hard palate (yellow dots in Figure 2b).

Additionally, the deep structure of the epithelium is categorized into "homogeneous" and "inhomogeneous" by regarding the local tissue reflectivity within a single B-scan. According to former studies that presented healthy oral mucosa [25–27], epithelium is expected to be less scattering than the highly reflecting collagen network within the lamina propria. If hypo- or hyperreflective areas are not identified, the epithelium is classified as homogeneous as shown in Figure 2a. In comparison, the masticatory mucosa of the hard palate in Figure 2b shows an inhomogeneous epithelium containing a hyperreflective surface of the ridges (yellow dots in Figure 2b).

Since OCT is an interferometric technique allowing the depth-resolved distance measurement, the optical path length (OPL) of the epithelium (EP, from the surface to the basement membrane BM, Figure 2) is measured at five evenly distributed positions throughout each cross section (red bars in Figure 2c). For this purpose, the OCT cross section was visualized with ImageJ using a 23"-screen. By drawing a vertical line with the straight line tool of Image J, the distance from the top of the epithelial surface to the visually undermost pixel of the hypointense epithelial layer was measured. Here, the position of the basement membrane was determined by eye. Considering the vertical length of the pixel of l = 5 µm and the refractive index of the epithelium of n = 1.37 [25,39] at a center wavelength of λ = 840 nm, the corresponding mean value of the geometrical length is determined for each B-scan. Combining the results of each specific measurement point, sex- and age-specific reference values of healthy oral mucosa are obtained within the investigated regions (see Appendix A).

Furthermore, the basement membrane (BM), defined as junction between the epithelium (EP) and the underlying lamina propria (LP), is visually verified for integrity. The class "intact" is used to characterize a continuous basement membrane without any gaps (cp. Figure 2a). A reduced demarcation of the border is described as "unsharp". The term "not assessable" is used for the case that the basement membrane could not be depicted due to the reduced penetration depth. Consequently, the evaluation of the lamina propria and the measurement of the epithelial thickness is not possible.

Corresponding to the approach of OCT angiography, the grade of tissue vascularization is estimated by measuring the luminal area of larger vessels and relating the result to the avascular epithelial layer (also referred to as mean vessel density) [40,41]. For this, single or multiple yellow-colored elliptic shapes mark regions of vascularization , as shown in Figure 2c. The sum of the segmented areas is divided by the total area of the detected epithelium determined by a polygonal shape. Depending on the ratio, the vascular supply by major vessels is classified as "low" (<0.10), "moderate" (0.10–0.30) or "high" (>0.30).

Additional characteristic features of the lamina propria, such as minor salivary glands (SG in Figure 3a) or lymphoid follicles (LF in Figure 3b), are considered in the last criterion. Salivary glands, which consist of a few lobules and an excretory duct (cp. asterisk in Figure 2b), emerge as round hyporeflective elements [42], embedded within the hyperreflective connective tissue. Lymphoid follicles appear hyporeflective with an inner germinal centre [43].

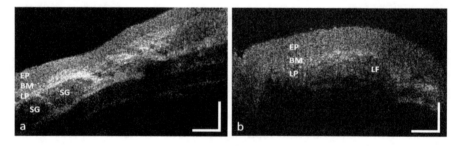

Figure 3. Exemplary OCT images of the oropharynx (**a**) and the palatine tonsil (**b**). The connective tissue of the oropharynx contains minor salivary glands whereas the palatine tonsil includes multiple lymphoid follicles. EP: epithelium, BM: basement membrane, LP: lamina propria, SG: salivary gland, LF: lymphoid follicle. Scale bar: 200 µm.

2.5. Statistical Analysis

In order to compare the investigation areas (Figure 1), the percentage distribution of the results of the qualitative evaluation criteria (Table 1) is determined for each measurement point. Concerning the epithelial thickness, a mean value is calculated for each series of five B-scans representing the individual epithelial thickness of the volunteer at the corresponding measurement point. Subsequently, these individual values are used to determine the mean value and standard deviation for the final determination of the epithelial thickness at each measurement point (see Appendix A, Table A1). A similar approach is done for the sex- and age-related groups with the objective to generate an initial data set of reference values. The results for each measurement point and every investigation area are summarized in box plots. The grade of tissue vascularization is analyzed in the same way by calculating mean values for the series of five B-scans of each volunteer and presenting them in box plots depending on the location within the oral cavity.

Table 2 summarized details about the study population and the number of OCT cross sections. Altogether, 3560 OCT images of 47 healthy adult volunteers ($N_{male} = 25$ and $N_{female} = 22$) form the basis for the described analysis. The whole sample consisted of fair-skinned participants without oral pigmentation in the visual examination. The mean age corresponds to 29.4 years (range: 20–56 years). Concerning the age groups, 30 subjects (63.8%) were assigned to the mean one (25–45 years). None of the volunteers showed suspicious lesions in the visual examination or described oral symptoms within the anamnesis. Moreover, there was no report of alcohol intake or smoking above the tolerance levels.

Table 2. Statistics on the study population and the amount of the OCT cross sections.

Study Population		OCT Cross Sections	
Nb. of volunteers	47	Investigation area	Nb. of images
Male	25 (53.2%)		
Female	22 (46.8%)	Labial mucosa	705
Mean age (years)	29.36	Alveolar mucosa	470
<25 years	14 (29.8%)	Buccal mucosa	705
25–45 years	30 (63.8%)	Sublingual mucosa	705
>45 years	3 (6.4%)	Hard palate	235
Oral symptoms/lesions	0	Soft palate & oropharynx	570
Alcohol intake > TL [1]	0	Palatine tonsils	170
Never drinking	19 (40.4%)		
Tobacco consumption > TL [1]	0	*Total*	3,560
Never smoking	20 (42.6%)		

[1] Tolerance level.

The measurement of the anterior oral cavity was feasible in all cases resulting in 235 OCT images for each measurement point (MP1-MP12). The soft palate (MP13) as well as the uvula (MP14) have been accessible in 45 (95.7%) and 40 (85.1%) volunteers, respectively. In addition, the oropharynx (MP15) and the palatine tonsil (MP16) have been able to detect in 29 (61.7%) and 34 (72.3%) volunteers. In 38.4% of the cases, the first of two image stacks (à 64 B-scans) provided visually appropriate B-scans for the OCT image analysis. Using OCT images out of the second stack was especially required for the analysis of the labial and alveolar mucosa due to the flexible soft tissue alongside these regions.

2.6. Histological Analysis

Histological correlation was implemented by means of hematoxylin and eosin (HE) stained cross sections [44] of human oral soft tissue, which have been provided by the Institute of Anatomy, Faculty of Medicine, Technische Universitaet Dresden, Germany. Consequently, histological images have not been collected from subjects recruited to the study. A total of seventy histological cross sections, including ten for each investigation area, have been used for the juxtaposition of OCT and histology. Exemplary slides were integrated within a collection of OCT cross sections for characteristic oral sites.

3. Results

In the following subsections, the results of the OCT image analysis of the defined investigation areas are described in detail based on the evaluation criteria presented in Section 2.4. A summary of the results concerning the qualitative criteria is depicted in the percentage bar chart in Figure 4.

The epithelial thickness at each measurement point is outlined by means of box plots in Figure 5 providing information about the age- and sex-independent mean value, the sample median and the interquartile range. The coloration of the boxes corresponds to the investigation areas according to the measurement plan (cp. Figure 1). Focusing on the grade of tissue vascularization by means of the calculated mean vessel density (see Section 2.4), a graphical representation is realized by box plots in Figure 6.

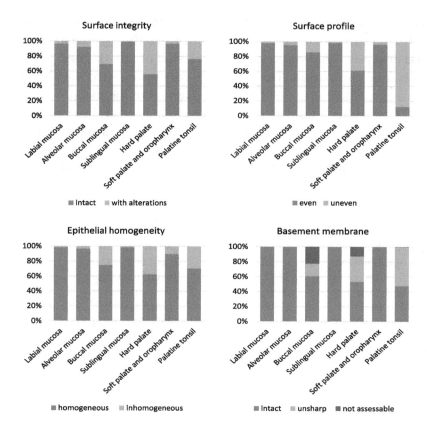

Figure 4. Results of the evaluation of the OCT cross sections within seven oral investigation areas. The image analysis contained the assessment of surface integrity, surface profile, epithelial homogeneity and basement membrane. Percentage values of the qualitative evaluation of the different criteria are presented by the colored bars.

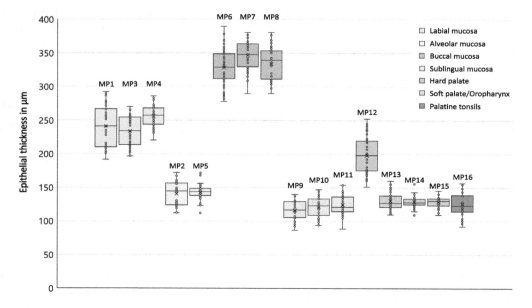

Figure 5. Box plots of the epithelial thickness (age- and gender-independent). The results for all measurement points are presented by colored boxes in accordance with the corresponding investigation areas (cp. Figure 1). The sample median is depicted as central line inside the boxes, the sample mean value corresponds to the cross. The individual mean values are illustrated by circles. The width of the box is equivalent to the interquartile range. Maximum and minimum of the sample are shown by the whiskers.

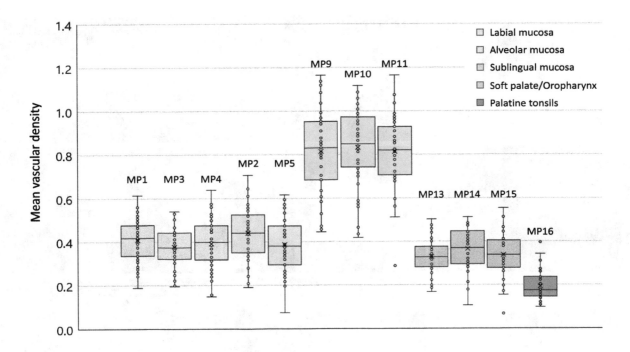

Figure 6. Box plot of the mean vascular density. Due to the limited penetration depth of the probing light within the buccal region and the hard palate, resulting in the limited visualization of the lamina propria and embedded vessels, reference values for the vascularization by major vessels of both regions could not be provided.

3.1. Labial and Alveolar Mucosa

With regard to the surface integrity and profile, labial mucosa has been evaluated as intact in 96.4% and even in 98.0% of the OCT cross sections (Figure 7b–f, Figure 4). The epithelial layer has been classified as homogeneous (98.5%) correlating to a regular epithelial structure in accordance with exemplary histological images. The total value of the labial mucosa was measured to be 243 ± 25 µm (Table A1). The basement membrane has been assessed as intact in all OCT cross sections and histological slides (e.g., Figure 7a), respectively (Figure 4). Tissue vascularization was mainly high (60.3%) with a mean ratio of 0.39 ± 0.10 (Figure 6) due to an existing network of larger vessels [45,46]. Looking at the additional components, minor salivary glands occurred within the lamina propria in 34.5%. Although, these glands are spread over the whole oral cavity, the highest density is found within the labial, buccal, palatal and sublingual areas [42,47].

Summarizing the results of two measurement points of the alveolar region (MP2 und MP5), epithelial surface of the alveolar mucosa has been defined as intact in 92.2% and even in 95.4% (Figure 7h–i, Figure 4). The epithelial layer has been classified as homogeneous in 96.6%. The mean thickness was 142 ± 15 µm (Table A1) with no deviation between the upper and the lower alveolar area. A continuous decrease from the labial to the alveolar mucosa is already well described by histology [46] and previous OCT studies [27]. An intact basement membrane was noticed in all OCT images confirmed by exemplary histological slides (e.g., Figure 7g). The grade of tissue vascularization by means of major vessels was classified as high in 62.1% of the detected OCT cross sections with a mean ratio of 0.41 ± 0.13 (Figure 6) being highly correlated to the mean vessel density in the labial mucosa. Moreover, clusters of salivary glands were observed in 47.4% ensuring the moistening of the alveolar region as described in histology [46].

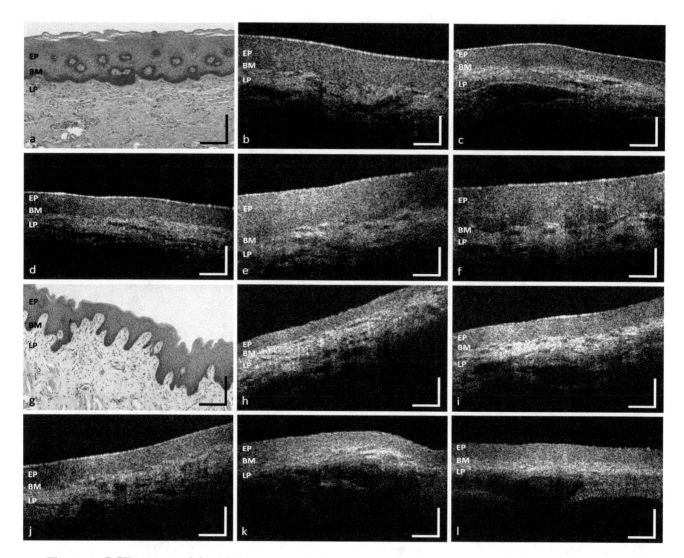

Figure 7. OCT images of the labial mucosa (**b**–**f**) and the alveolar mucosa (**h**–**l**). The sample pictures represent the upper (MP1) (**b**,**c**) and the lower lip (MP3,MP4) (**d**–**f**) as well as the upper (MP2) (**h**,**i**) and lower alveolar region (MP5) (**j**–**l**). Exemplary HE stained histological cross sections depicting the labial and the alveolar mucosa (**a**,**g**) ([44] modified). EP: epithelium, BM: basement membrane, LP: lamina propria. Scale bars: 200 µm.

3.2. Buccal Mucosa

OCT image analysis of the buccal mucosa (Figure 8b–f) was realized by means of three measurement points depicting the anterior, the central and the posterior part. At these points, 30.6% of the OCT cross sections (Figure 8b,c arrows) showed a surface with alterations while surface profile was categorized as uneven due to a raised surface in about 14.2% (Figure 8f yellow dots). In 74.6%, the epithelium was classified as homogeneous with a mean thickness of 336 ± 25 µm (Figure 5), being slightly thicker among the male volunteers (Table A1: MP6-8, Figure A2). Comparing the measurement points of the buccal side, epithelium was thickest at the central part. The basement membrane was intact in 60.8%, however, an amount of 22.4% was stated as not assessable due to the increased epithelial thickness and the limited imaging depth in biological tissue [36]. With regard to future studies, automated segmentation of the epithelium of the buccal mucosa could be challenging due to hyperkeratinization and a reduced visibility of the basement membrane. The grade of vascular supply by larger vessels was moderate (67.7%) with a mean ratio of 0.21 ± 0.14 (Figure 6). Further characteristic features were not able to be detected as salivary glands are beyond the imaging depth and surrounded by fat tissue in the submucosa [46].

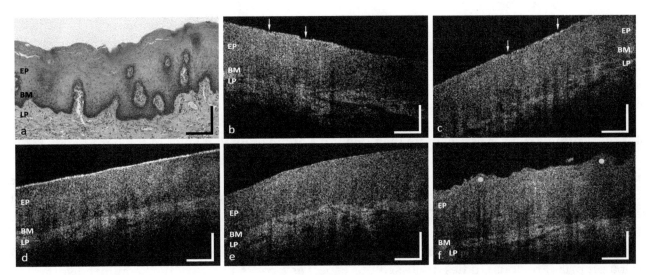

Figure 8. OCT images of the buccal mucosa (**b–f**). The sample pictures represent the anterior (MP6) (**b,c**), the central (MP7) (**d**) and the posterior buccal region (MP8) (**e,f**). Exemplary HE stained histological cross sections depicting the buccal mucosa (**a**) ([44] modified). EP: epithelium, BM: basement membrane, LP: lamina propria; Arrows: epithelial surface alteration, Yellow dots: uneven surface profile. Scale bars: 200 µm.

3.3. Sublingual Mucosa

Regarding the sublingual mucosa, OCT images (Figure 9b–f) were taken from the ventral tongue (MP9, MP10) and the neighboring mouth floor (MP11), respectively. The epithelial surface appeared intact (98.9%) and even (98.2%) in agreement with all of the histological slides (e.g., Figure 9a). The epithelial structure was classified as homogeneous in 98.3% of all cases with a mean thickness of 120 ± 15 µm (Table A1). Statistical analysis revealed significantly higher values in male participants (Table A1: MP9-11, Figures A1 and A2). There were no unsharp stages determined in the course of the basement membrane. Compared to the other measurement points, the most extensive grade of vascular supply was found, because of the large sublingual arteries and veins within the lamina propria in this oral region [46]. In the present study, 86.6% of the OCT sections were evaluated as highly vascularized with a mean ratio of 0.82 ± 0.17 (Figure 6). Beyond this, OCT images did not show any supplementary local features.

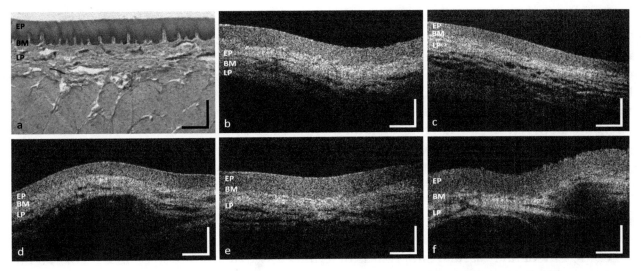

Figure 9. OCT images of the ventral tongue (**b,c**) and the mouth floor (MP11) (**d–f**). The sample pictures represent the anterior (MP9) (**b**) and posterior sublingual region (MP10) (**c**). Exemplary HE stained histological cross sections depicting the sublingual mucosa (**a**) ([44] modified). EP: epithelium, BM: basement membrane, LP: lamina propria. Scale bars: 200 µm.

3.4. Hard Palate

As exemplarily illustrated in (Figure 10b), in 44.6% of the detected OCT cross sections of the hard palate, multiple alterations of the epithelial surface have been detected. Moreover, the surface profile contained single or groups of convex ridges (38.8%) matching with the transverse palatal folds, as characteristic regional feature [38], which can be more or less pronounced for the selected measurement region (MP12 in Figure 1). Since hyperreflective areas have been detected below the folds, indicating a denser tissue, more than one third of the epithelial layer of the hard palate (37.5%) were classified as inhomogeneous (Figure 4). Mean epithelial thickness was $198 \pm 26\,\mu m$ (Table A1) being up to 40% higher inside the convex areas. Altogether, these findings represent a physiological adaptation to the masticatory function [46]. The mean value among female volunteers ($175 \pm 11\,\mu m$) was lower compared to the male ($218 \pm 19\,\mu m$) (Table A1: MP12, Figures A1 and A2) in accordance with former histological studies [48]. In about 34.5% of all cases, the basement membrane was assessed as unsharp due to a reduced contrast of the hyperreflective epithelial layer compared to the subsequent lamina propria. Previous studies discussed this aspect as a consequence of the keratinized surface [27]. Minor salivary glands appeared as additional components in 15.0% of the OCT cross sections, which is confirmed by histology [46].

3.5. Soft Palate and Oropharynx

Combining the results alongside the soft palate (MP13), the uvula (MP14) and the oropharynx (MP15), the epithelial surface was intact (96.7%) and even (96.4%), as depicted in the OCT images (Figure 10e–i) and the epithelium appeared homogeneous (89.6%). Among the measurement points, there were no significant differences in the epithelial thickness and the mean value resulted in $130 \pm 11\,\mu m$ (Table A1: MP13-15, Figure A2). The basement membrane was visible and evaluated as intact in all of the OCT cross sections and the histological slides (e.g., Figure 10d), respectively. Vascularization by major vessels was rated as high in the majority of cases (56.1%) with a mean ratio of 0.34 ± 0.09 due to a distinct vessel network in the reticular layer of the lamina propria [46]. Moreover, packets of minor salivary glands, surrounded by connective tissue, occurred in 61.1% of all cases. This feature has been also seen in histological images and described in the literature [47].

3.6. Palatine Tonsils

Image analysis of the palatine tonsil was performed by using OCT cross sections (Figure 10k,l) by means of a single measurement point (MP16 in Figure 1). In 76.1% of all cases, epithelial surface was categorized as intact in correspondence to the histological slides (e.g., Figure 10j). The surface profile was classified as uneven (87.5%) with concave pits that are equal to the tonsillar crypts [43]. A homogeneous (70.6%) epithelium was found with a mean thickness of $125 \pm 17\,\mu m$ (Table A1) being similar to the neighboring soft palate. Looking at age-related changes, thickness was lower in the participants between 25 and 45 years compared to younger volunteers (Table A1). Confirming this aspect, an age-dependent decrease in the parenchymal lymphatic tissue combined with an increase in tissue fibrosis and fatty degeneration was reported by former histological investigations [49]. Due to a lower contrast between the epithelium and the lamina propria, the basement membrane was evaluated as unsharp in 52.2%. This finding is caused by a more permeable epithelial junction resulting in huge numbers of lymphocytes between the regularly arranged epithelial cells and in the underlying connective tissue to ensure a sufficient defense of exogenous infections [50]. In 60.3% of all cases, a moderate vascular supply was determined with a mean ratio of 0.19 ± 0.07 (Figure 6). Regarding additional characteristic features, 86.4% of the OCT images and all histological slides showed groups of lymphoid follicles within the lamina propria as part of the primary immune function [43].

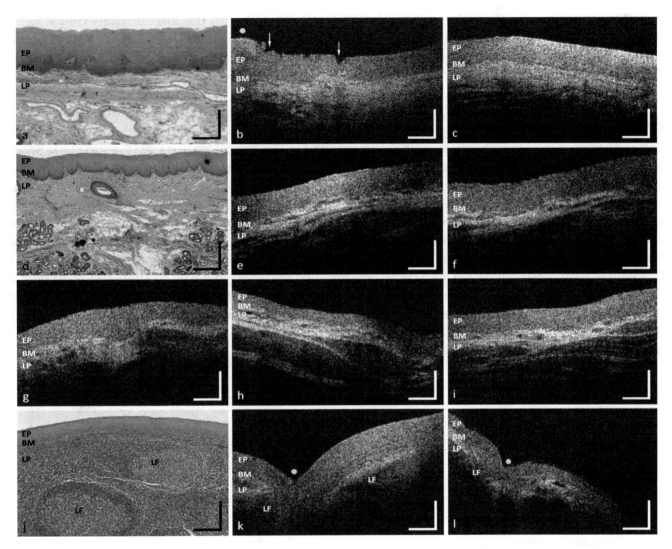

Figure 10. OCT images of the hard palate (MP12) (**b,c**), the soft palate (MP13) (**e,f**), the uvula (MP14) (**g**), the oropharynx (MP15) (**h,i**) and the palatine tonsil (MP16) (**k,l**). Exemplary HE stained histological cross sections depicting the hard palate (**a**), the soft palate (**d**) and the palatine tonsil (**j**) ([44] modified). EP: epithelium, BM: basement membrane, LP: lamina propria, LF: lymphoid follicle; Arrows: epithelial alteration, Yellow dots: palatal ridges and tonsillar crypts. Scale bars: 200 μm.

4. Discussion

With reference to the limited number of freely accessible OCT images concerning the healthy human oral mucosa, this study aimed to examine a representative sample of disease-free volunteers by means of an endoscopic OCT system. Looking at the study population (Table 2), the distribution between both sexes was balanced, especially within the age groups. Moreover, most participants were younger than 45 years and none of them exceeded the tolerance levels of smoking and alcohol intake or possessed visually suspicious lesions. Thus, oral soft tissue among the study population can be stated as healthy while leaving out invasive biopsies. By using the endoscopic OCT system, all of the measurement points of the oral cavity could be reached. Although some volunteers reported an uncomfortable feeling during the examination process for measurement points within the posterior oral cavity and the oropharynx, at least 60% of the cases have been accessible and therefore image data were sufficient for a representative analysis. Previous studies concerning healthy oral soft tissue concentrated on the imaging of the anterior oral mucosa [17,25–27], so detailed information about the accessibility of the posterior areas have not been reported before. However, the presented data suggest that this aspect should be considered for the determination of the sample size.

Regarding the results of the epithelial thickness measurement, the lowest mean values were determined for the sublingual mucosa ($120 \pm 15\,\mu m$) in accordance with the reference values of the mouth floor ($100 \pm 14\,\mu m$) by Stasio et al. [27]. Additionally, Stasio et al. provided comparable results for the labial mucosa ($271 \pm 36\,\mu m$) and Prestin et al. [25] presented similar data for the anterior mouth floor ($99 \pm 22\,\mu m$), the uvula ($144 \pm 30\,\mu m$) and the hard palate ($239 \pm 57\,\mu m$). The highest mean value within the presented study was calculated for the buccal mucosa with about $336 \pm 25\,\mu m$. At this point, Stasio et al. reported a mean value of $374 \pm 62\,\mu m$ agreeing with the reference value of Prestin et al. ($294 \pm 68\,\mu m$). One should consider, that the results for the buccal mucosa by Prestin et al. were received by measurements with direct contact containing the influence of tissue stretching. In this study, measurement process was performed contact-free for which reason local tissue compression could be avoided. On the other hand, the penetration depth of the probing light was limited by a thick epithelium reducing the visibility of the basement membrane and the subsequent lamina propria. Thus, the thickness measurement of the buccal epithelium by the presented EOCT system is limited. Histological investigations reported a mean value of $480 \pm 90\,\mu m$ for the buccal mucosa [51]. Deviations between in vivo OCT and histology could be reasoned in tissue fixation and histological preparation of the physiological oral mucosa [52]. In compliance with our expectations, the epithelial thickness of the measurement points did not show notable differences within the investigation areas (MP6-MP8), and thus, reference values can be defined by means of a reduced number of recommended measurement points as shown in the diagram (Figure 11).

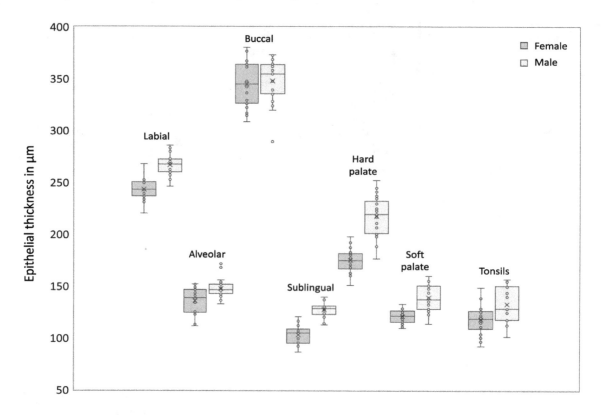

Figure 11. Box plot of the gender-specific epithelial thickness of recommended measurement points. The limited selection of distinctive measurement points is conceivable to serve as prospective parameter for assessing oral health. Labial: MP4, Alveolar: MP5, Buccal: MP7, Sublingual: MP9, Hard palate: MP12, Soft palate: MP13, Tonsils: MP16

The assessment of tissue vascularization was realized by calculating the mean vascular density by means of major vessels. Considering the anatomical structure of the oral mucosa, the luminal cross-sectional area of larger vessels was related to the avascular epithelium. Apart from the buccal mucosa and the hard palate where measurement was restricted due to a limited penetration depth, a moderate to high grade of vascularization was found within the defined investigation areas (Figure 1). Setting these results in a wider context, previous OCT studies used different approaches to quantify vascular supply [40,45]. Tsai et al. [40] calculated an average vessel density by using en-face projections of OCT angiographic images. At a depth of 250 to 500 μm, a high vascularization was determined for the labial mucosa, the buccal mucosa and the sublingual mucosa, respectively. For future research on pathologies, the combination of intensity-based OCT and functional imaging , e.g., Doppler OCT and OCT angiography, is recommended while concentrating on both, capillaries and large blood and lymphatic vessels.

Looking at the qualitative image criteria, the evaluation of the OCT cross sections provided similar results for the labial mucosa, the alveolar mucosa, the sublingual mucosa and the soft palate, respectively. There, OCT cross sections displayed an even and homogeneous epithelial layer without surface alterations that is clearly demarcated by a visually consistent basement membrane. With reference to previous histological descriptions [46], these findings correlate with the anatomical structure of the lining mucosa, which includes an intact and regular epithelium with a smooth border to the adjacent lamina propria. The appearance of lining mucosa in OCT was analyzed by Ridgway et al. [26] using sample pictures of the lower lip, the ventral side of the tongue and the mouth floor showing a homogeneous hyporeflective epithelium and a hyperreflective lamina propria. Gentile et al. [17] presented a similar characterization in the context of a systematic review as reference for future investigations. However, epithelial surface has not been widely examined by means of OCT before due to the absence of established criteria. Although the buccal mucosa is histologically classified as lining mucosa as well, in vivo OCT images showed an epithelium containing numerous alterations and inhomogeneous areas. According to former histologic reports [46], this feature can be explained as a consequence of mechanical stress leading to epithelial damage and local reactive keratinization. Concerning the epithelial homogeneity, Stasio et al. [27] described regional changes in the epithelial layer as a result of surface keratinization. OCT cross sections of the hard palate displayed an epithelium with multiple alterations and a keratinized surface as typical feature of the masticatory mucosa in agreement with histological examinations [46]. For the first time, the presented study provided detailed information about the surface profile by delivering in vivo OCT pictures of the transverse palatal folds.

Concerning the depiction of minor salivary glands, the used OCT system allowed the identification of clusters that are located close to the basement membrane [53]. The appearance in the OCT images was accordant with the description of Grulkowski et al. [42] in the form of round hyporeflective elements with an excretory duct surrounded by connective tissue. However, for the depiction of deeper-lying clusters of minor salivary glands, the usage of an OCT system with a center wavelength of 1300 nm is recommended.

5. Summary and Conclusions

In the presented clinical study, in vivo OCT cross sections of the healthy human oral mucosa were obtained with the aim of generating a standardized image analysis of intensity-based OCT cross sections. Concentrating on cancer-relevant parts of the oral cavity and the oropharyngeal isthmus, a total of 47 volunteers was examined gathering more than 3500 OCT images out of seven investigation areas by means of an EOCT system. In extension to former OCT studies, information about the not readily accessible posterior areas, such as the oropharynx and the palatine tonsil, was achieved. Concerning the image evaluation, a list of seven criteria was implemented especially considering the integrity and the profile of the epithelial surface as well as the grade of vascular supply by major vessels as future indicators for the detection of suspicious oral lesions. Moreover, the extent of freely available OCT cross sections was enlarged by creating a collection of sample pictures demonstrating regional characteristics to expand the current state of knowledge about the healthy adult oral soft tissue. In order to prevent unnecessary biopsies, histological correlation was realized using HE stained image material out of a virtual database of human tissue. Altogether, there was a good correlation between the OCT cross sections and the histological slides as diagnostic gold standard.

To the best of our knowledge, for the first time mean values for the epithelial thickness of the alveolar mucosa, the palatine tonsil and the oropharynx were obtained from OCT images. Comparing the results of different investigation areas, epithelium of the sublingual mucosa was found to be thinnest in contrast to a maximum alongside the buccal region. Furthermore, the influence of sex and age on the epithelium was examined by dividing the sample into groups. Within the sublingual and the palatal region, mean epithelial thickness was increased in male subjects while age-related variations were found at the palatine tonsil. According to the anatomical configuration, mean vascular density was measured in relation to the avascular epithelium. Focusing on major vessels, a moderate to high tissue vascularization was determined within the observed regions including a maximum alongside the sublingual area. In a wider context, the assessment might be extended by quantifying the number of capillaries by means of imaging techniques like OCT angiography.

Concerning the analysis of the qualitative criteria, areas of lining mucosa appeared similar in the OCT cross sections possessing an even and homogeneous epithelium without alterations followed by a visually intact basement membrane. Within the buccal region, the hard palate and the palatine tonsil, respectively, oral mucosa showed local features representing physiological adaptations to mechanical stress or immune functions. Altogether, the findings suggest that an appropriate characterization of the healthy oral soft tissue can be achieved with a few measurement points.

Looking at disease-free individuals without alcohol or tobacco consumption above the tolerance levels, this study also indicates fields of further research. As an example, visually normal oral soft tissue in subjects with increased alcohol and tobacco intake need to be investigated for reaching a better understanding of early changes. Beyond that, the results should be the basis for future clinical studies aiming to improve the differentiation of suspicious lesions into benign and malignant.

With regard to the examination process, image analysis confirmed that future in vivo measurements can be simplified by gathering short series of OCT cross sections from a limited number of sites inside the investigation areas. In addition, there is a potential for the automatic epithelial thickness measurement based on the presented data in combination with future studies with an increased number of image data sets and analysts. In clinical practice, OCT might serve as adjunctive screening tool that is used to complement the visual evaluation and to facilitate the determination of the biopsy site. Against this background, the presented study offers a recommendation for the selection of the measurement points and comprehensive data about the expected appearance in OCT images.

Author Contributions: Conceptualization, M.A and J.W.; methodology, M.A., C.S. and J.W..; investigation, C.S. and J.W.; custom software development, C.S., J.M. and J.G.; formal analysis, J.W.; resources, J.W. and E.K.; data curation, M.A., J.M. and J.W.; writing—original draft preparation, M.A. and J.W.; writing—review and editing, C.S., J.G. and E.K.; visualization, J.W.; supervision, J.W.; project administration, J.W.; funding acquisition, J.W. and E.K. All authors have read and agreed to the published version of the manuscript.

Acknowledgments: We would like to thank Karl Storz GmbH & Co. KG, Tuttlingen, Germany for provision of the rigid NIR endoscopes and corresponding components. Histological cross sections were thankfully provided by the Institute of Anatomy, TU Dresden, Carl Gustav Carus Faculty of Medicine, Dresden, Germany.

Appendix A

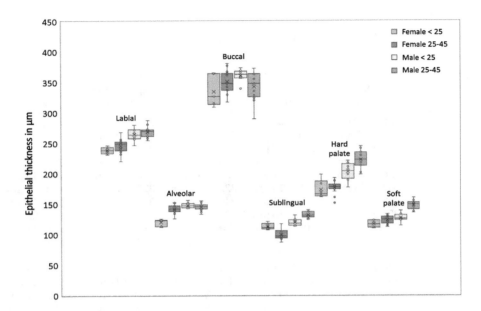

Figure A1. Box plot of the gender- and age-specific epithelial thickness of selected distinctive measurement points. Labial: MP4, Alveolar: MP5, Buccal: MP7, Sublingual: MP9, Hard palate: MP12, Soft palate: MP13 (cp. Figure 1).

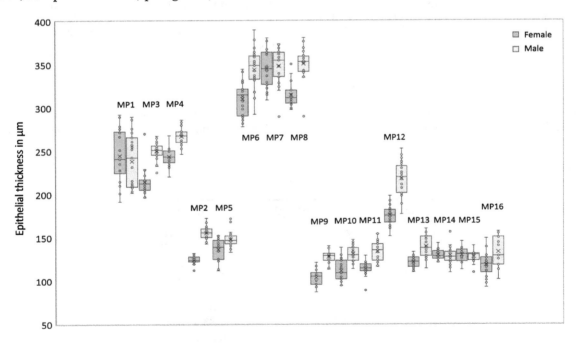

Figure A2. Box plot of the gender-specific epithelial thickness according to the location. Labial: MP1/MP3/MP4, Alveolar: MP2/MP5, Buccal: MP6-MP8, Sublingual: MP9/MP10, Mouth floor: MP11, Hard palate: MP12, Soft palate: MP13, Uvula: MP14, Oropharynx: MP15, Tonsils: MP16 (cp. Figure 1).

Table A1. Mean epithelial thickness ($\pm$ standard deviation) of individual measurement points and defined regions adjusted by sex and age.

Measurement Point/Region	Sex Distribution		Age Group			Total
	Male	Female	< 25	25–45	> 45	
MP 1	238 ± 30 μm	244 ± 30 μm	250 ± 32 μm	236 ± 28 μm	250 ± 37 μm	241 ± 30 μm
MP 2	155 ± 7 μm	124 ± 5 μm	140 ± 15 μm	140 ± 17 μm	147 ± 31 μm	141 ± 17 μm
MP 3	250 ± 10 μm	214 ± 15 μm	232 ± 18 μm	231 ± 23 μm	264 ± 7 μm	233 ± 22 μm
MP 4	267 ± 9 μm	244 ± 10 μm	253 ± 16 μm	258 ± 15 μm	253 ± 9 μm	256 ± 15 μm
MP 5	148 ± 9 μm	136 ± 12 μm	136 ± 15 μm	144 ± 7 μm	162 ± 13 μm	142 ± 12 μm
MP 6	344 ± 23 μm	310 ± 19 μm	327 ± 34 μm	327 ± 24 μm	341 ± 18 μm	328 ± 27 μm
MP 7	348 ± 20 μm	345 ± 21 μm	349 ± 22 μm	347 ± 21 μm	333 ± 10 μm	347 ± 21 μm
MP 8	351 ± 18 μm	315 ± 13 μm	336 ± 24 μm	333 ± 24 μm	331 ± 28 μm	334 ± 24 μm
MP 9	128 ± 8 μm	103 ± 9 μm	116 ± 7 μm	116 ± 18 μm	121 ± 14 μm	116 ± 15 μm
MP 10	131 ± 9 μm	110 ± 12 μm	124 ± 7 μm	120 ± 17 μm	119 ± 14 μm	121 ± 15 μm
MP 11	134 ± 11 μm	114 ± 8 μm	121 ± 5 μm	127 ± 17 μm	117 ± 5 μm	124 ± 14 μm
MP 12	218 ± 19 μm	175 ± 11 μm	190 ± 21 μm	199 ± 26 μm	220 ± 43 μm	198 ± 26 μm
MP 13	139 ± 12 μm	121 ± 7 μm	122 ± 8 μm	135 ± 14 μm	131 ± 7 μm	131 ± 13 μm
MP 14	129 ± 12 μm	129 ± 6 μm	126 ± 7 μm	129 ± 7 μm	148 ± 14 μm	129 ± 9 μm
MP 15	128 ± 8 μm	130 ± 8 μm	131 ± 7 μm	128 ± 7 μm	122 ± 12 μm	129 ± 8 μm
MP 16	133 ± 17 μm	118 ± 14 μm	142 ± 15 μm	115 ± 11 μm	141 ± 3 μm	125 ± 17 μm
Labial mucosa	252 ± 22 μm	234 ± 24 μm	245 ± 25 μm	242 ± 25 μm	256 ± 20 μm	243 ± 25 μm
Alveolar mucosa	152 ± 9 μm	130 ± 11 μm	138 ± 15 μm	142 ± 13 μm	155 ± 23 μm	142 ± 15 μm
Buccal mucosa	348 ± 20 μm	323 ± 24 μm	338 ± 28 μm	336 ± 24 μm	335 ± 18 μm	336 ± 25 μm
Sublingual mucosa	131 ± 10 μm	109 ± 11 μm	121 ± 7 μm	121 ± 18 μm	119 ± 10 μm	120 ± 15 μm
Hard palate	218 ± 19 μm	175 ± 11 μm	190 ± 21 μm	199 ± 26 μm	220 ± 43 μm	198 ± 26 μm
Soft palate and oropharynx	133 ± 12 μm	126 ± 8 μm	126 ± 8 μm	131 ± 11 μm	134 ± 15 μm	130 ± 11 μm
Palatine tonsils	133 ± 17 μm	118 ± 14 μm	142 ± 15 μm	115 ± 11 μm	141 ± 3 μm	125 ± 17 μm

Table A2. Mean vascular density of specific oral measurement points and regions. Due to the limited visualization of the lamina propria for the inner cheek and the hard palate, vascularization by major vessels of both regions could not be determined.

Measurement Point/Region	Vascularization
MP1	0.42 ± 0.10
MP2	0.44 ± 0.12
MP3	0.38 ± 0.09
MP4	0.39 ± 0.11
MP5	0.39 ± 0.12
MP9	0.81 ± 0.20
MP10	0.83 ± 0.17
MP11	0.81 ± 0.16
MP13	0.33 ± 0.08
MP14	0.37 ± 0.10
MP15	0.34 ± 0.11
MP16	0.19 ± 0.07
Labial mucosa	0.39 ± 0.10
Alveolar mucosa	0.41 ± 0.13
Sublingual mucosa	0.82 ± 0.17
Soft palate and oropharynx	0.34 ± 0.09
Palatine tonsils	0.19 ± 0.07

Table A3. Success rate of OCT data collection per measurement point, participant and investigation area.

Participant Number	Age Group	Sex	1	3	4	2	5	6	7	8	9	10	11	12	13	14	15	16	Success Rate (%)
1	(1)	m	x	x	x	x	x	x	x	x	x	x	x	x	x	x	x	x	100
2	(1)	m	x	x	x	x	x	x	x	x	x	x	x	x	x	x	x	x	100
3	(1)	m	x	x	x	x	x	x	x	x	x	x	x	x	x	x	x	x	100
4	(1)	m	x	x	x	x	x	x	x	x	x	x	x	x	x	x	x	x	100
5	(1)	m	x	x	x	x	x	x	x	x	x	x	x	x	x	x	0	x	93.8
6	(1)	m	x	x	x	x	x	x	x	x	x	x	x	x	x	x	0	0	87.5
7	(1)	m	x	x	x	x	x	x	x	x	x	x	x	x	x	x	0	0	87.5
8	(1)	m	x	x	x	x	x	x	x	x	x	x	x	x	x	0	0	0	81.3
9	(2)	m	x	x	x	x	x	x	x	x	x	x	x	x	x	x	x	x	100
10	(2)	m	x	x	x	x	x	x	x	x	x	x	x	x	x	x	x	x	100
11	(2)	m	x	x	x	x	x	x	x	x	x	x	x	x	x	x	x	x	100
12	(2)	m	x	x	x	x	x	x	x	x	x	x	x	x	x	x	x	x	100
13	(2)	m	x	x	x	x	x	x	x	x	x	x	x	x	x	x	x	x	100
14	(2)	m	x	x	x	x	x	x	x	x	x	x	x	x	x	x	x	x	100
15	(2)	m	x	x	x	x	x	x	x	x	x	x	x	x	x	x	x	x	100
16	(2)	m	x	x	x	x	x	x	x	x	x	x	x	x	x	x	0	x	93.8
17	(2)	m	x	x	x	x	x	x	x	x	x	x	x	x	x	x	0	x	93.8
18	(2)	m	x	x	x	x	x	x	x	x	x	x	x	x	x	x	0	0	87.5
19	(2)	m	x	x	x	x	x	x	x	x	x	x	x	x	x	x	0	0	87.5
20	(2)	m	x	x	x	x	x	x	x	x	x	x	x	x	x	x	0	0	87.5
21	(2)	m	x	x	x	x	x	x	x	x	x	x	x	x	x	0	0	0	81.3
22	(2)	m	x	x	x	x	x	x	x	x	x	x	x	x	0	0	0	0	75.0
23	(2)	m	x	x	x	x	x	x	x	x	x	x	x	x	0	0	0	0	75.0
24	(3)	m	x	x	x	x	x	x	x	x	x	x	x	x	x	x	x	x	100
25	(3)	m	x	x	x	x	x	x	x	x	x	x	x	x	x	x	x	x	100
26	(1)	f	x	x	x	x	x	x	x	x	x	x	x	x	x	x	x	x	100
27	(1)	f	x	x	x	x	x	x	x	x	x	x	x	x	x	x	x	x	100
28	(1)	f	x	x	x	x	x	x	x	x	x	x	x	x	x	x	x	x	100
29	(1)	f	x	x	x	x	x	x	x	x	x	x	x	x	x	x	0	x	93.8
30	(1)	f	x	x	x	x	x	x	x	x	x	x	x	x	x	0	0	0	81.3
31	(2)	f	x	x	x	x	x	x	x	x	x	x	x	x	x	x	x	x	100
32	(2)	f	x	x	x	x	x	x	x	x	x	x	x	x	x	x	x	x	100
33	(2)	f	x	x	x	x	x	x	x	x	x	x	x	x	x	x	x	x	100
34	(1)	f	x	x	x	x	x	x	x	x	x	x	x	x	x	x	x	x	100
35	(2)	f	x	x	x	x	x	x	x	x	x	x	x	x	x	x	x	x	100
36	(2)	f	x	x	x	x	x	x	x	x	x	x	x	x	x	x	x	x	100
37	(2)	f	x	x	x	x	x	x	x	x	x	x	x	x	x	x	x	x	100
38	(2)	f	x	x	x	x	x	x	x	x	x	x	x	x	x	x	x	x	100
39	(2)	f	x	x	x	x	x	x	x	x	x	x	x	x	x	x	x	x	100
40	(2)	f	x	x	x	x	x	x	x	x	x	x	x	x	x	x	x	x	100
41	(2)	f	x	x	x	x	x	x	x	x	x	x	x	x	x	x	x	x	100
42	(2)	f	x	x	x	x	x	x	x	x	x	x	x	x	x	x	x	x	100
43	(2)	f	x	x	x	x	x	x	x	x	x	x	x	x	x	x	0	x	93.8
44	(2)	f	x	x	x	x	x	x	x	x	x	x	x	x	x	x	0	0	87.5
45	(2)	f	x	x	x	x	x	x	x	x	x	x	x	x	x	x	0	0	87.5
46	(2)	f	x	x	x	x	x	x	x	x	x	x	x	x	x	0	0	0	100
47	(3)	f	x	x	x	x	x	x	x	x	x	x	x	x	x	x	x	x	100

Investigation area	Labial mucosa		Alveolar mucosa		Buccal mucosa		Sublingual mucosa		Hard palate	Soft palate/ oropharynx			Palatine tonsil
Success rate %	100		100		100		100		100	95.7	85.1	61.7	72.3

Age group: (1): <25; (2): 25–45; (3): >45. Sex: m: male; f = female. Success rate: Percentage of measurement points reached (x: OCT data collected, 0: no OCT data).

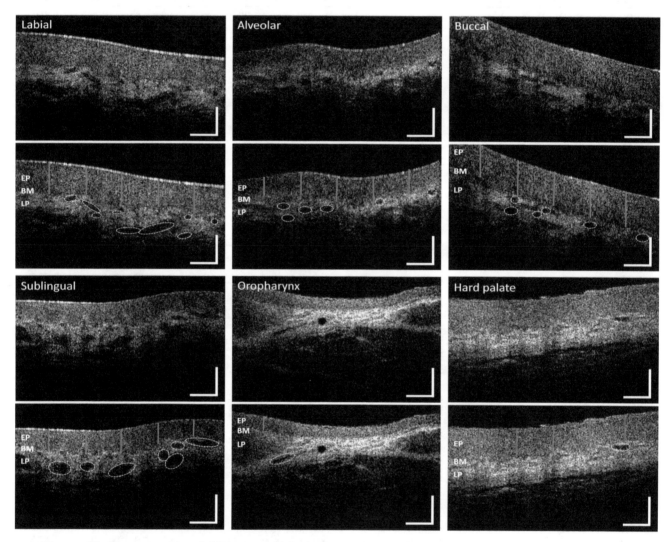

Figure A3. Representative OCT images of the human oral mucosa in vivo of the labial, alveolar, buccal and sublingual region as well as the oropharynx and the hard palate demonstrating the principle of the visual image analysis. EP: epithelium, BM: basement membrane, LP: lamina propria; Vertical lines: epithelial thickness measurement, Ellipsoidal shapes: marked regions of vascularization. Scale bars: 200 μm.

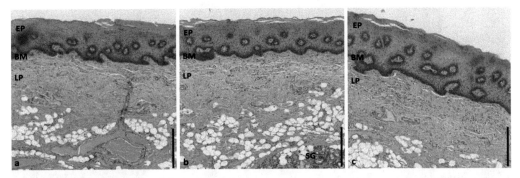

Figure A4. Supplementary HE stained histological cross sections of the human labial oral mucosa [44]. EP: epithelium, BM: basement membrane, LP: lamina propria, SG: salivary gland. Scale bar: 200 μm.

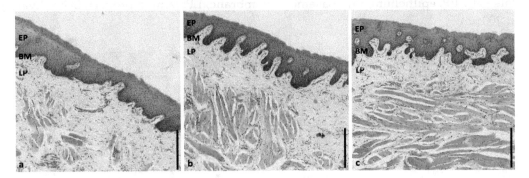

Figure A5. Supplementary HE stained histological cross sections of the human alveolar mucosa [44]. EP: epithelium, BM: basement membrane, LP: lamina propria, Scale bar: 200 μm.

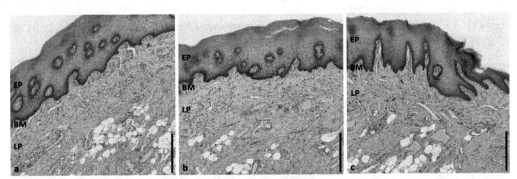

Figure A6. Supplementary HE stained histological cross sections of the human buccal mucosa [44]. EP: epithelium, BM: basement membrane, LP: lamina propria, Scale bar: 200 μm.

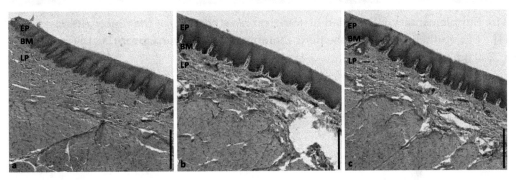

Figure A7. Supplementary HE stained histological cross sections of the human sublingual mucosa [44]. EP: epithelium, BM: basement membrane, LP: lamina propria, Scale bar: 200 μm.

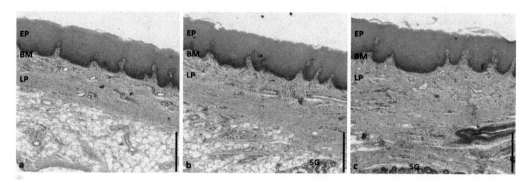

Figure A8. Supplementary HE stained histological cross sections of the mucosal tissue of the human hard palate [44]. EP: epithelium, BM: basement membrane, LP: lamina propria, SG: salivary gland. Scale bar: 200 μm.

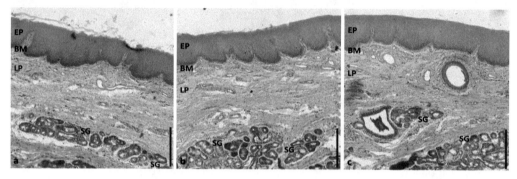

Figure A9. Supplementary HE stained histological cross sections of the mucosal tissue of the human soft palate [44]. EP: epithelium, BM: basement membrane, LP: lamina propria, SG: salivary gland. Scale bar: 200 μm.

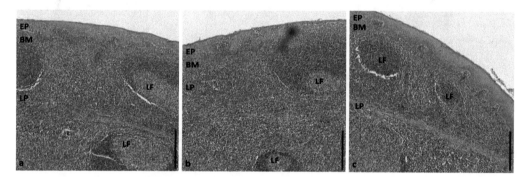

Figure A10. Supplementary HE stained histological cross sections of the mucosal tissue of the human tonsil [44]. EP: epithelium, BM: basement membrane, LP: lamina propria, LF: lymphoid follicle. Scale bar: 200 μm.

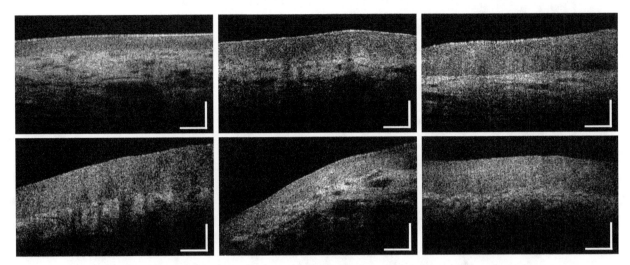

Figure A11. Supplementary intensity-based OCT cross sections of the mucosal tissue of the inner upper lip (MP1, Figure 1). Scale bars: 200 μm.

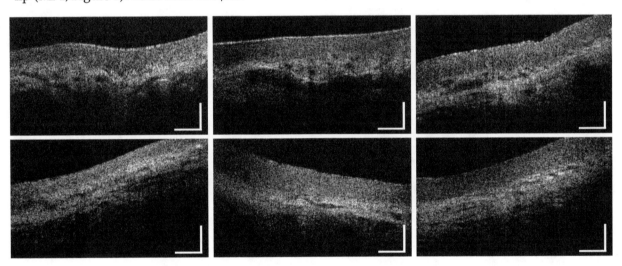

Figure A12. Supplementary intensity-based OCT cross sections of the alveolar mucosa of the upper vestibular region (MP2, Figure 1). Scale bars: 200 μm.

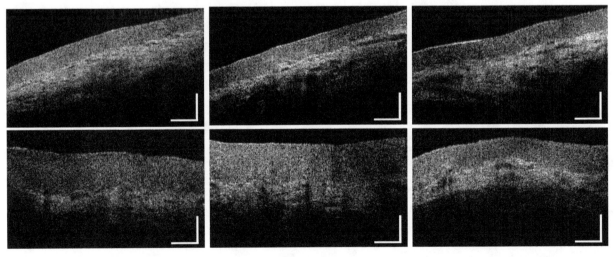

Figure A13. Supplementary intensity-based OCT cross sections of the mucosal tissue of the central inner lower lip (MP3, Figure 1). Scale bars: 200 μm.

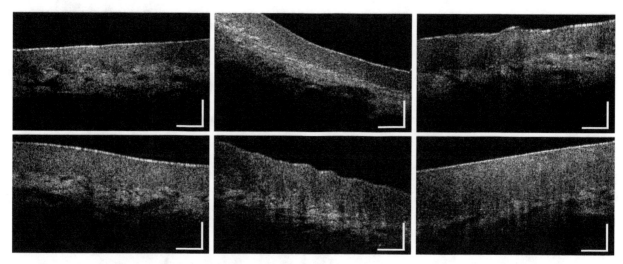

Figure A14. Supplementary intensity-based OCT cross sections of the mucosal tissue of the lateral inner lower lip (MP4, Figure 1). Scale bars: 200 μm.

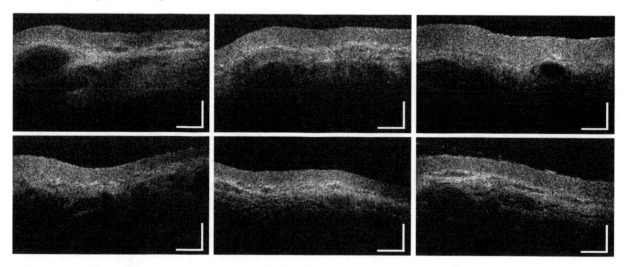

Figure A15. Supplementary intensity-based OCT cross sections of the alveolar mucosa of the lower vestibular region (MP5, Figure 1). Scale bars: 200 μm.

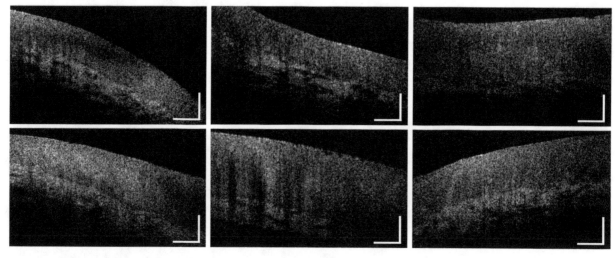

Figure A16. Supplementary intensity-based OCT cross sections of the buccal mucosa of the anterior inner cheek (MP6, Figure 1). Scale bars: 200 μm.

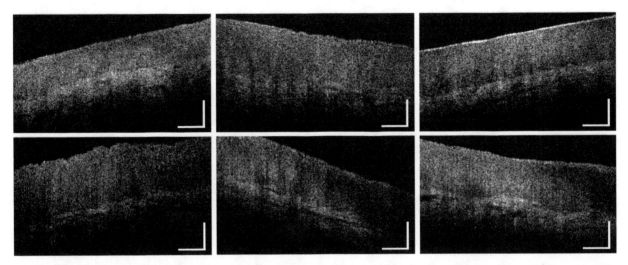

Figure A17. Supplementary intensity-based OCT cross sections of the buccal mucosa of the central inner cheek (MP7, Figure 1). Scale bars: 200 μm.

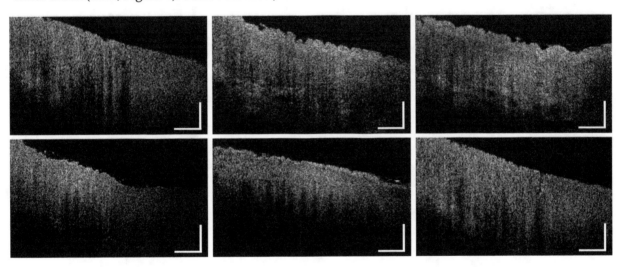

Figure A18. Supplementary intensity-based OCT cross sections of the buccal mucosa of the posterior inner cheek (MP8, Figure 1). Scale bars: 200 μm.

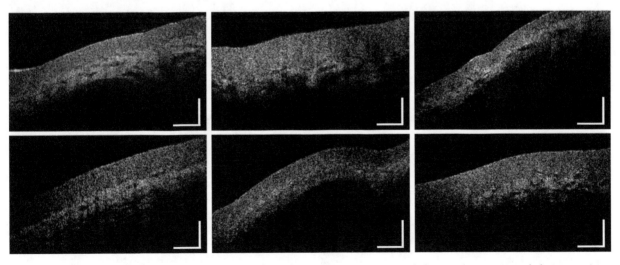

Figure A19. Supplementary intensity-based OCT cross sections of the oral mucosa of the anterior ventral tongue (MP9, Figure 1). Scale bars: 200 μm.

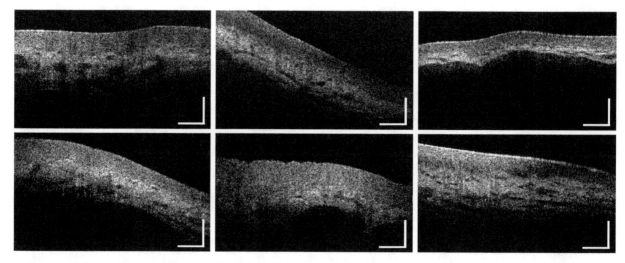

Figure A20. Supplementary intensity-based OCT cross sections of the oral mucosa of the central ventral tongue (MP10, Figure 1). Scale bars: 200 μm.

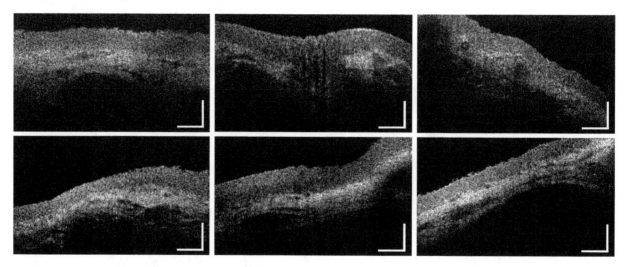

Figure A21. Supplementary intensity-based OCT cross sections of the mucosal tissue of the mouth floor (MP11, Figure 1). Scale bars: 200 μm.

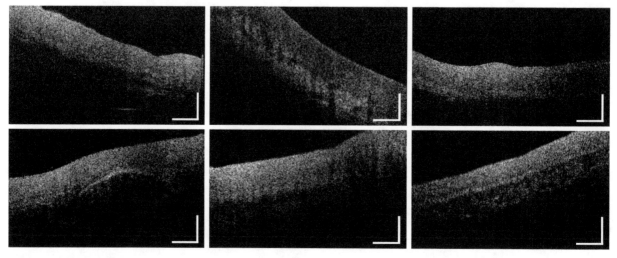

Figure A22. Supplementary intensity-based OCT cross sections of the oral muucosa of the hard palate (MP12, Figure 1). Scale bars: 200 μm.

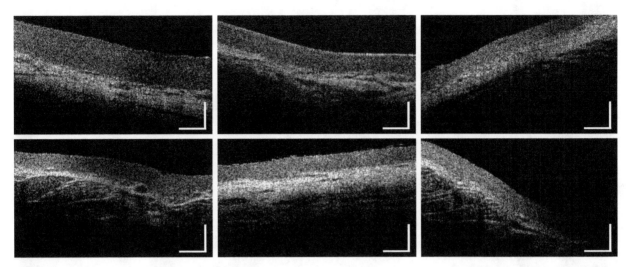

Figure A23. Supplementary intensity-based OCT cross sections of the mucosal tissue of the soft palate (MP13, Figure 1). Scale bars: 200 μm.

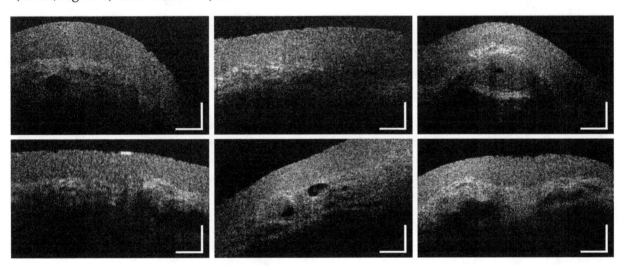

Figure A24. Supplementary intensity-based OCT cross sections of the oral mucosa of the uvula (MP14, Figure 1). Scale bars: 200 μm.

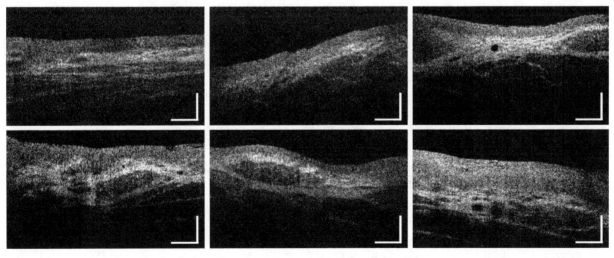

Figure A25. Supplementary intensity-based OCT cross sections of the mucosal tissue of the oropharynx (MP15, Figure 1). Scale bars: 200 μm.

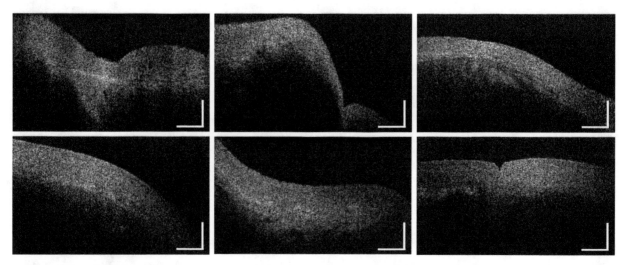

Figure A26. Supplementary intensity-based OCT cross sections of the mucosal tissue of the palatine tonsil (MP16, Figure 1). Scale bars: 200 μm.

References

1. World Health Organization (WHO). *Cancer Today—Data Visualization Tools for Exploring the Global Cancer Burden in 2018*; World Health Organization (WHO): Geneva, Switzerland.
2. Montero, P.H.; Patel, S.G. Cancer of the Oral Cavity. *Surg. Oncol. Clin. N. Am.* **2015**, *24*, 491–508. . [CrossRef] [PubMed]
3. Rivera, C.; Venegas, B. Histological and molecular aspects of oral squamous cell carcinoma. *Oncol. Lett.* **2014**, *8*, 7–11. [CrossRef] [PubMed]
4. Robert Koch-Institut; die Gesellschaft der epidemiologischen Krebsregister in Deutschland e.V. *Krebs in Deutschland für 2015/2016*; Technical report; 2020. Available online: https://www.krebsdaten.de/ Krebs/DE/Content/Publikationen/Krebs_in_Deutschland/krebs_in_deutschland_inhalt.html (accessed on 15 October 2020).
5. Shield, K.D.; Ferlay, J.; Jemal, A.; Sankaranarayanan, R.; Chaturvedi, A.K.; Bray, F.; Soerjomataram, I. The global incidence of lip, oral cavity, and pharyngeal cancers by subsite in 2012. *CA Cancer J. Clin.* **2017**, *67*, 51–64. [CrossRef] [PubMed]
6. de Martel, C.; Georges, D.; Bray, F.; Ferlay, J.; Clifford, G.M. Global burden of cancer attributable to infections in 2018: A worldwide incidence analysis. *Lancet Glob. Health* **2020**, *8*, e180–e190. [CrossRef]
7. Deutsche Krebsgesellschaft; Deutsche Krebshilfe; AWMF. *Konsultationsfassung S3-Leitlinie Diagnostik und Therapie des Mundhöhlenkarzinoms*; Leitlinienprogramm Onkologie: Berlin, Germany, 2019; Volume 3.01, pp. 26–37. Available online: https://www.leitlinienprogramm-onkologie.de/fileadmin/user_upload/ Downloads/Leitlinien/Mundhoehlenkarzinom/Version_3/LL_Mundhoehlenkarzinom_Langversion_ Konsultationsfassung_3.01.pdf (accessed on 15 October 2020).
8. Rivera, C. Essentials of oral cancer. *Int. J. Clin. Exp. Pathol.* **2015**, *8*, 11884–11894. [CrossRef]
9. Avon, S.L.; Klieb, H.B. Oral soft-tissue biopsy: An overview. *J. Can. Dent. Assoc.* **2012**, *78*, 1–9.
10. Kumaraswamy, K.L.; Vidhya, M.; Rao, P.K.; Mukanda, A. Oral biopsy: Oral pathologist's perspective. *J. Cancer Res. Ther.* **2012**, *8*, 192–198. [CrossRef]
11. Herranz González-Botas, J.; Varela Vázquez, P.; Vázquez Barro, C. Second primary tumours in head and neck cancer. *Curr. Oncol. Rep.* **2016**, *67*, 123–129. [CrossRef]
12. Bhatia, N.; Lalla, Y.; Vu, A.N.; Farah, C.S. Advances in optical adjunctive aids for visualisation and detection of oral malignant and potentially malignant lesions. *Int. J. Dent.* **2013**, *2013*. [CrossRef]
13. Huang, D.; Swanson, E.A.; Lin, C.P.L.; Schuman, J.S.; Stinson, W.G.; Chang, W.; Hee, M.R.; Flotte, T.; Gregory, K.; Puliafito, C.A.; et al. Optical coherence tomography (OCT). *Science* **1991**, *254*, 1178–1181. [CrossRef]

14. Wilder-Smith, P.; Holtzman, J.; Epstein, J.; Le, A. Optical diagnostics in the oral cavity: An overview. *Oral Dis.* **2010**, *16*, 717–728. [CrossRef] [PubMed]

15. Gora, M.J.; Suter, M.J.; Tearney, G.J.; Li, X. Endoscopic optical coherence tomography: Technologies and clinical applications [Invited]. *Biomed. Opt. Express* **2017**, *8*, 2405–2444. [CrossRef] [PubMed]

16. Higgins, L.M.; Pierce, M.C. Design and characterization of a handheld multimodal imaging device for the assessment of oral epithelial lesions. *J. Biomed. Opt.* **2014**, *19*, 086004. [CrossRef] [PubMed]

17. Gentile, E.; Maio, C.; Romano, A.; Laino, L.; Lucchese, A. The potential role of in vivo optical coherence tomography for evaluating oral soft tissue: A systematic review. *J. Oral Pathol. Med.* **2017**, *46*, 864–876. [CrossRef] [PubMed]

18. Matheny, E.S.; Hanna, N.M.; Jung, W.G.; Chen, Z.; Wilder-Smith, P.; Mina-Araghi, R.; Brenner, M. Optical coherence tomography of malignancy in hamster cheek pouches. *J. Biomed. Opt.* **2004**, *9*, 978. [CrossRef]

19. Wilder-Smith, P.; Lee, K.; Guo, S.; Zhang, J.; Osann, K.; Chen, Z.; Messadi, D. In vivo diagnosis of oral daysplasia and malignancy using optical coherence tomography: Preliminary studies in 50 Patients. *Lasers Surg. Med.* **2009**, *41*, 353–357. [CrossRef]

20. Hamdoon, Z.; Jerjes, W.; Upile, T.; McKenzie, G.; Jay, A.; Hopper, C. Optical coherence tomography in the assessment of suspicious oral lesions: An immediate ex vivo study. *Photodiagnosis Photodyn. Ther.* **2013**, *10*, 17–27. [CrossRef]

21. Volgger, V.; Stepp, H.; Ihrler, S.; Kraft, M.; Leunig, A.; Patel, P.M.; Susarla, M.; Jackson, K.; Betz, C.S. Evaluation of optical coherence tomography to discriminate lesions of the upper aerodigestive tract. *Head Neck* **2012**, *35*, 1558–1566. [CrossRef]

22. Tsai, M.T.; Lee, C.K.; Lee, H.C.; Wang, Y.M.; Yang, C.C.; Chiang, C.P. Effective indicators for oral cancer diagnosis based on optical coherence tomography. *Opt. Infobase Conf. Pap.* **2008**, *16*, 15847–15862. [CrossRef]

23. Tsai, M.T.; Lee, C.K.; Lee, H.C.; Chen, H.M.; Chiang, C.P.; Wang, Y.M.; Yang, C.C. Differentiating oral lesions in different carcinogenesis stages with optical coherence tomography. *J. Biomed. Opt.* **2009**, *14*, 044028. [CrossRef]

24. Lee, C.K.; Chi, T.T.; Wu, C.T.; Tsai, M.T.; Chiang, C.P.; Yang, C.C.C.C. Diagnosis of oral precancer with optical coherence tomography. *Biomed. Opt. Express* **2012**, *3*, 1632. [CrossRef] [PubMed]

25. Prestin, S.; Rothschild, S.I.; Betz, C.S.; Kraft, M. Measurement of epithelial thickness within the oral cavity using optical coherence tomography. *Head Neck* **2012**, *34*, 1777–1781. [CrossRef] [PubMed]

26. Ridgeway, J.M.; Armstrong, W.B.; Guo, S.; Mahmood, U.; Su, J.; Jackson, R.P.; Shibuya, T.; Crumley, R.L.; Gu, M.; Chen, Z.; et al. In vivo optical coherence tomography of the human oral cavity and oropharynx. *Arch. Otolaryngol.—Head Neck Surg.* **2006**, *132*, 1074–1081. [CrossRef] [PubMed]

27. Di Stasio, D.; Lauritano, D.; Iquebal, H.; Romano, A.; Gentile, E.; Lucchese, A. Measurement of oral epithelial thickness by optical coherence tomography. *Diagnostics* **2019**, *9*, 1–8. [CrossRef] [PubMed]

28. Pande, P.; Shrestha, S.; Park, J.; Serafino, M.J.; Gimenez-Conti, I.; Brandon, J.; Cheng, Y.S.; Applegate, B.E.; Jo, J.A. Automated classification of optical coherence tomography images for the diagnosis of oral malignancy in the hamster cheek pouch. *J. Biomed. Opt.* **2014**, *19*, 086022. [CrossRef]

29. Goldan, R.N.; Lee, A.; Cahill, L.C.; Liu, K.Y.; MacAulay, C.E.; Poh, C.F.; Lane, P.M. Automated Segmentation of Oral Mucosa from Wide-Field OCT Images (Conference Presentation). In *Advanced Biomedical and Clinical Diagnostic and Surgical Guidance Systems XIV*; International Society for Optics and Photonics: Bellingham, WA, USA, 2016; p. 25. [CrossRef]

30. Wei, W.; Choi, W.J.; Wank, R.K. Microvascular imaging and monitoring of human oral cavity lesions in vivo by swept-source OCT based angiography. *Lasers Med Sci.* **2018**, *33*, 123–134. [CrossRef]

31. de Boer, J.F.; Hitzenberger, C.K.; Yasuno, Y. Polarization sensitive optical coherence tomography—A review [Invited]. *Biomed. Opt. Express* **2017**, *8*, 1838–1873. [CrossRef]

32. Walther, J.; Golde, J.; Kirsten, L.; Tetschke, F.; Hempel, F.; Rosenauer, T.; Hannig, C.; Koch, E. In vivo imaging of human oral hard and soft tissues by polarization-sensitive optical coherence tomography. *J. Biomed. Opt.* **2017**, *22*, 1–17. [CrossRef]

33. Walther, J.; Li, Q.; Villiger, M.; Farah, C.S.; Koch, E.; Karnowski, K.; Sampson, D.D. Depth-resolved birefringence imaging of collagen fiber organization in the human oral mucosa in vivo. *Biomed. Opt. Express* **2019**, *10*, 1942. [CrossRef] [PubMed]

34. Burger, M.; Brönstrup, A.; Pietrzik, K. Derivation of tolerable upper alcohol intake levels in Germany: A systematic review of risks and benefits of moderate alcohol consumption. *Prev. Med.* **2004**, *39*, 111–127. [CrossRef]

35. Hashibe, M.; Brennan, P.; Benhamou, S.; Castellsague, X.; Chen, C.; Curado, M.P.; Maso, L.D.; Daudt, A.W.; Fabianova, E.; Wünsch-Filho, V.; et al. Alcohol drinking in never users of tobacco, cigarette smoking in never drinkers, and the risk of head and neck cancer: Pooled analysis in the international head and neck cancer epidemiology consortium. *J. Natl. Cancer Inst.* **2007**, *99*, 777–789. [CrossRef] [PubMed]

36. Walther, J.; Schnabel, C.; Tetschke, F.; Rosenauer, T.; Golde, J.; Ebert, N.; Baumann, M.; Hannig, C.; Koch, E. In vivo imaging in the oral cavity by endoscopic optical coherence tomography. *J. Biomed. Opt.* **2018**, *23*, 071207. [CrossRef]

37. Walther, J.; Krüger, A.; Cuevas, M.; Koch, E. Effects of axial, transverse, and oblique sample motion in FD OCT in systems with global or rolling shutter line detector. *J. Opt. Soc. Am.* **2008**, *25*, 2791. [CrossRef]

38. Abràmoff, M.D.; Magalhães, P.J.; Ram, S.J. Image processing with imageJ. *Biophotonics Int.* **2004**, *11*, 36–41. [CrossRef]

39. Curl, C.L.; Bellair, C.J.; Harris, T.; Allman, B.E.; Harris, P.J.; Stewart, A.G.; Roberts, A.; Nugent, K.A.; Delbridge, L.M. Refractive index measurement in viable cells using quantitative phase-amplitude microscopy and confocal microscopy. *Cytom. Part A* **2005**, *65*, 88–92. [CrossRef]

40. Tsai, M.T.; Chen, Y.; Lee, C.Y.; Huang, B.H.; Trung, N.H.; Lee, Y.J.; Wang, Y.L. Noninvasive structural and microvascular anatomy of oral mucosae using handheld optical coherence tomography. *Biomed. Opt. Express* **2017**, *8*, 5001–5012. [CrossRef]

41. Maslennikova, A.V.; Sirotkina, M.A.; Moiseev, A.A.; Finagina, E.S.; Ksenofontov, S.Y.; Gelikonov, G.V.; Matveev, L.A.; Kiseleva, E.B.; Zaitsev, V.Y.; Zagaynova, E.V.; et al. In-vivo longitudinal imaging of microvascular changes in irradiated oral mucosa of radiotherapy cancer patients using optical coherence tomography. *Sci. Rep.* **2017**, *7*, 16505. [CrossRef] [PubMed]

42. Grulkowski, I.; Nowak, J.K.; Karnowski, K.; Zebryk, P.; Puszczewicz, M.; Walkowiak, J.; Wojtkowski, M. Quantitative assessment of oral mucosa and labial minor salivary glands in patients with Sjögren's syndrome using swept source OCT. *Biomed. Opt. Express* **2014**, *5*, 259–274. [CrossRef] [PubMed]

43. Pahlevaninezhad, H.; Lee, A.M.; Rosin, M.; Sun, I.; Zhang, L.; Hakimi, M.; MacAulay, C.; Lane, P.M. Optical coherence tomography and autofluorescence imaging of human tonsil. *PLoS ONE* **2014**, *9*, e115889. [CrossRef] [PubMed]

44. Institute of Anatomy, Faculty of Medicine, Technische Universitaet Dresden. *Virtual Database—Histological Cross Sections of the Healthy Human Oral Mucosa*; Institute of Anatomy, Faculty of Medicine, Technische Universitaet Dresden: Dresden, Germany, 2020.

45. Otis, L.L.; Piao, D.; Gibson, C.W.; Zhu, Q. Quantifying labial blood flow using optical Doppler tomography. *Oral Surg. Oral Med. Oral Pathol. Oral Radiol. Endodontol.* **2004**, *98*, 189–194. [CrossRef]

46. Squier, C.; Brogden, K.A. *Human Oral Mucosa—Development, Structure & Function*; John Wiley & Sons, Ltd.: Hoboken, NJ, USA, 2011. [CrossRef]

47. Kessler, A.T.; Bhatt, A.A. Review of the Major and Minor Salivary Glands, Part 1: Anatomy, Infectious, and Inflammatory Processes. *J. Clin. Imaging Sci.* **2018**, *8*, 47. [CrossRef] [PubMed]

48. Lee, Y.J.; Kwon, Y.H.; Park, J.B.; Herr, Y.; Shin, S.I.; Heo, S.J.; Chung, J.H. Epithelial Thickness of the Palatal Mucosa: A Histomorphometric Study in Koreans. *Anat. Rec.* **2010**, *293*, 1966–1970. [CrossRef] [PubMed]

49. Harada, K. The histopathological study of human palatine tonsils—Especially age changes. *Nihon Jibiinkoka Gakkai Kaiho* **1989**, *92*, 1049–1064. [CrossRef] [PubMed]

50. Pai, S.I.; Westra, W.H. Molecular Pathology of Head and Neck Cancer: Implications for Diagnosis, Prognosis, and Treatment. *Annu. Rev. Pathol.* **2009**, *4*, 49–70. [CrossRef]

51. Landay, M.A.; Schroeder, H.E. Quantitative electron microscopic analysis of the stratified epithelium of normal human buccal mucosa. *Cell Tissue Res.* **1977**, *177*, 383–405. [CrossRef]

52. Singhal, P.; Singh, N.N.; Sreedhar, G.; Banerjee, S.; Batra, M.; Garg, A. Evaluation of histomorphometric changes in tissue architecture in relation to alteration in fixation protocol—An invitro study. *J. Clin. Diagn. Res.* **2016**, *10*, ZC28–ZC32. [CrossRef]

53. Hand, A.R.; Pathmanathan, D.; Field, R.B. Morphological features of the minor salivary glands. *Arch. Oral Biol.* **1999**, *44*, S3–S10. [CrossRef]

3

Fabrication of Coaxial and Confocal Transducer Based on Sol-Gel Composite Material for Optical Resolution Photoacoustic Microscopy

Masayuki Tanabe [1],*⊙, Tai Chieh Wu [2], Makiko Kobayashi [1]⊙ and Che Hua Yang [2]

[1] Faculty of Advanced Science and Technology, Kumamoto University, Kumamoto 8608555, Japan; kobayashi@cs.kumamoto-u.ac.jp
[2] College of Mechanical and Electrical Engineering, National Taipei University of Technology, Taipei 10608, Taiwan; djwu1224@gmail.com (T.C.W.); chyang@ntut.edu.tw (C.H.Y.)
* Correspondence: mtanabe@cs.kumamoto-u.ac.jp

Abstract: We have newly developed coaxial and confocal optical-resolution photoacoustic microscopy based on sol-gel composite materials. This transducer contains a concave-shaped piezoelectric layer with a focus depth of 5 mm and a hole with a diameter of 3 mm at the center to pass a laser beam into a phantom. Therefore, this system can directly detect an excited photoacoustic signal without prisms or acoustic lenses. We demonstrate the capability of the system through pulse-echo and photoacoustic imaging experiments. The center frequency of the fabricated transducer is approximately 7 MHz, and its relative bandwidth is 86%. An ex-vivo experiment is conducted, and photoacoustic signals are clearly obtained. As a result, 2- and 3-dimensional maximum amplitude projection images are reconstructed.

Keywords: ultrasonic transducer; photoacoustic imaging; optical-resolution photoacoustic microscopy; sol-gel composite material

1. Introduction

Photoacoustic (PA) imaging is a novel visualization method that provides optical resolution and acoustic penetration. A PA imaging system employs a pulsed laser to generate acoustic waves at a focal point and an ultrasonic transducer to detect emitted acoustic waves [1–7]. Optical resolution PA microscopy (OR-PAM) is a PA imaging method where the optical focal size is considerably smaller than that of ultrasound, and thus, the spatial resolution of OR-PAM is generally determined by optical diffraction. The signal-to-noise ratio (SNR) and sensitivity of PA signals mainly depend on energy power required to transmit a pulsed laser and the receiving performance of an optic-acoustic transmitter (OAT), which transmits a pulsed laser and receives PA signals.

In OR-PAM, various designs of the OAT have been proposed to improve the efficiency of receiving PA signals. For example, prisms are used as a customized optical-acoustic combiner with an unfocused ultrasonic transducer, as shown in Figure 1a [1]. In this design, a silicone oil layer sandwiched by two prisms is utilized to achieve the confocal and coaxial alignment of optical and acoustic beams. The silicone layer is optically transparent but acoustically reflective. However, in this system, there is acoustic energy loss at the boundary between an acoustic lens, a silicone oil layer, and a medium. In addition, it is difficult to maintain a uniform thickness of the silicone oil layer because the thickness is easily influenced by the holder of prisms. Wang et al. have developed a different PA imaging system using a reflective objective and an ultrasonic transducer, as shown in Figure 1b [2]. The reflective objective has a long working distance and a large numerical aperture to achieve almost diffraction-limited optical focusing. A commercial transducer fabricated from a polyvinylidene fluoride (PVDF) polymer is placed underneath the objective to directly detect excited acoustic waves. This system can directly receive acoustic waves without obstacles. However, the sensitivity of PVDF is inferior to that of ceramic-type transducers such as $Pb(Zr_xTi_{1-x})O_3$ ($0 \leq x \leq 1$) (PZT). Furthermore, an optical reflective mirror blocks the center part of an optical beam. This decreases the optical energy at the zero-order diffraction bright spot and degrades the resolution of PA images. In another design, a PZT transducer with a hole is used with an acoustic lens, as shown in Figure 1c [3]. This transducer can transmit a laser beam through the hole and receive a PA signal without a reflective objective. The acoustic lens is placed before the transducer to focus on PA signals. However, this system still experiences energy loss in the acoustic lens.

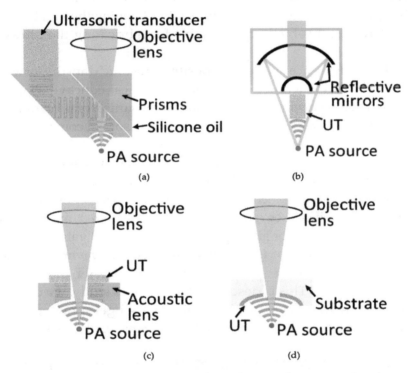

Figure 1. Optical-acoustic combinations in optical-resolution photoacoustic microscopy (OR-PAM). (a) Piston ultrasonic transducer (UT) is used with a two-prism acoustic reflector separated with a layer of silicone oil for reflecting the acoustic beam. (b) Piston UT is used with two reflective mirrors to reflect the laser beam. (c) Ring-shaped UT with an acoustic lens is used with a hole to transmit a laser beam. (d) Proposed concave transducer created using sol-gel composite spray technique. $Pb(Zr_xTi_{1-x})O_3$ ($0 \leq x \leq 1$) (PZT)/PZT layer is fabricated on a curved substrate with a hole for transmitting a laser beam.

An OAT should satisfy the following requirements to improve the sensitivity and SNR of PA imaging: (1) the optical-acoustic arrangement should be aligned, (2) the shapes of an ultrasonic receiving surface and the wavefront of a PA signal should be the same to obtain PA signals in phase at each point on the receiving surface, and (3) the obstacles for optical and acoustic beams should be eliminated. Therefore, the objective of this study was to fabricate an optimized OAT for OR-PAM. The proposed OAT system is broadly illustrated in Figure 1d. This OAT can transmit lasers and directly receive acoustic waves.

Curved ultrasonic transducers with a hole at the center [8–11], which satisfy the above-mentioned requirements, have been mainly manufactured as high intensity focused ultrasound sensors [10,11]. However, they are difficult to manufacture and expensive. In this study, we fabricated an ultrasonic transducer suitable for PA imaging for the first time using a sol-gel composite material [12–17], which makes it easy to create a sensor with a curved shape, and evaluated its fundamental performance

The sol-gel composite transducer is based on a sol-gel spraying technique, and it has been investigated in nondestructive testing applications [12,13]. The conventional sol-gel spraying technique uses only a sol-gel solution [18–20], whereas our method utilizes a sol-gel composite material, which is a mixture of a ferroelectric powder and a dielectric sol-gel solution. The piezoelectric layer fabricated by the sol-gel composite spraying method is composed of three phases: the ferroelectric powder phase, dielectric sol-gel phase, and air phase. The air phase is generated when the alcohol and water included in the sol-gel solution vaporizes during the firing process. This is described later. This method provides several advantages over conventional bulk PZT, PZT composites, and conventional sol-gel transducers in terms of the fabrication of the OAT. First, the concave piezoelectric layer can be fabricated by directly spraying the sol-gel composite material on the surface of a curved metal substrate. Second, backing and matching layers are not required because the PZT layer consists of tiny pores that decrease acoustic impedance. Third, the center frequency can be controlled by changing the number of spraying processes. Owing to these characteristics, this method is suitable for fabricating the ultrasonic transducer for PA imaging.

In a previous study, a flat surface sol-gel composite ultrasonic transducer was attached to a steel buffer rod. A probing end was machined into a hemispherical concave shape for the purpose of focusing, resulting in high spatial resolution with a lateral resolution of 0.19 mm and a focusing depth of 1.31 mm in the water at 23 °C [16]. However, curved surface sol-gel composite spraying transducers have never been fabricated for the purpose of focusing beams.

In another study, an ultrasonic sensor was fabricated on a stainless-steel plate with a hole in the center using the sol-gel spraying method, and laser irradiation and echo reception were performed simultaneously [14]. However, the distance from a focal point to each point of the sensor surface was inconsistent, resulting in long-tail echoes of approximately 5 μs. Next, another sensor with a curved surface was fabricated. Using the sensor and a preamplifier of 70 dB gain, an echo with a duration of approximately 0.5 μs and an amplitude of 4.7 V_{p-p} was obtained. However, the sensor size was 2.4 mm^2, much smaller than that of the previous sensor, 300 mm^2 [14]. Thereafter, the design was improved and a stronger echo was obtained [17]. This is described later. In this study, we developed an alternative method for fabricating a curved surface transducer using the sol-gel spraying method. We conducted experiments using a tissue phantom and performed three-dimensional maximum amplitude projection (MAP) to present the performance of the sensor.

The rest of this paper is organized as follows: Section 2 briefly describes the fabrication process of the transducer, its ultrasonic performance testing, and the experimental setup of PA imaging. The results are presented in Section 3. The discussion of the results is provided in Section 4.

2. Materials and Methods

2.1. Transducer Fabrication

We apply the sol-gel composite spraying technique to develop a concave-shaped single ultrasonic transducer. The general fabrication process of the sol-gel composite ultrasonic transducer is described below. First, a commercial PZT powder (Hizirco PZT L, Hayashi Chemical Industry Co., Ltd., Kyoto, Japan) [21] and a PZT sol-gel solution created in our laboratory are mixed at 1:2 ratio by weight using a ball milling machine for at least 24 h. Subsequently, the composite material is sprayed on a thin stainless-steel plate using a customized automatic coating machine at 25 °C. The thin stainless-steel plate is also used as a bottom electrode. After spraying, drying is performed at 150 °C for 10 min and firing is performed at 650 °C for 5 min. The spraying, drying, and firing processes are repeated until the PZT/PZT layer reaches a desirable thickness. After the PZT/PZT layer fabrication process, polarization is performed for 5 min at room temperature using a corona discharge device. After polarization, the piezoelectric d constant, d_{33}, is measured using a d33 m (ZJ-3B, IACAS) to evaluate the fundamental performance of the transducer. The flowchart of the fabrication process is shown in Figure 2.

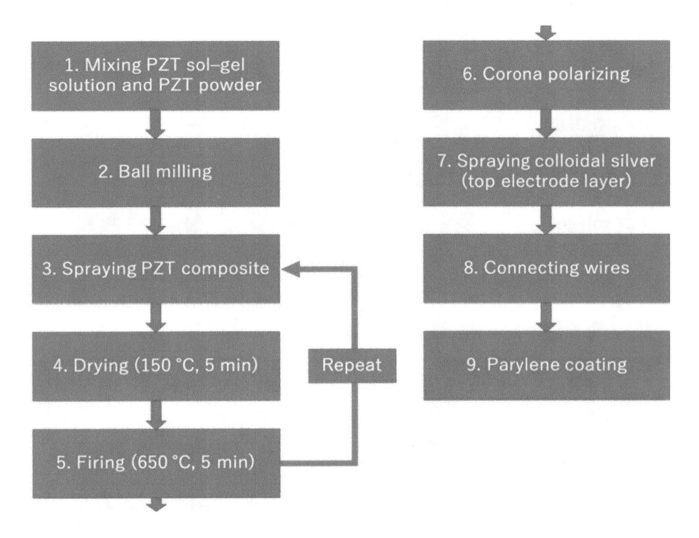

Figure 2. Flowchart of the fabrication process of a sol-gel composite PZT/PZT transducer.

The sol-gel composite ultrasonic transducer is fabricated as follows to achieve the coaxial and confocal ability: Figure 3 shows the entire design of the transducer. The diameter of the rod is 13 mm, the height is 5 mm, and the rod consists of a hole with a diameter of 3 mm for transmitting a laser beam and scanning a small area. The concave surface with a curvature radius of 5 mm, which is sandwiched between colloidal silver and the stainless-steel rod, is the active transducer area. The distance between each point on the surface and the focal point is 5 mm, and the depth from the bottom of the transducer to the focal point is 3 mm. The optical and acoustic focal points are set at the same position to achieve coaxial and confocal alignment. Figure 4a shows the piezoelectric layer of the transducer. The piezoelectric constant, d_{33}, is approximately 76 pC/N. The top electrode layer is fabricated by spraying colloidal silver on the piezoelectric layer using an airbrush. After spraying colloidal silver, the substrate is dried at 150 °C for 1 min using a heat gun. Next, two wires are bonded on the bottom and top electrodes by utilizing an electrically conductive adhesive. The stainless-steel rod is used as a substrate. Consequently, the transducer is coated with parylene for waterproofing [22]. Figure 4b shows the finished transducer.

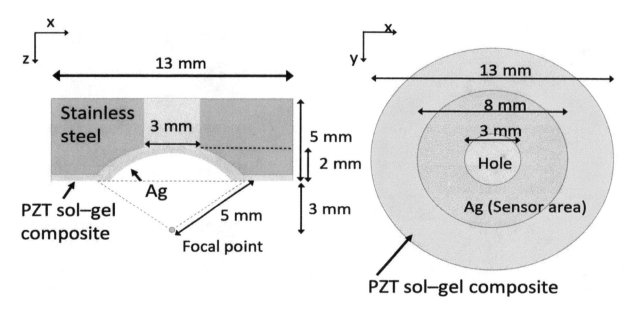

Figure 3. Design of fabricated transducer.

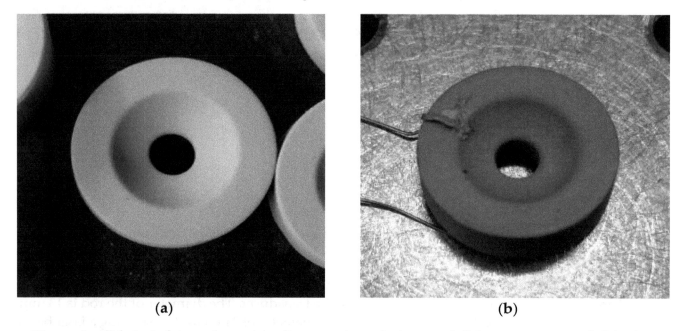

Figure 4. Fabricated transducer (**a**) after spraying, drying, and firing processes and (**b**) after connecting wires.

2.2. Pulse-Echo Experimental Design

The diagram of a pulse-echo experimental setup is shown in Figure 5. In the experiment, the fabricated transducer was fixed by a clamp with a 3-axis stage and moved to perform scans in the lateral and axial directions. A pulser/receiver (MODEL 5800, Olympus Corp., Tokyo, Japan) was used for transmitting and receiving ultrasound. The stage and pulser/receiver were controlled using LABVIEW (National Instruments, Austin, TX, USA). Ensemble average processing was applied to the obtained echo signals, with 100 times at each spatial point. In receiving, preamp gain was set as 40 dB, high-pass filter frequency was set as 1 MHz, and low-pass filter frequency was set as 10 MHz.

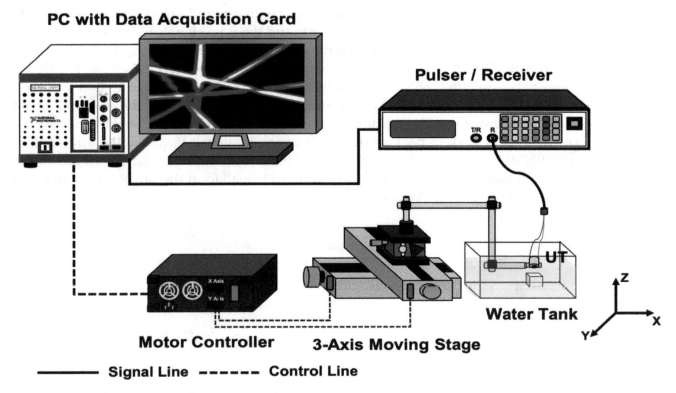

PC with Data Acquisition Card

Pulser / Receiver

Water Tank

Motor Controller   **3-Axis Moving Stage**

───── **Signal Line** ────── **Control Line**

Figure 5. Setup of the pulse-echo experiment using fabricated transducer. The fabricated transducer is moved by the three-dimensional stage and ultrasonic pulses are excited at each point. The moving pitch is approximately 13.3 μm and 500 μm in the lateral and axial directions, respectively.

3. Results

3.1. Fundamental Performance of Fabricated Transducer

To evaluate the performance of the fabricated transducer, its electrical impedance was measured using a network analyzer (E5061B, Keysight Technologies, Inc., Santa Rosa, CA, USA). The measured frequency characteristic of the electrical impedance is shown in Figure 6. According to this figure, the resonant frequency is 7 MHz. However, an antiresonant frequency is not seen below 30 MHz. Therefore, it can be predicted that the antiresonant frequency is considerably higher than 30 MHz.

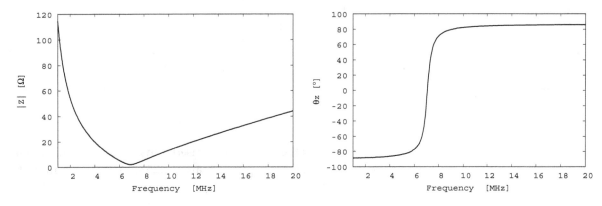

Figure 6. Electrical impedance of the fabricated transducer. Resonant frequency is approximately 7.0 MHz.

A pulse-echo experiment was conducted with the experimental setup as described in Figure 5 to characterize the acoustic resolution performance of the fabricated transducer. In the experiment, the fabricated transducer was fixed by a clamp with a 3-axis stage and moved to perform scans in the lateral and axial directions. A transparent phantom was constructed, which consisted of a copper wire with a diameter of 0.15 mm embedded in transparent agar with a sound velocity of approximately 1500 m/s. The agar phantom was placed in a water tank, and the echo signals from the copper wire were collected. An example of an echo signal from the copper wire is shown in Figure 7. The center frequency is approximately 7 MHz, and its −6 dB frequency bandwidth is 6 MHz (3.5–9.5 MHz). Hence, the relative frequency bandwidth is 86%. This bandwidth is fairly broad considering that matching and backing layers were omitted in the fabricated transducer. Figure 8 illustrates the axial and lateral resolution obtained by measuring the amplitudes of the echoes from the copper wire by moving the 3-axis stage. The maximum peak-to-peak amplitude is approximately 4 V$_{p-p}$, and the full width at half maximum (FWHM) is approximately 1.25 mm and 0.2 mm in the axial and lateral directions, respectively. It is found that a satisfactory large amplitude and small focal size are obtained owing to the curved shape of the fabricated transducer.

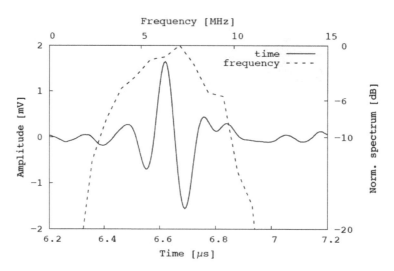

Figure 7. Pulse-echo signal obtained from copper wire using fabricated focused transducer through pulse-echo testing in time (solid line) and frequency (dashed line) domains.

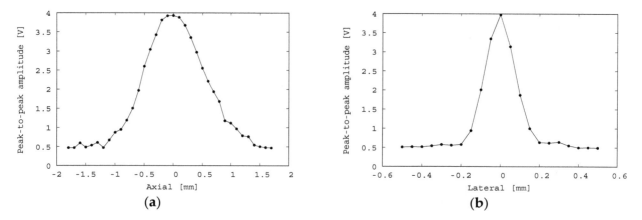

Figure 8. (a) Axial and (b) lateral intensity profiles of the fabricated focused transducer in the pulse-echo experiment. The full width at half maximum (FWHM) is approximately 1.25 mm and 0.2 mm in the axial and lateral directions, respectively.

3.2. Photoacoustic Visualization

The experimental setup for PA imaging is shown in Figure 9. In this experiment, a pulsed fiber laser (GLPM-10, IPG Photonics Corp., Massachusetts, Japan) with a wavelength of 532 nm and an input beam diameter of 5 mm was used. The focal length of the objective lens was 30 mm. The theoretical spot size of the laser was 5.5 μm. The pulse energy out of the objective lens was set as 0.6 μJ. This energy is significantly lower compared to previous studies. This is described in detail later. The pulse repetition frequency (PRF) of the emitted pulse was set as 50 kHz. A pulsed laser was generated, and it passed through a beam splitter, which was used for obtaining a trigger signal. Subsequently, the laser was reflected at a mirror, propagated through an achromatic lens (AC254-030-A, Thorlabs, Inc., Newton, NJ, USA), and finally focused at a point in a specimen. The emitted PA signals were received by the fabricated transducer. A conventional OAT consisting of an acoustic lens with a focal length of 12.7 mm, reflecting prisms, and an unfocused transducer (V384, Olympus Inc.) with a center frequency of 3.5 MHz was used as a reference, as shown in Figure 1a. The obtained signals were amplified by a pulser/receiver (MODEL 5800, Olympus Inc.) and a preamp (MODEL 5678, Olympus Inc.). The total gain was 60 dB, the cutoff frequency of the high-pass filter was 1 MHz, and the cutoff frequency of the low-pass filter was 10 MHz. The obtained signals were digitized at a sampling rate of 400 MHz and transferred to a computer, where an image was formed. In addition, ensemble average processing was applied to 20 signals to obtain smooth signals. As a specimen, a copper wire with a diameter of 0.15 mm and a human hair with a diameter of approximately 50 μm were separately embedded in transparent agar and fixed in the water tank. The signals obtained using the fabricated transducer and conventional OAT are shown in Figure 10. As shown in Figure 10a,b, the amplitude of the PA signal obtained using the fabricated focused transducer is 2.8 V_{p-p} for the copper wire and 4.4 V_{p-p} for the human hair. On the other hand, no peak is observed in the waveform obtained using the conventional OAT, as shown in Figure 10c,d.

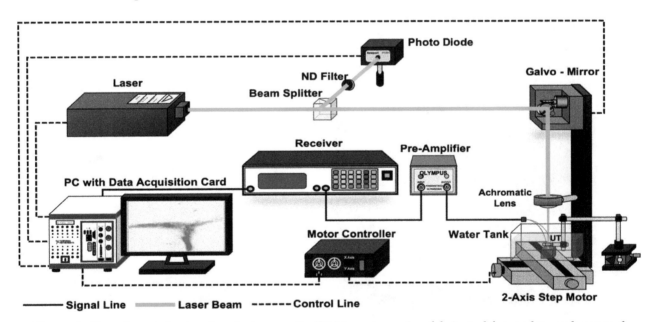

Figure 9. Experimental setup for photoacoustic (PA) imaging using fabricated focused transducer and conventional optic-acoustic transmitter (OAT).

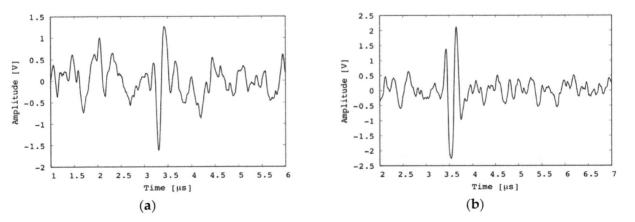

(a)   (b)

Figure 10. *Cont.*

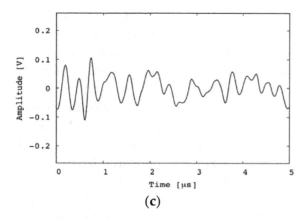

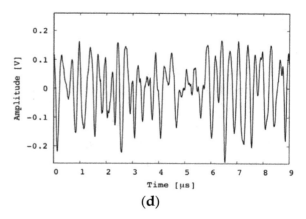

(c)   **(d)**

Figure 10. PA signals obtained from (**a**) copper wire and (**b**) hair using fabricated focused transducer, (**c**) copper wire and (**d**) hair using conventional OAT.

Although the waveform obtained by the fabricated focused transducer has a larger amplitude of noise signal than that of the conventional OAT, the ratio of the PA signal to the noise is 1.6 for copper wire and 3.4 for human hair. On the other hand, the SNR of the conventional OAT must be below unity because the conventional OAT could not obtain a PA signal.

A chicken testicle was used as a specimen to evaluate the transducer for biomaterial imaging, as shown in Figure 11. The scanning area was set as 1×1 mm^2 (the number of pixels was 100×100). The blood vessels on the surface with a diameter of less than 75 μm were visualized. Figure 12 illustrates an example of the PA signal obtained from the blood vessels. The peak-to-peak amplitude is approximately 4.5 V, and the SNR is 13 dB.

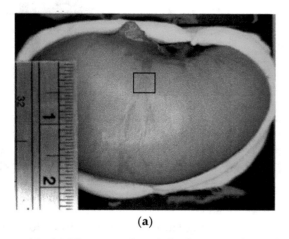

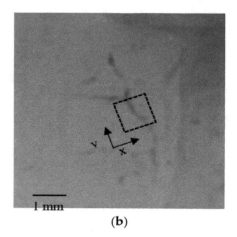

(a)   **(b)**

Figure 11. (**a**) Photographs of chicken testicle and (**b**) magnified view of the region bounded by the solid black line in (**a**). Black-dashed box in (**b**) indicates a scan area with a size of 1×1 mm^2 (pixel size: 100×100). Vessel diameter is less than 75 μm.

In the imaging process, MAP was applied to the obtained PA signals. The maximum amplitude (z-coordinate) of a PA signal at each position scanned in x-y coordinates was calculated as

$$\mathrm{MAP}(x, y) = \max_{0 \leq i \leq N} s(x, y, i), \tag{1}$$

where s is the PA signal obtained from the specimen, x and y are the coordinates, i is discrete time, and N is discrete measured time. First, one maximum value at each pixel was selected for the entire measurement time range to create a two-dimensional MAP image, which is illustrated in Figure 13. The MAP image captures the branching of a blood vessel, which is similar to the shape in the optical image shown in Figure 11. Subsequently, to visualize the specimen three-dimensionally, the obtained PA signal was divided at intervals of 0.125 mm and 20 planes were obtained. Each maximum value was stacked and visualized three-dimensionally. The two-dimensional MAP image obtained at each depth and the three-dimensional MAP image obtained by stacking these images are shown in Figure 13a,b, respectively. Even though the conventional OAT with the transducer (V384, Olympus Inc.) was used for measurement as a reference, the PA signal could not be obtained owing to significantly low signal energy that was below the noise level.

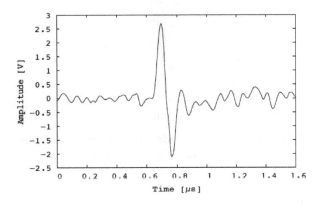

Figure 12. Example of PA signal obtained from chicken testicle.

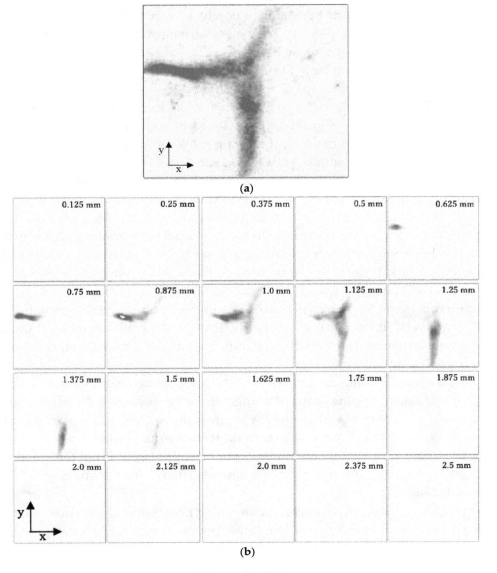

Figure 13. *Cont.*

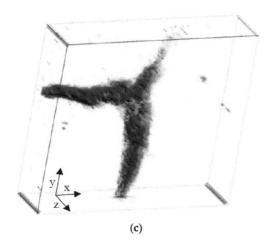

(c)

Figure 13. Reconstructed maximum amplitude projection (MAP) images of chicken testicle. (**a**) Two-dimensional MAP image, (**b**) two-dimensional MAP at each depth, and (**c**) three-dimensional MAP image.

4. Discussion and Conclusions

In this study, a sol-gel composite ultrasonic transducer was successfully fabricated on a curved-surface stainless-steel substrate to produce a newly designed OAT. The substrate was machined into a concave shape to focus at a point 5 mm from each surface point, and a 3-mm-diameter hole was drilled in the center of the substrate to allow the focused laser beam to pass through.

Using the fabricated sol-gel composite ultrasonic transducer in the pulse-echo mode, the duration of the echo obtained was approximately 0.2 μs, significantly shorter than the 5 μs duration of the previously fabricated flat-type transducer. The FWHM was 1.25 mm in the lateral direction and 0.2 mm in the axial direction. This is much larger than the laser focal zone. In particular, the transducer can visualize in the axial range of 1.25 mm without moving the laser focus in the depth direction.

PA signals were obtained by using the fabricated sol-gel composite ultrasonic transducer. Since the lateral FWHM of the transducer (0.2 mm) was larger than the spot size of the laser (5.25 μm), the laser beam can tilt in the range of the lateral FWHM of the transducer using the Galvano-mirror. However, to obtain PA images with a diameter larger than 0.2 mm, the OAT was fixed with the stage to align the ultrasonic and laser beams on the same axis, and the phantom was moved by a 2-axis step motor. As a result, we succeeded in visualizing a blood vessel with a diameter of 75 μm within a collected image range of 1×1 mm^2. The branching of the blood vessel can be observed in different depth and stacked as a 3D image.

On the other hand, using the conventional OAT in which combined the acoustic lens, reflecting prisms, and the commercial ultrasonic transducer, the PA signal for the same blood vessel was buried in noise, and could not be acquired. In addition, it may hurt the specimen when transmit more energy to obtain the stronger PA signal.

The advantages of this system are as follows: the axes of the laser beam and ultrasonic beam can be aligned with the focus point without using reflective devices such as prisms and mirrors, the fabricated transducer is curved so that the PA signals can be collected with the same phase from the focal point so an acoustic lens is not necessary, and the transducer can be placed closer to the focal point so that the ultrasonic propagating attenuation can be suppressed. From these aspects, the sol-gel composite ultrasonic transducer has potential as a new alternative for PA imaging to PVDF and other piezoelectric transducers.

With respect to ease of fabrication, only the machining processing of the substrate is unique to the fabrication process of the transducer presented in this paper. The other processes are the same as for other sol-gel composite ultrasonic transducers. This means that many different types and shapes of sol-gel composite ultrasonic transducers can be sprayed and manufactured together, thereby reducing production costs.

However, the technique has drawbacks in real-time visualization. Three-dimensional MAP images are obtained by calculating the MAP at regular intervals in the depth direction. If the horizontal resolution of the proposed system is significantly smaller than the region of interest, the number of scans increases considerably, and the process becomes time-consuming. This problem must be resolved to perform real-time visualization using the proposed transducer.

Widening the acquisition area of the sol-gel composite ultrasonic transducer is an alternative method of achieving real-time visualization. The curvature of the transducer surface can be optimized to extend the focal zone of the transducer, and hence, the acquisition area can be widened. However, this decreases the amplitude of the PA signals obtained from each point. To compensate for this, the sensitivity of the sol-gel composite ultrasonic transducer should be further improved to increase the acquisition area of PA signals. If the acquisition area is wide, scanning a laser beam only within the acquisition area at high speed will lead to real-time visualization. Annular and two-dimensional arrays are good alternatives for efficiently obtaining PA signals. An array can be created for our transducer by patterning the top electrodes. However, the fine patterning of the top electrodes and extensive wiring are required for performing real-time PA imaging. In the future, the fabrication of various shapes of the array transducer will be investigated.

Author Contributions: Conceptualization, C.H.Y. and M.K.; methodology, M.T. and T.C.W.; sensor fabrication, M.T.; writing—original draft preparation, M.T.; writing—review and editing, M.T., M.K., and C.H.Y.; visualization, M.T. and T.C.W; supervision, C.H.Y.; project administration, C.H.Y.; funding acquisition, M.T., M.K, and C.H.Y. All authors have read and agreed to the published version of the manuscript.

Acknowledgments: We thank T. Yamakawa from Kumamoto University for helping us with the parylene coating. We also thank Shinwa Seiko for the fabrication of stainless-steel rods.

References

1. Hu, S.; Wang, L.V. Optical-resolution photoacoustic microscopy: Auscultation of biological systems at the cellular level. *Biophys. J.* **2013**, *105*, 841–847. [CrossRef] [PubMed]
2. Wang, H.; Yang, X.; Liu, Y.; Jiang, B.; Luo, Q. Reflection-mode optical-resolution photoacoustic microscopy based on a reflective objective. *Opt. Exp.* **2013**, *21*, 24210–24218. [CrossRef] [PubMed]
3. Estrada, H.; Turner, J.; Kneipp, M.; Razansky, D. Real-time optoacoustic brain microscopy with hybrid optical and acoustic resolution. *Laser Phys. Lett.* **2014**, *11*, 045601. [CrossRef]
4. Wang, L.; Maslov, K.; Yao, J.; Rao, B.; Wang, L.V. Fast voice-coil scanning optical-resolution photoacoustic microscopy. *Opt. Lett.* **2011**, *36*, 139–141. [CrossRef] [PubMed]
5. Strohm, E.M.; Moore, M.J.; Kolios, M.C. Single cell photoacoustic microscopy: A review. *IEEE J. Select. Top. Quantum Electron.* **2016**, *22*, 680121. [CrossRef]
6. Yao, J.; Wang, L.V. Photoacoustic microscopy. *Laser Photonics Rev.* **2013**, *7*, 758–778. [CrossRef] [PubMed]
7. Yao, J.; Wang, L.V. Sensitivity of photoacoustic microscopy. *Photoacoustics* **2014**, *2*, 87–101. [CrossRef] [PubMed]
8. Cheng, C.; Chao, C.; Shi, X.; Leung, W.W.F. A flexible capacitive micromachined ultrasonic transducer (CMUT) array with increased effective capacitance from concave bottom electrodes for ultrasonic imaging applications. In Proceedings of the IEEE International Ultrasonics Symposium, Rome, Italy, 20–23 September 2009; pp. 996–999.
9. Fei, C.; Yang, Y.; Guo, F.; Lin, P.; Chen, Q.; Zhou, Q.; Sun, L. PMN-PT single crystal ultrasonic transducer with half-concave geometric design for IVUS imaging. *IEEE Trans. Biomed. Eng.* **2018**, *65*, 2087–2092. [CrossRef] [PubMed]
10. Igarashi, S.; Morishita, T.; Takeuchi, S. Experimental evaluation of high intensity ultrasound source system using acoustic waveguide and concave transducer with 100 mm diameter for calibration of hydrophone. In Proceedings of the IEEE International Ultrasonics Symposium, Kobe, Japan, 22–25 October 2018; pp. 1–4.

11. Woo, J.; Roh, Y. Design and fabrication of an annular array high intensity focused ultrasound transducer with an optimal electrode pattern. *Sens. Actuator. A Phys.* **2019**, *290*, 156–161. [CrossRef]

12. Kobayashi, M.; Jen, C.K.; Levesque, D. Flexible Ultrasonic Transducers. *IEEE Trans. Ultrason. Ferroelectr. Freq. Control.* **2006**, *53*, 1478–1486. [CrossRef] [PubMed]

13. Fujimoto, S.; Namihira, T.; Iwata, K.; Kobayashi, M. Curie temperature and high temperature behavior of Pb (Zr,Ti)O_3/Pb (Zr,Ti)O_3 Sol-gel composites. *Jpn. J. Appl. Phys.* **2015**, *54*, 07HB04. [CrossRef]

14. Tanabe, M.; Wu, T.C.; Hirata, K.; Kobayashi, M.; Nishimoto, M.; Yang, C.H. A Sol-gel PZT/PZT transducer for coaxial photoacoustic imaging. In Proceedings of the IEEE International Ultrasonic Symposium, Tours, France, 18–21 September 2016; pp. 1–4.

15. Tanabe, M.; Wu, T.C.; Hirata, K.; Kobayashi, M.; Nshimoto, M.; Yang, C.H. Development of transducer for photoacoustic imaging employing Sol-Gel composite spraying technique. In Proceedings of the Symposium on Ultrasonic Electronics, Busan, Korea, 16–18 November 2016.

16. Ono, Y.; Kobayashi, M.; Moisan, O.; Jen, C.K. High-temperature and broadband immersion ultrasonic probes. *IEEE Sens. J.* **2006**, *6*, 580–587. [CrossRef]

17. Liu, S.H.; Wu, T.C.; Tanabe, M.; Kobayashi, M.; Yang, C.H. Fiber laser based optical-resolution photoacoustic microscopy. In Proceedings of the 15th Asia Pacific Conference for Non-Destructive Testing, Singapore, 13–17 November 2017; p. 293.

18. Luginbuhl, P.; Racine, G.-A.; Lerch, P.; Romanowicz, B.; Brooks, K.G.; de Rooij, N.F.; Renaud, P.; Setter, N. Piezoelectric cantilever beams actuated by PZT Sol-gel thin film. *Sens. Actuator A Phys.* **1996**, *54*, 530–535. [CrossRef]

19. Lefki, K.; Dormans, G.J.M. Measurement of piezoelectric coefficients of ferroelectric thin films. *J. Appl. Phys.* **1994**, *76*, 1764–1767. [CrossRef]

20. Ren, W.; Zhou, H.-J.; Wu, X.-Q.; Zhang, L.-Y.; Yao, X. Measurement of piezoelectric coefficients of lead zirconate titanate thin films by the normal load method using a composite tip. *Mater. Lett.* **1997**, *31*, 185–188. [CrossRef]

21. Hayashi Chemical Industry Co. Ltd. Available online: https://www.hayashi-chemical.co.jp/en/product/fine_ceramic/#fc_02 (accessed on 7 November 2019).

22. Piedade, A.P.; Nanes, J.; Vieira, M.T. Thin films with chemically graded functionality based on fluorine polymers and stainless steel. *Acta Biomater.* **2008**, *4*, 1073–1080. [CrossRef] [PubMed]

4

Raman Spectroscopy of Changes in the Tissues of Teeth with Periodontitis

Elena Timchenko [1,*], Pavel Timchenko [1], Larisa Volova [2], Oleg Frolov [3], Maksim Zibin [4] and Irina Bazhutova [5]

[1] Department of Laser and Biotechnical Systems, Samara National Research University, 443086 Samara, Russia; Timpavel@mail.ru
[2] Research and Production Center "Samara Tissue Bank", Samara State Medical University, 443079 Samara, Russia; volovalt@yandex.ru
[3] Department of Physics, Samara National Research University, 443086 Samara, Russia; owl-63@ya.ru
[4] «DIAMANT» Dental Clinic, 443090 Samara, Russia; zybin_m.a@mail.ru
[5] Department of Dentistry, Samara State Medical University, 443079 Samara, Russia; docba@mail.ru
*   Correspondence: laser-optics.timchenko@mail.ru

Abstract: The results of experimental studies of the tissues of teeth with periodontitis, using the Raman spectroscopy method, are presented in this work. Spectral changes in the tissues of teeth with periodontitis were identified, and the results can be used for the correction of treatment of this disease in dental practice. Criteria for the noninvasive diagnosis of periodontitis, based on changes in tooth enamel spectral properties, were developed.

Keywords: raman spectroscopy; optical diagnostic; periodontitis; tooth tissues; biophotonics; calculus

1. Introduction

Chronic periodontitis is a serious and widespread periodontal pathology that causes significant impairment to dentoalveolar system functions, with damage to supporting tooth structures and the loss of teeth [1]. Periodontitis is mostly spread (60–65%) among people over age 30 [2]. However, the percentage of young patients with a severe form of chronic periodontitis has increased to 11.2%, and among people over age 65, it is 30% [3]. Current data indicate that periodontitis is a polyethiological disease [4]. Periodontitis is an insidious disease because the initial signs of inflammatory processes often remain unnoticed, and the chronic condition causes serious consequences not only for the dentoalveolar system, but for the patient as a whole.

Prompt diagnosis and prevention through the treatment of patients with periodontal diseases is essential. To improve this process and allow for a noninvasive diagnosis of periodontitis, it is necessary to identify the structural changes that occur in the tissues of teeth with this disease. Most studies that have investigated changes caused by this disease have not focused on changes in hard dental tissues, but have investigated the surrounding soft tissues [5,6], oral fluid [6–8], or osseous tissue regeneration during periodontitis treatment [9]. Few studies have focused on the tissues of teeth with periodontitis. The authors of [10] showed that the main structural change in the tissues of teeth with generalized periodontitis is dentin mineralization, and the process of root canal treatment of such teeth is recommended as an additional means of avoiding progression to dentin demineralization. The authors of [11] noted an increase in the micro-hardness of enamel in cases involving progression to periodontitis. Meanwhile, the authors of [10] showed that there are no apparent structural changes in the enamel in generalized periodontitis.

An analysis of the literature data showed that, for chronic periodontitis, the changes in hard dental tissues, especially in enamel, are unconfirmed, and having information about the changes in the composition of tooth enamel could allow the development of a noninvasive method to diagnose this disease and provide a correct treatment plan. Therefore, research of the tissues of teeth with periodontitis is urgently needed.

Biochemical analysis, scanning electron microscopy [10], fluorescence [7], and spectroscopy [10] are well-known current methods used for tooth tissue research. Biochemical analysis and scanning electron microscopy (SEM) provide quality images of the tooth tissue microstructure and are the most widely used for assessing tooth structure, but they require destructive preparation of the sample [9,10,12,13]. Fluorescence diagnosis in dentistry is based on the analysis of the spectra of fluorescence of hard dental tissues. While the main studied substance is hydroxyapatite, of which teeth are composed, detailed analysis of the composition of teeth is not possible [7]. The limitations of these hard dental tissue research methods could be overcome with the use of Raman spectroscopy. This is a simple, noninvasive, and rapid way of assessing dental tissue [9,12,13].

In [12], with the use of traditional routine histological methods and Raman spectroscopy, comparative research on mineralized tissues of the human jaw was carried out, and it was shown that the joint use of these methods allows significantly more data about pathological processes in the mineralized tissues (in the case of caries) to be collected, as well as allowing the features of mineralization under the conditions of directed bone regeneration to be defined. The authors of [9] studied the processes of bone healing and regeneration in periodontitis treatment using Raman spectroscopy. In our previous work [13], we used Raman spectroscopy to analyze the structure of teeth compared with synthetic apatites. Spectral lines related to the hard and soft tissues of teeth that provide important data for understanding the chemical structural properties of dentin and enamel were discussed. In [6,14–16], attention was paid to the study of the periodontal ligament after the application of orthodontic force and gingival slit fluid in periodontal disease. The authors showed the possibility of using Raman spectroscopy to monitor the periodontal condition at the biochemical level in subjects undergoing orthodontic treatment.

The aim of this work is to study the changes in the tissues of teeth with periodontitis using the Raman spectroscopy method for early, rapid diagnosis and the correction of treatment.

2. Materials and Methods

A randomized study design was used. Forty-two teeth (molars, premolars, and canines) from European patients aged 35–70 of both genders, that were removed due to chronic periodontitis (26 teeth) or for orthodontic reasons (control group, 16 teeth), were used as the materials of the study. Diagnosis of periodontitis was done clinically and after cone beam computed tomography (CT) analysis (the code of the disease according to ICD-10 (1997)—K05.3). The teeth removed due to severe chronic periodontitis with periodontal pockets of at least 6 mm deep and pathologic tooth mobility of grades III–IV were selected for the main group of study. Computed tomography showed a decrease in the bone tissue around the roots of removed teeth of more than half of the root length.

The study was carried out in accordance with the Declaration of Helsinki. The protocol was approved by the Ethics Committee (extract 20.05.2020 No. 207 of minutes of the meeting of the Committee on Bioethics of Samara State Medical University). The samples were collected within a period of 2 months. Measurements were taken immediately after the sampling.

The surfaces of teeth in 5 different areas were studied: enamel (a), dentin (b), in longitudinal slices), cementum (c), and dental calculus localized in the outer part of the teeth. The degree of intensity of the surface formation of the studied teeth corresponded to distinct under-gum (e) and above-gum (d) calculus [17].

Three spectra were investigated (with subsequent averaging) in every studied area at 3–5 different points of the surface of every tissue of each tooth. Samples were divided into 2 main groups: the control group (Figure 1I) and the group with periodontitis (Figure 1II).

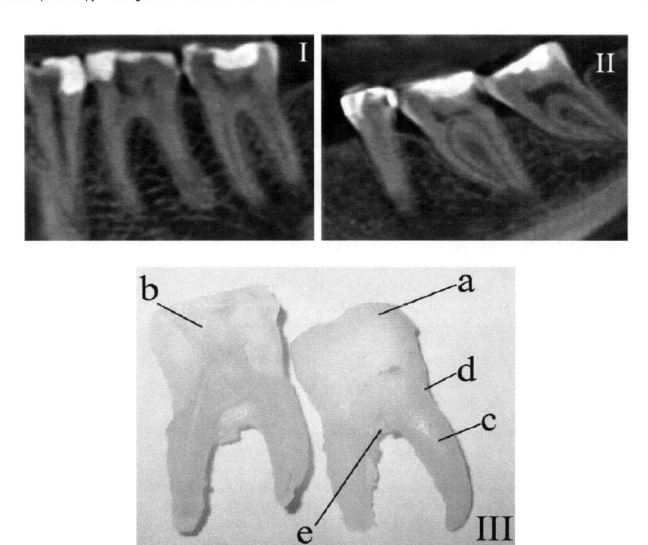

Figure 1. The fragments of teeth following computed tomography that were (**I**) healthy and (**II**) diagnosed with periodontitis. (**III**) Photo of a tooth with the researched areas indicated: a—enamel, b—dentin, c—cementum, d—above-gum dental calculus, and e—under-gum dental calculus.

An in vivo study of the enamel of 22 teeth (molars, premolars, and canines) of one female volunteer patient was also carried out. One of the patient's teeth was diagnosed with localized periodontitis (disease code according to ICD-10 (1997)—K05.3).

The study was carried out using Raman spectroscopy, implemented using the process described in detail in [18].

The experimental process included the use of a semiconductor laser (LML-785.0RB-04, California, USA), an optical module for Raman spectroscopy (RPB-785, Changchun, China), a spectrograph (Sharmrock SR-303i, www.andor.oxinst.com) with an integrated digital camera (ANDOR DV-420A-OE, www.andor.oxinst.com) that was cooled to −60 °C, and a computer.

The use of this spectrograph provided a wavelength resolution of 0.15 nm with a low level of inherent noise. The method of subtracting the fluorescence component of polynomial approximation with additional filtration of random noise effects was used to exclude autofluorescence from the Raman spectrum. Analysis of the Raman spectra was carried out in the range of 350–2200 cm^{-1} in this work. The power of the laser radiation, 400 mW, within the used exposure time (30 s) did not cause any changes to the samples. The optical probe, positioned over the subject at a distance of 7 mm, was used for Raman spectrum registration [19].

3. Results

We considered the characteristic average normalized Raman spectra of surface formations on teeth with this disease (Figure 2). This is often the reason for this disease.

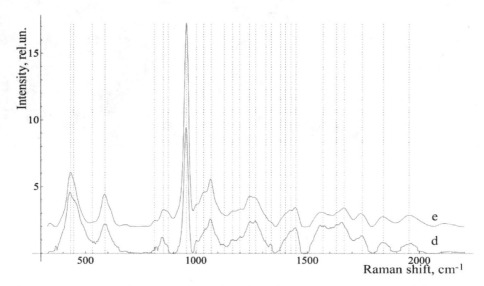

Figure 2. The average Raman spectra, normalized to the average intensity of the studied samples. d—above-gum dental calculus and e—under-gum dental calculus.

Figure 2 shows that the Raman spectra of the under-gum and above-gum calculi have certain spectral features that are apparently related to different periods of disease formation. In the initial stage of dental calculus formation, the above-gum calcareous deposits are composed primarily of organic components, as can be seen from the more intense lines in the ranges of 1550–1565 cm^{-1} (Amide II) and 1600–1665 cm^{-1} (Amide I) and the less intense line at 956 cm^{-1} (PO$_4^{3-}$ (ν_1), hydroxyapatite), compared with the under-gum calculus spectrum. At the same time, the under-gum calculus spectrum is characterized by the explicit intensity of the lines of mineral components (PO$_4^{3-}$ (ν_1), hydroxyapatite).

Figures 3 and 4 show the averaged spectra of the tissues of teeth with periodontitis and healthy teeth from the in vitro study (Figure 3) and the in vivo study (Figure 4).

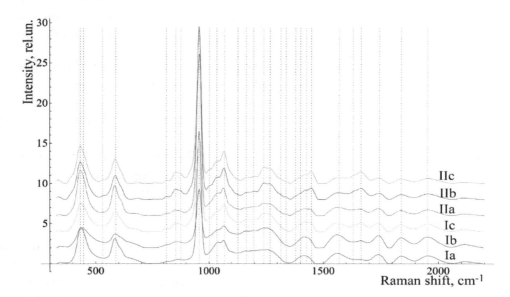

Figure 3. The average Raman spectra, normalized to the average intensity, for two groups of samples studied in vitro: a—enamel, b—denti and c—cementum. I = healthy, while II = diagnosed with periodontitis.

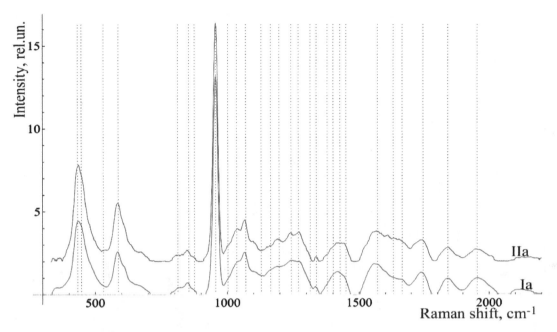

Figure 4. The average Raman spectra, normalized to the average intensity, of two in vivo studied groups of teeth of the volunteer: Ia—healthy enamel and IIa—enamel of the teeth with periodontitis.

The analysis of the healthy tooth tissues and the tissues of teeth with periodontitis showed that the main spectral features of tissues of teeth with periodontitis are changes in the intensity of organic compound lines at 852, 873 cm^{-1} (C–C stretching, proline, and hydroxyproline (collagen assignment)) [20], 1664 (Amide I), 1242 (Amide III) [21], and 1446 cm^{-1} (lipids and proteins) [22], as well as changes in the intensity of the lines of mineral compounds of the teeth at 956 cm^{-1} (P–O symmetrical valence fluctuation PO_4^{3-} (ν_1)) [23].

The comparative analysis shown in Figures 2–4 highlights many spectral changes in all tissues of teeth with periodontitis. These changes mainly occur in the same Raman lines as those related to calculus.

These spectral features are likely to be related to biochemical processes that take place during the formation of surface deposits during periodontitis (e.g., dental calculus and plaques), which affect all tooth tissues. The etiology of calculus formation is related to the mechanism of mineralization of the tooth surface deposits that consist of hydrocarbons and proteins (30% of each), as well as about 15% of lipids. The other components are extracellular bacterial products (plaques), remnants of their cytoplasm, and cell membranes (extracellular polysaccharides) [17].

To make the received Raman spectra more informative, a nonlinear regressive analysis of the Raman spectra was conducted, including an investigation of their spectral line decomposition. Figure 5 shows the results of decomposition of the spectral contours on the sum of distribution of the Gaussian lines. The Gaussian test function is described by the formula in [24].

The composition of the spectral lines was determined by literature analysis and multi-iteration modeling of 392 Raman spectra using MagicPlotPro 2.5.1 software. When modeling the spectral contours at the lines used as a template, the position x_0 and the width of the line (HWHM—half width at half) dx were fixed. Only the intensity of the line was selected when modeling. This allowed us to achieve highly stable results when modeling the contours. The amplitude of the lines a, which depended on the values of the independent regressors dx and x_0, as defined in the initial terms of the analysis, was used as a criterion variable.

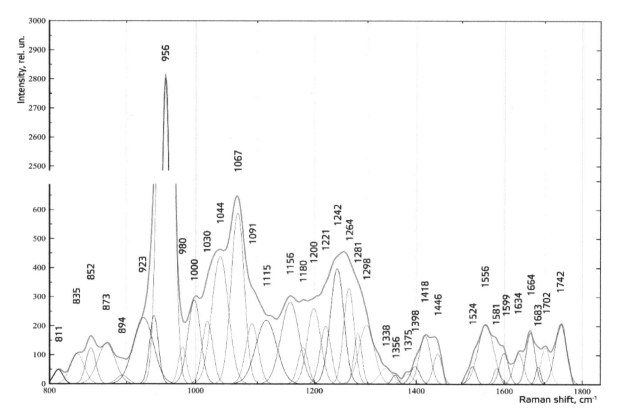

Figure 5. Spectral contour distribution of the enamel samples. The blue line is the original spectrum.

The average value of the coefficient of determination for the initial result spectrum in the range of 780–1780 cm^{-1} was R^2 = 0.998, the relative spectral line intensity assessment error a was less than 8%, the average standard deviation of the coordinate of a line x_0 was 1.4 cm^{-1}, and the average standard deviation of the width of the Gaussian line (HWHM) dx was 2.3 cm^{-1}.

For the relative quantitative analysis of the component composition, the relative coefficient k was introduced, where the Raman line of amide I ~1664 cm^{-1} was used as a denominator:

$$k_i = \frac{I_i}{I_{1664}}, \tag{1}$$

where I_i represents the values of intensity of the spectral lines of the analyzed components.

The analysis of the received data was done with IBM SPSS Statistics software through linear discriminant analysis (LDA).

The analysis of the relationships among groups with a pathology or relation to a certain tooth tissue is shown in Figure 6. It can be seen that most of the dispersion between the studied groups of samples can be described by the LD-1 function (58.5%). The common sampling size was 392 Raman spectra. The discriminant function LD-2 was able to describe 29.1% of the dispersion. This function has the physical meaning of the relationship of tooth tissue to the healthy group or to the group with periodontitis.

Positive values of LD-1 were found to mainly characterize the Raman spectra received from the enamel samples, and vice versa; the negative values characterized the samples of cementum, dentine, and dental calculus. The areas of the groups showed intersections, which influenced the rate of correctly classified subjects. The LD-1 function has the physical meaning of the difference between spectral compositions of tooth tissues. Positive values of LD-2 characterized the Raman spectra of the tooth tissue with periodontitis, and the negative values characterized the Raman spectra of healthy tooth tissue.

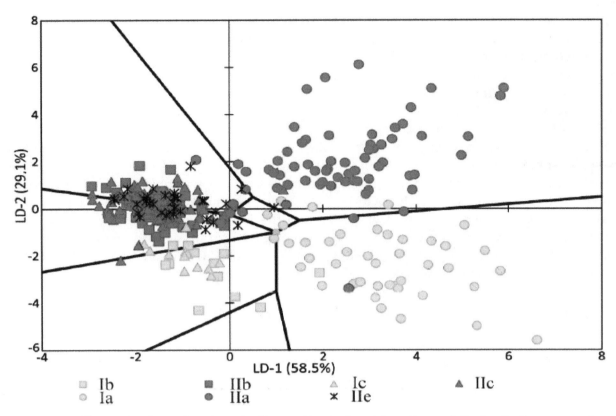

Figure 6. Chart of values showing the linear discriminant functions of the tooth tissue samples. a—enamel, b—dentin, and c—cementum. I = healthy tissue, II = tissue diagnosed with periodontitis.

Figures 6 and 7 show that the difference between healthy tissues and tissues with periodontitis can be described by the LD-2 function. It can be noted that the spectral composition of dental calculus showed similar changes to the spectra of dentin and cementum, which confirms the earlier hypothesis that calculus influences the internal structures of tooth tissue.

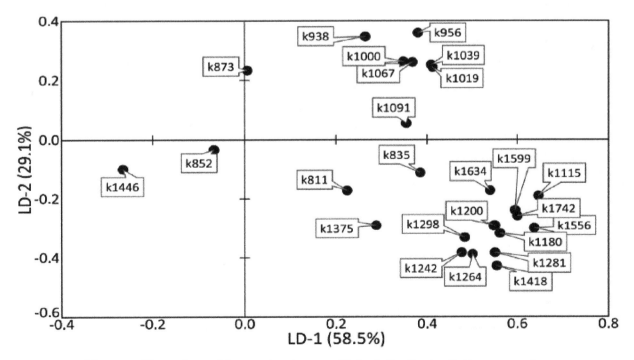

Figure 7. The values of factor structure coefficients for the tooth tissue samples.

High relative intensity values were observed for the lines ~1446 (CH_2 scissoring and CH_3 bending fluctuations of lipids and proteins), ~852 (C–C stretching benzene ring of proline), and ~873 cm^{-1} (C–C stretching benzene ring of hydroxyproline), with the rest of the lines having low spectral lines. These values characterize the tooth tissues—dentin, cementum with periodontitis, as well as calculus—compared with enamel, which indicates the differences in the organic–mineral compositions of these tissues.

Study of the changes in the enamel of teeth with periodontitis was further carried out. Figures 8 and 9 show a comparison of the LDA results of the enamel of healthy teeth and teeth with periodontitis. Sixty-seven spectra of the enamel of teeth with periodontitis and 43 Raman spectra of the enamel of healthy teeth were analyzed. The discriminant function LD-1 was able to describe 100% of the dispersion. Positive LD-1 values characterized the Raman spectra of the healthy enamel samples (the average LD-1 value of the group was 1.95, and the standard deviation was 0.912), and vice versa; negative values characterized the Raman spectra of the group of pathologic enamel samples (the average LD-1 value of the group was −1.25, and the standard deviation was 1.052). The areas of the groups had a minor intersection in the range of LD-1 = (−0.25; 2.25).

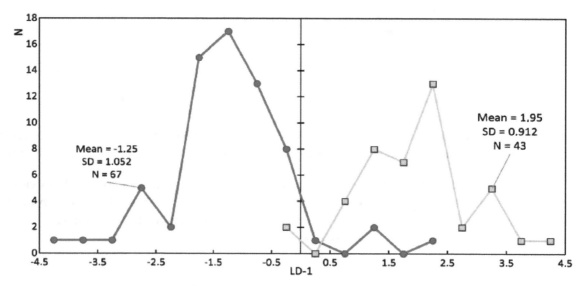

Figure 8. Chart of the linear discriminant function values of the enamel samples. The red line is the enamel of teeth with periodontitis (damaged enamel), and the blue line is the enamel of healthy teeth.

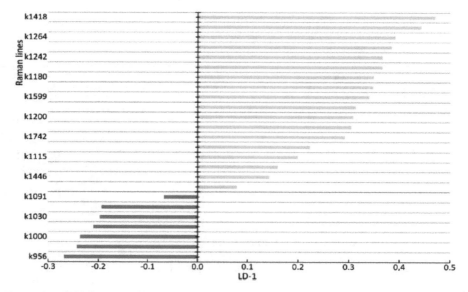

Figure 9. The values of factor structure coefficients for the enamel samples. Negative values are highlighted in red and positive values are highlighted in blue.

Figure 9 shows the coefficients of the factor structure matrix, with a correlation between the variables in the model and the discriminant function. In the analysis, these correlation coefficients were considered to be the factor loadings of the variables for each discriminant function.

The higher the absolute value of LD-1 for the variable is, the more strongly it determined the difference between the groups of samples in the received model of discriminant analysis. For example, the values of the introduced coefficients k873, k956, k1000, k1039, k1044, k1067, and k1091 were higher in the group of enamel samples with periodontitis, which indicates an increase in the relative intensity of the corresponding lines in tissue with periodontitis.

The increase in the relative intensity of the lines for hydroxyapatite 956 (P–O symmetrical valence fluctuation PO_4^{3-} (v_1)), ~1044 (PO_4^{3-} (v_3) (P–O asymmetrical valence fluctuation)), 1067 (C–O planar valence fluctuation CO_3^{2-} (v_1) B-type substitution), and 1091 cm^{-1} (C–O planar valence fluctuation CO_3^{2-} (v_1) A-type substitution) may be related to the presence of a water–mineral metabolism disorder in the tissues of teeth with periodontitis, which leads to more intensive substitution of the hydroxide ion OH by apatite ions CO_3^{2-} in the structure.

The change in the relative intensity of the lines at 1000 cm^{-1} and 1039 cm^{-1}, corresponding to fluctuations in the phenylalanine molecule, and 873 cm^{-1} (C–C stretching, proline and hydroxyproline (collagen assignment)) are apparently related to collagen synthesis disorder, which can also be seen in osteoporotic changes of bone tissues, as we showed earlier in [25].

We also observed a reduction in the relative intensity of the lines at ~1742 (phospholipids), ~1556 (Amide II Parallel/Antiparallel β-sheet structure), 1200–1300 (Amide III), ~1418, and ~1446 cm^{-1} (CH_2 scissoring and CH_3 bending fluctuations of lipids and proteins) in the tissues of teeth with periodontitis compared with healthy tissues. This effect may have been caused by the dehydration of peptide groups of amides that are sensitive to structural changes in the molecules of collagen [26].

In [6,16], chemical and structural changes were shown in the periodontal ligament after the application of orthodontic force and gingival slit fluid in teeth with periodontitis. Violation of the ligamentous apparatus leads to the development of periodontitis and changes in tooth tissues. Raman spectroscopy analysis of enamel can be used for the early diagnosis of periodontitis.

As a result of the discriminant analysis, we built a discriminant model of the enamel of healthy teeth and the enamel of teeth with periodontitis, taking into account characteristic changes in the relative intensity of the Raman lines. The number of true positive (TP) results was 64, while there were 3 false negative (FN) results. The number of true negative (TN) results was 41, and there were 2 false positive (FP) results.

The calculated sensitivity and specificity values of the method are

$$Sen = \frac{TP}{TP + FN} = \frac{64}{64 + 3} = 95.5\% \tag{2}$$

$$Spe = \frac{TN}{TN + FP} = \frac{41}{41 + 2} = 95.3\%. \tag{3}$$

Figure 10 shows the results of the receiver operator characteristic (ROC) analysis of the developed algorithm for diagnosing periodontitis. The discriminant adequacy of the method had an area under the curve (AUC) value of 0.983, which indicates the great quality of the diagnostic tool. The standard error (SE) was 0.01, and the 95% confidence interval of the AUC was in the range of 0.963–1. The optimal cut-off point for the presented algorithm, determined according to the condition of balance between sensitivity and specificity, was 0.55 (Figure 11). The values of sensitivity and specificity for the diagnostic model at that cut-off point were 95.5% and 95.3%, respectively.

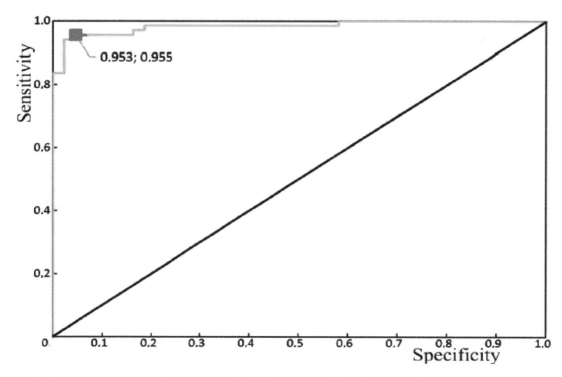

Figure 10. Receiver operator characteristic (ROC) analysis of the algorithm for periodontitis assessment, using the Raman spectroscopy method: green line—ROC-curve, the red square is the optimal cut-off point.

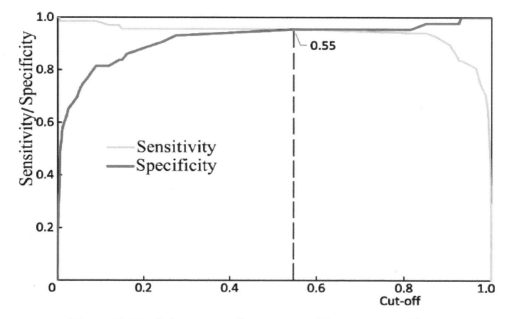

Figure 11. The balance point between sensitivity and specificity.

Therefore, if the received spectrum of enamel is classified as the spectrum of enamel with periodontitis, it could be a reason for including the patient in the at-risk group and may determine the treatment given.

4. Discussion

The main spectral changes in the tissues of teeth with periodontitis were identified in this work. The etiology of these changes is connected to the formation of calculus on the surface of teeth which, in turn, results in structural changes to all tooth tissues with periodontitis. These changes occur due to the presence of a water–mineral metabolism disorder in the tooth tissues (intensive substitution of hydroxide ion OH by apatite ions CO_3^{2-} in the structure) or collagen synthesis disorder. Similar changes occur in bone tissues with osteoporosis, as we presented earlier in [25].

The spectral changes found in this work that occur in periodontitis do not occur in other widespread dental diseases (e.g., caries). We previously carried out studies [27] that showed a decrease in the concentration of ions $(PO_4)^{3-}$ in caries, as also shown in [28].

Diagnosing the spectral changes in tooth enamel, as well as developing an algorithm to identify enamel with periodontitis, will allow at-risk patients to be identified and treated with hydroxyapatite. The sensitivity and specificity values of the developed algorithm were 95.5% and 95.3%, respectively.

The received results are a prerequisite for creating an express device for the noninvasive (in vivo) assessment of periodontitis, based on changes in tooth enamel spectral values. These studies have already been carried out in vivo in this work and have shown good results, similar to the results of in vitro studies.

Author Contributions: Conceptualization, E.T. and L.V.; methodology, P.T. and L.V.; software, O.F. and P.T.; validation, P.T. and L.V.; formal analysis, P.T. and O.F.; investigation, O.F., M.Z. and I.B.; resources, E.T., L.V., M.Z. and I.B.; data curation, M.Z. and I.B.; writing—original draft preparation, E.T.; writing—review and editing, P.T. and L.V.; visualization, O.F. and P.T.; supervision, E.T., L.V. and I.V.B.; project administration, E.T.; All authors have read and agreed to the published version of the manuscript.

References

1. Epifanova:, Y.V.; Avanesov, A.M. The estimation of levels of bioamines in the blood cells at patients with parodontitis. *Electronniy Nauchno-Obraz. Vestnic Zdorovie i Obraz. v XXI veke-2012 [Electron. Sci. Educ. Bull. Health Educ. XXI Century—2012]* **2012**, *14*, 114–115.

2. Shashmurina, V.R.; Devlikanova, L.I.; Chumachenko, E.N. Biochemical characteristics of pulp removal in cases of periodontal diseases. *Ross. Stomatol. Vestn. [Russ. Dent. Bull.]* **2017**, *21*, 64–67. [CrossRef]

3. Papapanou, P.N.; Susin, C. Periodontitis epidemiology: Is periodontitis under-recognized, over-diagnosed, or both? *Periodontol. 2000* **2017**, *75*, 45–51. [CrossRef] [PubMed]

4. Cepov, L.M.; Cepova, E.L.; Cepov, A.L. Periodontitis: Local focus serious problems (literature review). *Parodontologiya* **2014**, *3*, 3–6.

5. Khaydar, D.A.; Kulchenko, A.G. Hypoxia of periodontium tissues with chronic periodontitis, Special issue. In Proceedings of the Materials of the XIX International Congress "Health and Education in the XXI Century", Moscow, Russia, 18–20 December 2017.

6. Camerlingo, C.; D'Apuzzo, F.; Grassia, V.; Perillo, L.; Lepore, M. Micro-Raman Spectroscopy for Monitoring Changes in Periodontal Ligaments and Gingival Crevicular Fluid. *Sensors* **2014**, *14*, 22552–22563. [CrossRef]

7. Sukhinina, A.V. The Methods of Optical Spectroscopy for Dental Disease Diagnosis. Ph.D Thesis, Abstract National Research Nuclear University MEPh, Moscow, Russia, 2014.

8. Gonchukov, S.; Sukhinina, A.; Bakhmutov, D.; Minaeva, S. Raman spectroscopy of saliva as a perspective method for periodontitis diagnostics. *Laser Phys. Lett.* **2011**, *9*, 73–77. [CrossRef]

9. Gatin, E.; Nagy, P.; Paun, I.; Dubok, O.; Bucur, V. Windisch Raman Spectroscopy: Application in Periodontal and Oral Regenerative Surgery for Bone Evaluation. *IRBM* **2019**, *40*, 279–285. [CrossRef]

10. Tsimbalistov, A.V.; Pikhur, O.L.; Dubova, M.A.; Sadikov, R.A.; Frank-Kamenetskaya, O.V.; Golovanova, O.A.; Belskaya, L.V. Morphology and Composition of Human Dental Hard Tissues and Dental Stones with the General Parodontite. *Vestn. St. -Peterbg. Univ. [St.-Petersburg Univ. Bull.]* **2006**, *11*, 128–135.

11. Remizov, S.M. Measuring microhardness for comparative assessment of dental tissues of human healthy and affected teeth. *Stomatologiya* **1965**, *3*, 33–37.

12. Minaeva, S.A.; Mikhaylovskiy, A.A.; Bukharova, T.B.; Antonov, E.N.; Goldshteyn, D.V.; Popov, V.K.; Volkov, A.V. Morphological study of hard tissues of facial skeleton using the Raman spectroscopy. *Ross. Stomatol.* **2005**, *1*, 3–10.

13. Ramakrishnaiah, R.; Rehman, G.U.; Basavarajappa, S.; Al Khuraif, A.A.; Durgesh, B.H.; Khan, A.S.; Rehman, I.U. Applications of Raman Spectroscopy in Dentistry: Analysis of Tooth Structure. *Appl. Spectrosc. Rev.* **2014**, *50*, 332–350. [CrossRef]

14. Kapoor, P.; Kharbanda, O.P.; Monga, N.; Miglani, R.; Kapila, S. Effect of orthodontic forces on cytokine and receptor levels in gingival crevicular fluid: A systematic review. *Prog. Orthod.* **2014**, *15*, 1–21. [CrossRef] [PubMed]

15. D'Apuzzo, F.; Perillo, L.; Delfino, I.; Portaccio, M. Monitoring early phases of orthodontic treatment by means of Raman spectroscopies. *J. Biomed. Opt.* **2017**, *22*, 1. [CrossRef]

16. Perillo, L.; d'Apuzzo, F.; Ilario, M.; Laino, L.; Di Spigna, G.; Lepore, M.; Camerlingo, C. Monitoring Biochemical and Structural Changes in Human Peridontal Ligaments during Orthodontic Treatment by Means of Micro-Raman Spectroscpy. *Sensors* **2020**, *20*, 497. [CrossRef]

17. Borodovitsina, S.I.; Saveleva, N.A.; Tabolina, E.S. *Dental Disease Prevention*; Ryazan State Medical University: Ryazan, Russia, 2019; p. 264.

18. Timchenko, E.V.; Timchenko, P.E.; Pisareva, E.V.; Vlasov, M.Y.; Volova, L.T.; Frolov, O.O.; Fedorova, Y.V.; Tikhomirova, G.P.; Romanova, D.A.; Daniel, M.A. Spectral Analysis of Rat Bone Tissue During Long Antiorthostostatic Hanging and at Introduction of Allogen Hydroxyapatitis. *Opt. Spectrosc.* **2020**, *128*, 989–997. [CrossRef]

19. Timchenko, E.V.; Timchenko, P.E.; Taskina, L.A.; Volova, L.T.; Miljakova, M.N.; Maksimenko, N.A. Using Raman spectroscopy to estimate the demineralization of bone transplants during preparation. *J. Opt. Technol.* **2015**, *82*, 153–157. [CrossRef]

20. Raghavan, M. Investigation of Mineral and Collagen Organization in Bone Using Raman Spectroscopy. Ph.D. Thesis, University of Michigan, Ann Arbor, MI, USA, 2011.

21. Ager, J.; Nalla, R.K.; Breeden, K.L.; Ritchie, R.O. Deep-ultraviolet Raman spectroscopy study of the effect of aging on human cortical bone. *J. Biomed. Opt.* **2005**, *10*, 034012. [CrossRef]

22. Gyeong Bok, J.; In Soon, K.; Young Ju, L.; Dohyun, K.; Hun-Kuk, P.; Gi-Ja, L.; Chaekyun, K. Label-free noninvasive characterization of osteoclast differentiation using raman spectroscopy coupled with multivariate analysis. *Curr. Opt. Photonics* **2017**, *1*, 412–420.

23. Ionita, I. Diagnosis of tooth decay using polarized micro-Raman confocal spectroscopy. *Rom. Rep. Phys.* **2009**, *61*, 567–574.

24. Motulsky, H.J.; Christopoulos, A. *Fitting Models to Biological Data Using Linear and Nonlinear Regression*; A practical guide to curve fitting; GraphPad Software Inc.: San Diego, CA, USA, 2003.

25. Timchenko, E.V.; Timchenko, P.E.; Pisareva, E.V.; Vlasov, M.Y.; Volova, L.T.; Fedotov, A.A.; Fedorova, Y.V.; Tyumchenkova, A.S.; Romanova, D.A.; Daniel, M.A.; et al. Optical analysis of bone tissue by Raman spectroscopy in experimental osteoporosis and its correction using allogeneic hydroxyapatite. *J. Opt. Technol.* **2020**, *87*, 161–167. [CrossRef]

26. Sukhodub, L.; Moseke, C.; Sulkio-Cleff, B.; Maleev, V.; Semenov, M.; Bereznyak, E.; Bolbukh, T. Collagen–hydroxyapatite–water interactions investigated by XRD, piezogravimetry, infrared and Raman spectroscopy. *J. Mol. Struct.* **2004**, *704*, 53–58. [CrossRef]

27. Timchenko, E.V.; Zherdeva, L.A.; Volova, L.T.; Burda, A.G.; Timchenko, P.E. Use of Raman spectroscopy for diagnosis of disease in dental tissue. *J. Opt. Technol.* **2016**, *83*, 313. [CrossRef]

28. Mandra, Y.V.; Ivashov, A.S.; Votjakov, S.L.; Kiseleva, D.V. Possibilities of Raman microspectrometry imaging for structural investigation of human enamel and dentin. *Eksperimentalnaya Klin. Stomatol.* **2011**, *1*, 24–28.

5

Micro-Droplet Detection Method for Measuring the Concentration of Alkaline Phosphatase-Labeled Nanoparticles in Fluorescence Microscopy

Rufeng Li [1], Yibei Wang [1], Hong Xu [1], Baowei Fei [2] and Binjie Qin [1,*

[1]   School of Biomedical Engineering, Shanghai Jiao Tong University, Shanghai 200240, China; brave_lee@sjtu.edu.cn (R.L.); wangyibei@sjtu.edu.cn (Y.W.); xuhong@sjtu.edu.cn (H.X.)

[2]   Emory University School of Medicine, Georgia Institute of Technology, Atlanta, GA 30329 USA; bfei@emory.edu

*   Correspondence: bjqin@sjtu.edu.cn

Abstract: This paper developed and evaluated a quantitative image analysis method to measure the concentration of the nanoparticles on which alkaline phosphatase (AP) was immobilized. These AP-labeled nanoparticles are widely used as signal markers for tagging biomolecules at nanometer and sub-nanometer scales. The AP-labeled nanoparticle concentration measurement can then be directly used to quantitatively analyze the biomolecular concentration. Micro-droplets are mono-dispersed micro-reactors that can be used to encapsulate and detect AP-labeled nanoparticles. Micro-droplets include both empty micro-droplets and fluorescent micro-droplets, while fluorescent micro-droplets are generated from the fluorescence reaction between the APs adhering to a single nanoparticle and corresponding fluorogenic substrates within droplets. By detecting micro-droplets and calculating the proportion of fluorescent micro-droplets to the overall micro-droplets, we can calculate the AP-labeled nanoparticle concentration. The proposed micro-droplet detection method includes the following steps: (1) Gaussian filtering to remove the noise of overall fluorescent targets, (2) a contrast-limited, adaptive histogram equalization processing to enhance the contrast of weakly luminescent micro-droplets, (3) an red maximizing inter-class variance thresholding method (OTSU) to segment the enhanced image for getting the binary map of the overall micro-droplets, (4) a circular Hough transform (CHT) method to detect overall micro-droplets and (5) an intensity-mean-based thresholding segmentation method to extract the fluorescent micro-droplets. The experimental results of fluorescent micro-droplet images show that the average accuracy of our micro-droplet detection method is 0.9586; the average true positive rate is 0.9502; and the average false positive rate is 0.0073. The detection method can be successfully applied to measure AP-labeled nanoparticle concentration in fluorescence microscopy.

Keywords: fluorescence microscopy; micro-droplet; spot detection; alkaline phosphatase (AP); nanoparticles

---

1. Introduction

Advances in microscopy and fluorescence tools have pushed the quantitative biological research for biomolecules at nanometer and sub-nanometer scales [1–3]. Among these fluorescence tools, nanoparticles on which alkaline phosphatase (AP) was immobilized (AP-labeled nanoparticles for short) [4] are widely used as signal markers for tagging biomolecules of interest due to their stabilization and convenience for operation. Covered with a specific antibody, the AP-labeled nanoparticle can label one target biomolecule and emit a fluorescent signal by catalyzing the corresponding substrates. Therefore, the biomolecular concentration can be directly obtained by measuring the AP-labeled nanoparticle concentration. Traditional methods for AP-labeled nanoparticle concentration measurement are to divide the amount of total fluorescent signals from the AP-labeled nanoparticles by the volume of solution in the fluorescence microscopy image. However, it is difficult to count AP-labeled nanoparticles directly from fluorescent images since AP-labeled nanoparticles are too small to detect and are closely clustered. To solve this problem, a widely-used technology called the droplet microfluidics technique has been used to encapsulate the individual AP-labeled nanoparticle in monodispersed micro-droplets [5]. Micro-droplets with a similar size are water-in-oil droplets, which can be used as micro-reactors to encapsulate and detect AP-labeled nanoparticles [6]. All the micro-droplets encapsulate fluorogenic substrates, but only a small portion of micro-droplets would carry AP-labeled nanoparticles. Only the micro-droplets encapsulating AP-labeled nanoparticles will emit remarkable fluorescent signals via the enzymatic reaction between the APs and the corresponding fluorogenic substrates within droplets. We call these micro-droplets fluorescent micro-droplets and the others empty micro-droplets. However, empty micro-droplets may emit weak fluorescent signals that result from a few APs scattered within the micro-droplet in practice. Since the process of encapsulating AP-labeled nanoparticles in micro-droplets follows a random Poisson distribution [6,7], the probability of occurrence of the micro-droplets encapsulating AP-labeled nanoparticles can be obtained via the percentage of the fluorescent micro-droplets. Therefore, we can detect the proportion of fluorescent micro-droplets to the overall micro-droplets to measure the AP-labeled nanoparticle concentration. To achieve this purpose, micro-droplet detection is necessary to analyze the AP-labeled nanoparticle concentration.

The micro-droplet detection usually consists of two steps: detection of the overall micro-droplets and detection of fluorescent micro-droplets. There are certain problems involved in the detection of the overall micro-droplets. The empty micro-droplets with weak luminance are hard to detect due to the weak difference between empty micro-droplets and their surroundings. The complex noise environment in the fluorescence images may also increase the difficulties of micro-droplet detection. There are two important types of noises: the intrinsic photon noises resulting from the random nature of photon emission and the background noises caused by the detector's electronics [8]. Moreover, the additional noises like small bright speckles and vesicles could also impede subsequent droplet detection. Furthermore, there is still a tough issue that most micro-droplets are closely connected in the fluorescence images.

Traditional fluorescent target detection methods have been reported in the literature [9–11]. In [12], the authors provide a thorough comparative evaluation of the most frequently-used spot detection methods. The study shows the superiority of the multiscale variance-stabilizing transform (MSVST) detector method [13] and the H-dome-based detector (HD) method [14]. The MSVST method combines the red variance stabilizing transform (VST) with the isotropic undecimated wavelet transform [13,15] and performs well in filtering mixed-Poisson-Gaussian noises and in detecting fluorescent particles. However, the bright speckles and vesicles in the image may lead to the false detection of micro-droplets. Being different from MSVST, the HD method detects spots by extracting peaks with an amplitude higher than a given height, called domes, in a Laplace-of-Gaussian (LoG) filtered or Gaussian-filtered image. Because the amplitude of the peaks in micro-droplets varies in a large range, the HD method may not work well in micro-droplet detection. To overcome this drawback, Rezatofighi et al. [16] proposed an improved method called the maximum possible height-dome method (MPHD) to adaptively extract the dome. However, it may not perform well when both the bright speckles and closely-connected micro-droplets appear in the image. To further improve the detection performance, Jaiswal et al. [17] proposed a multi-scale spot-enhancing filter method (MSSEF) to calculate the binary map, which is obtained by iteratively applying a threshold to the LoG filtered image with scale changing. This method can significantly improve the detection performance on multiple closely-connected particles. However, since the selected threshold with respect to the mean and variance of the image may be inaccurate, it may not perform well on the micro-droplet detection. Besides, Basset et al. [18–20] proposed methods to select the optimal LoG scale or multiple scales corresponding to the different spot sizes in the image, but test results on fluorescent micro-droplet images proved the ineffectiveness of this method for the micro-droplet detection. As explained by Smal et al. [12], most current methods follow a common detection scheme, which consists of denoising the image, enhancing the spots and, finally, extracting the target spots in a binary map to further count the micro-droplets or estimate the positions. In addition, these methods perform ineffectively for the detection of closely-connected micro-droplets by implementing a connect-component analysis method. Recently, an automatic hotspots detection framework [21] was proposed to successfully detect active areas inside cells that show changes in their calcium concentration. However, this automatic segmentation of intracellular calcium concentration in individual video frames is about 80% accurate and may not be suitable for precisely detecting a single active cell in the highly accurate concentration measurement. Therefore, there is a need to develop new approaches in order to improve the accuracy and robustness for detecting the micro-droplets.

To address these difficulties, we propose an overall micro-droplet detection method for fluorescent micro-droplet images (FMIs).

2. Methods

The proposed method includes the following steps: (1) The Gaussian filter first removes the noise in the red fluorescent micro-droplet image. (2) The contrast-limited adaptive histogram equalization (CLAHE) [22] method divides the whole filtered image into different blocks and adaptively adjusts the local histogram of each block to enhance the contrasts of the weak luminance regions of overall micro-droplets. (3) The red maximizing inter-class variance thresholding [23–25] method (OTSU) segments the enhanced image to get the binary map of the overall micro-droplets. (4) By performing on the segmented binary map, the circular Hough transform method (CHT) [26,27] perfectly detects the overall micro-droplets due to its advantage in detecting the micro-droplets that are closely connected with each other. With the combined strengths of CLAHE, OTSU thresholding and the CHT methods, our method shows significant performances on the overall micro-droplet detection. Finally, the fluorescent micro-droplet can be easily extracted via an intensity-mean-based thresholding segmentation method and be counted with the CHT method again. We have compared the performance of our method on FMIs with the performances of the state-of-the-art methods including MSVST [13], MPHD [16] and MSSEF [17]. The comparative results demonstrate that our method outperforms these state-of-the-art methods.

2.1. Overall Micro-Droplet Detection

Figure 1 shows the overview of the proposed method for overall micro-droplet detection. We begin by preprocessing an input image with a Gaussian filter. Then, CLAHE is performed on the local histogram of the filtered image to enhance the contrast of micro-droplets. After this image enhancement, the difference between micro-droplets and background increases, and an OTSU thresholding-based segmentation method is applied to obtain a binary map of the overall micro-droplets. Finally, the CHT method precisely detects the circular contour of the overall micro-droplets.

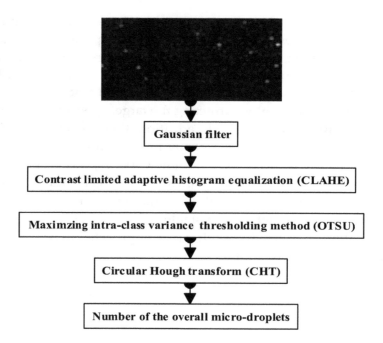

Figure 1. The framework of the proposed method for the overall micro-droplet detection.

2.1.1. Noise Reduction with the Gaussian Filter

The main noise sources in fluorescence microscopy images are the shot noise occurring in the photon counting in the imaging process and the additive Gaussian noise created by the electron characteristics of detectors [8,12]. The shot noise of the photons results from the random nature of photon emission and can be modeled as Poisson noise [8,28] when there is only a handful of photons emitted, whereas the noise can be considered as Gaussian noise when the number of photons is sufficient.

In most situations, the noise in fluorescent micro-droplet images can be approximately considered as Gaussian noise. Therefore, we simply use a normal Gaussian filter to remove the noise. In Figure 2, the signal-to-noise radio (SNR) of the denoised image is enhanced compared to that of the original images. We can see that the noises are eliminated effectively in the zoomed version of filtered image I.

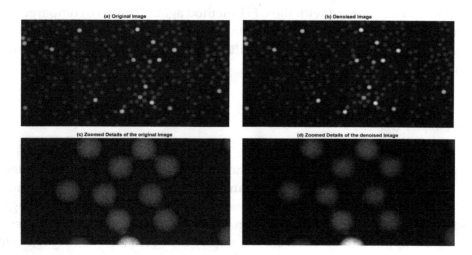

Figure 2. Original fluorescent image with SNR (signal-to-noise radio) of 7.1789 and the denoised image with SNR of 7.7489. (**a**) Original image. (**b**) Denoised image (I). (**c**) Zoomed details of the original image. (**d**) Zoomed details of the denoised image.

2.1.2. Contrast Limited Adaptive Histogram Equalization

In the filtered image, there are many micro-droplets with weak luminance. We then use the CLAHE [22] method to enhance the contrast of micro-droplets.

Firstly, the image I is divided into $N * N$ blocks (N is a user-defined constant, and N is by default set to 8) and local histogram of every block is calculated. Since the contrast amplification in the vicinity of a given pixel value is proportional to the histogram value at that pixel value, the local histogram is clipped at a predefined value T to limit the over-amplification of noise. The part of the histogram exceeding T is redistributed among all histogram bins to keep the area of the histogram unvarying. Then, histogram equalization uses the same transformation derived from the local histogram to transform all pixels in the block and enhance local contrasts. With these operations finished, we combine all the blocks together and apply bilinear interpolation to eliminate the block effect of images. Finally, the micro-droplets at low intensities are prominently enhanced. The output of this step is an enhanced image J, which is shown in Figure 3.

2.1.3. Maximizing inter-class Variance Thresholding Method

In Figure 3, the pixels in the enhanced image J can be grouped into two classes including background and micro-droplet pixels in terms of histogram distribution. Therefore, OTSU thresholding [23–25] is the most suited method to extract micro-droplets via histogram thresholding. The optimal threshold of this method is chosen by maximizing inter-class variance. The segmented binary map by the OTSU method effectively highlights the desired micro-droplets. However, there may be several falsely detected spots in the binary map due to the bright specks having a far smaller size than the micro-droplets in image J. In order to obtain accurate detection results, the morphological opening operation is used for post-processing to eliminate the influence of these abnormal spots. The output of this step is denoted as image K.

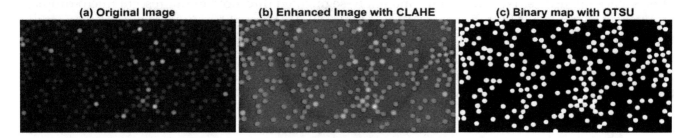

Figure 3. Intermediate results of contrast-limited adaptive histogram equalization (CLAHE) and OTSU on the overall micro-droplet detection: **(a)** Original image. **(b)** Enhanced image with CLAHE (J). **(c)** Binary map with OTSU (K).

2.1.4. Circle Detection via Circular Hough Transform

After getting the segmented binary map, we must count the number of overall micro-droplets to achieve a final detection result. The traditional fluorescent spot detection algorithms are usually based on connected component analysis (CCA). CCA-based methods perform well on detecting isolated micro-droplets, but poorly on detecting closely-connected micro-droplets. With further observation of micro-droplets, we found that all the micro-droplets appear as round spots with a similar radius. Therefore, we can employ CHT [26,27] to detect the spots with radii in a certain range. Moreover, CHT is insensitive to deformation, rotation and scaling of the circle in the image such that it can perfectly detect the incomplete round micro-droplets and closely-connected micro-droplets with lower false detection and higher accuracy. Furthermore, it has a low computational complexity, and the only parameter we need to set is the radius range of micro-droplets.

The CHT algorithm contains the following two essential steps:

- Accumulator array computation:

  The edge detection is carried out on the binary map to get an edge image (L). The edge pixels of L are designated as candidate pixels and are allowed to cast 'votes' in the accumulator array $A(a)$, which represents the weight of the circle with a fixed radius and the center of the circle. Here, $a = \{a, b, r\}$. (a, b) represents the space location of pixels, and r is the radius of the expected circle. At the beginning, all the elements of $A(a)$ are set to 0.

- Center and radius estimation:

  For every pixel x of the fluorescence image, we accumulate all the units of $A(a)$ that satisfy the function $f(x, a) = 0$. $f(x, a)$ is the analytical expression of circle:

$$f(x, a) = (x_1 - a)^2 + (x_2 - b)^2 - r^2 \tag{1}$$

Finally, the circular centers and radii are estimated by detecting the peaks in the accumulator array. We can get the number of micro-droplets by counting the centers of detected circles.

The overall micro-droplets can be detected with the method mentioned above. This method can accurately extract and count the overall micro-droplets on FMIs.

2.2. Fluorescent Micro-Droplet Detection

The fluorescent micro-droplets can be extracted by directly thresholding segmentation due to their high intensity and round shape. However, it is difficult to choose the segmental threshold (D) since the fluorescent micro-droplets in different images can appear to be very different in the fluorescence intensities. We collected the manually-segmented threshold of fluorescent micro-droplets and the intensity mean of the images. By analyzing the relationship of the manually-segmented threshold and the intensity mean of the image, we found that the segmental threshold has a significant linear correlation with the intensity mean of the image. Therefore, we model the relationship mentioned above with a linear fitting method and set up a linear function corresponding to the threshold D of the images:

$$D(m) = 1.3717 * m + 0.0126 \tag{2}$$

where m denotes the intensity mean of the image. After the binary map is obtained, the circular Hough transform (CHT) method (see the details in Section 2.1.4) is applied to count the fluorescent micro-droplets precisely. Figure 4 shows the detected result of this method.

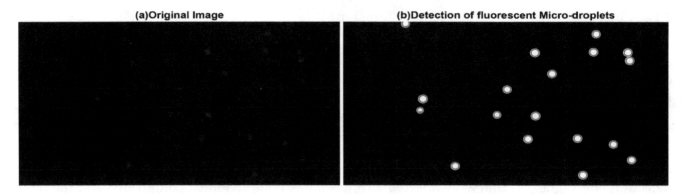

Figure 4. Detection of fluorescent micro-droplets. (**a**) Original image. (**b**) Detection of fluorescent micro-droplets.

2.3. Measurement of AP-Labeled Nanoparticle Concentration

Encapsulating AP-labeled nanoparticles delivered to the droplet-generation nozzle at random is a Poisson process. The probability of encapsulating k AP-labeled nanoparticles in a micro-droplet is then given by equation:

$$P(k) = e^{-\lambda} \frac{\lambda^k}{k!} \tag{3}$$

where λ is the average number of AP-nanoparticles per micro-droplet, e is the base of the natural logarithms, k is from natural numbers and $k!$ is the factorial of k.

After detecting the numbers of fluorescent and overall micro-droplets, we can obtain the probability $P(k \geq 1)$ by directly computing the proportion of the fluorescent micro-droplets to the overall micro-droplets. Then, the average number of AP-nanoparticles per micro-droplet λ can be calculated according to Equations (3) and (4):

$$P(k = 0) + P(k \geq 1) = 1 \tag{4}$$

Finally, λ is converted to the average amount of substance n (in moles) of a single micro-droplet; the AP-labeled nanoparticle concentration c is then measured by dividing the average amount of substance n (in moles) by the average volume V of a single micro-droplet. The concentration unit is given by fM, which corresponds to 10^{-15} mol/L.

2.4. Evaluation

The performance of the overall micro-droplet detection method can be evaluated in the following aspects: (1) Visual evaluations: The visual evaluations firstly give an intuitive performance comparison overview for all the detection methods. (2) TPR and FPR: The true positive rate (TPR) represents the number of true positives (TP) divided by the number of targets in ground truth data, and the false positive rate (FPR) represents the number of the false positives (FP) divided by the number of backgrounds in ground truth data. These two metrics can reflect the detection capability of an algorithm from different perspectives. (3) ROC and F-measure: For the overall evaluation of the detection method, the receiver operating characteristic (ROC curve) is used as a graph metric to uncover the detection power with different TPRs. The area under ROC (AUC) is an estimate of the area under ROC, which indicates the predictive power of the detector. Detectors with higher AUC have better detection power. Furthermore, we computed the F-measure defined by the harmonic mean of precision and recall $F = 2 * Prec * Rec / (Prec + Rec)$. The precision metric $Prec$ is defined as $Prec = TP / (TP + FP)$, and Rec is the index of recall defined as $Rec = TP / (TP + FN)$, where FN is the number of false negatives. The F-measure is a widely-used metric to measure the accuracy of the detection method. The higher F-measure score is related to the higher accuracy. (4) Overall number of micro-droplets detected: The purpose of our work is to precisely count micro-droplets. Therefore, the comparative results on the number of overall micro-droplets detected can directly reflect the superiority of our method.

The fluorescent micro-droplet detection method is evaluated by counting the number of fluorescent micro-droplets detected. We demonstrate the accuracy of this work via the relative error that is defined as the proportion of counting error to the true number counted manually. The counting error is the absolute value of the difference between the true number and the detected number. Low relative errors demonstrate high detection performances.

Finally, we calculate a test AP-labeled nanoparticle concentration with the results of micro-droplet detection and compute a reference concentration with the ground truth data. Then, we use the relative error again to compute the accuracy of our method for the AP-labeled nanoparticle concentration measurement. The comparative results of the test and the reference AP-labeled nanoparticle concentration further demonstrate the performance of our method.

2.5. Code

The source code for the proposed algorithm and associated MATLAB-based GUI are freely available on the author's website, along with instructions for installation and use: http://www.escience.cn/people/bjqin/research.html.

3. Results

This section gives the evaluation of the proposed method on the FMIs acquired from the Nano Biomedical Research Center (NBRC) in Shanghai Jiao Tong University, China. All the FMIs are acquired using an inverted fluorescence microscope (Olympus IX73, Olympus Ltd., Tokyo, Japan) at 100-times magnification when the fluorescence is fully developed. The size of FMI in pixels is 1080×1920, and the diameter of the micro-droplets in the image is approximately 30 μm. The relative experiment details are demonstrated as below. The APs encapsulated in the micro-droplet are obtained from calf intestine. Both APs and AP-labeled nanoparticles were synthesized by NBRC. The substrate concentration employed was 5 mM, where mM represents 10^{-3} mol/L.

3.1. Overall Micro-Droplet Detection

Quantitative evaluations of our method and the state-of-the-art methods mentioned above were carried out on the FMIs. The FMI data consist of a total of fifteen test images. The ground-truth of the overall micro-droplets on the FMIs was manually segmented by two experts at NBRC.

The three methods' parameters are set with the default parameters for achieving the best performances of these methods. As for our method, we set the stand variance σ of Gaussian filtering to one. The contrast enhancement threshold T is set to 0.05, and N is set to eight by default to make the CLAHE achieve the best performances. The search radius of circular Hough transform is set from 16 to 32. All the parameters of our method are set to make our method perform best.

3.1.1. Visual Evaluation

The visual evaluation of different methods is shown in Figure 5. We can see that the proposed method (Figure 5f) perfectly detects all the micro-droplets. Figure 5c also shows that MSVST may detect false micro-droplets. Moreover, Figure 5d,e demonstrates that MSSEF and MPHD may perform poorly on the overall micro-droplet detection.

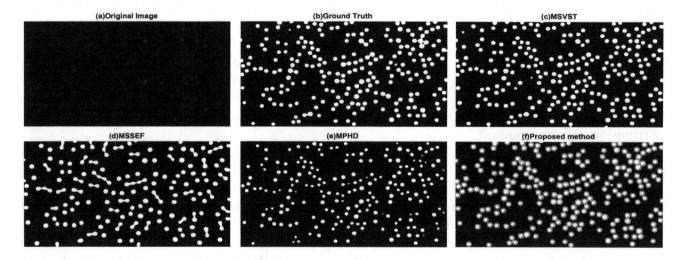

Figure 5. Comparative results of segmented binary maps of different methods: (**a**) Original image. (**b**) Ground truth. (**c**) Multiscale variance-stabilizing transform (MSVST). (**d**) Multiscale spot-enhancing filter method (MSSEF). (**e**) Maximum possible height-dome method (MPHD). (**f**) The proposed method.

3.1.2. TPR and FPR

The comparative evaluations of TPR and FPR are displayed in Figure 6. The TPR of our method is the highest TPR for all the test images, and the highest average TPR achieved by our method is 0.9502. The average FPR of our method is 0.0073. These performance metrics prove that the proposed method has achieved a satisfying micro-droplet detection compared with other methods.

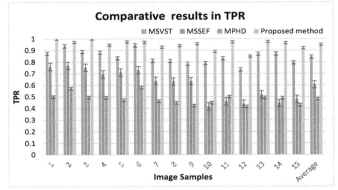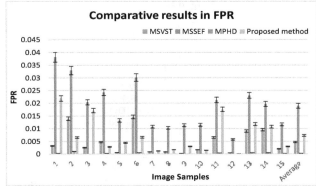

Figure 6. Comparison of TPR and FPR obtained with MSVST, MSSEF, MPHD and the proposed methods on fluorescent micro-droplet images (FMIs).

3.1.3. ROC and F-Measure

The ROC curve in Figure 7 is created by plotting the TPR against the FPR at various threshold settings. Since the AUC is used to evaluate the detecting power of the method, we can use this metric to further reveal the advantage of our method. As shown in Figure 7, the AUC of the proposed method is the highest in all comparative methods. Therefore, we conclude that the proposed method has achieved the best micro-droplet detection performance.

The F-measure is usually used as a detection accuracy metric to evaluate the comprehensive performance of the detector. The higher F-measure corresponds to the better detection. The evaluation results of the F-measure are listed in Table 1. The best average detection accuracy 0.9586 is achieved by our micro-droplet detection method. This highest F-measure score verifies the superiority of the proposed method over other methods.

Table 1. Comparison evaluation of the F-measure obtained with MSVST, MSSEF, MPHD and the proposed methods on FMIs.

Samples	MSVST	MSSEF	MPHD	The Proposed Method
Image1	0.9204	0.7414	0.6640	**0.9231**
Image 2	0.9306	0.7889	0.7250	**0.9674**
Image 3	0.9348	0.8127	0.6610	**0.9597**
Image 4	0.9260	0.7678	0.6591	**0.9656**
Image 5	0.9075	0.8038	0.6392	**0.9770**
Image 6	0.9343	0.7737	0.7318	**0.9677**
Image 7	0.8945	0.7607	0.6311	**0.9604**
Image 8	0.8931	0.7564	0.6183	**0.9663**
Image 9	0.8792	0.7569	0.5946	**0.9721**
Image 10	0.8810	0.5775	0.6183	**0.9402**
Image 11	0.8999	0.6082	0.6653	**0.9655**
Image 12	0.8462	0.6044	0.5859	**0.9186**
Image 13	0.9177	0.6545	0.6586	**0.9707**
Image 14	0.9202	0.5954	0.6555	**0.9692**
Image 15	0.8831	0.6368	0.5987	**0.9551**
Average	0.9046	0.7093	0.6471	**0.9586**

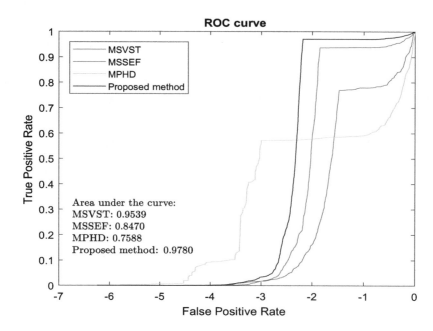

Figure 7. Comparison of the ROC curve obtained with MSVST, MPHD, MSSEF and the proposed methods.

3.1.4. Detected Number of Overall Micro-Droplets

Table 2 shows the final number of micro-droplets detected with different methods. The true number of overall micro-droplets is acquired manually by two experts. Compared with other methods, the proposed method performs stably in detecting capability of the overall micro-droplets in all 15 images, and the detected error is less than two for all the images.

Table 2. Comparison evaluation of the overall number of detected micro-droplets.

Samples	True Number	MSVST	MSSEF	MPHD	The Proposed Method
Image1	161	163	93	152	161
Image 2	222	232	142	202	222
Image 3	221	223	142	202	221
Image 4	223	227	135	198	222
Image 5	219	224	149	202	218
Image 6	229	235	152	210	229
Image 7	250	255	150	236	249
Image 8	239	245	149	224	240
Image 9	245	246	141	224	245
Image 10	381	393	155	350	381
Image 11	372	383	159	348	372
Image 12	381	386	175	345	381
Image 13	347	356	166	320	349
Image 14	414	422	175	371	412
Image 15	358	365	164	325	357

3.2. Fluorescent Micro-Droplet Detection

The detected results of fluorescent micro-droplets are shown in Table 3. The true number of fluorescent micro-droplets is obtained manually by two experts. For the total test images, the proposed method has obtained 100 percent detection accuracy for the thirteen test images with the relative errors in detecting the remaining two images achieving 6.25% and 6.06%. These detected results demonstrate the proposed method's capability in accurately detecting the fluorescent micro-droplets.

Table 3. Comparison evaluation of the number of detected fluorescent micro-droplets.

Samples	True Number	Detected Number of Fluorescent Micro-Droplets	Relative Error
Image1	21	21	0.00%
Image 2	18	18	0.00%
Image 3	18	18	0.00%
Image 4	16	17	6.25%
Image 5	13	13	0.00%
Image 6	24	24	0.00%
Image 7	27	27	0.00%
Image 8	26	26	0.00%
Image 9	9	9	0.00%
Image 10	36	36	0.00%
Image 11	28	28	0.00%
Image 12	30	30	0.00%
Image 13	33	35	6.06%
Image 14	32	32	0.00%
Image 15	31	31	0.00%

3.3. AP-Labeled Nanoparticle Concentration Measurement

Compared with the reference concentration (Table 4), the test AP-labeled nanoparticle concentration calculated with the detected results of micro-droplets has been measured with high accuracy in most samples. The low relative errors in Table 4 further demonstrate the high performance of our method in the measurement of AP-labeled nanoparticle concentration. fM in Table 4 corresponds to 10^{-15} mol/L.

Table 4. Comparison evaluation of the alkaline phosphatase (AP)-labeled nanoparticle concentration measurement.

Samples	True AP-Labeled Nanoparticle Concentration (fM)	Test AP-Labeled Nanoparticle Concentration (fM)	Relative Error
Image1	16.4222	16.4222	0.00%
Image 2	9.9356	9.9356	0.00%
Image 3	9.9825	9.9825	0.00%
Image 4	8.7483	9.3610	7.00%
Image 5	7.1905	7.2246	0.47%
Image 6	13.0088	13.0088	0.00%
Image 7	13.4291	13.4862	0.43%
Image 8	13.5327	13.4730	0.44%
Image 9	4.3976	4.3976	0.00%
Image 10	11.6625	11.6625	0.00%
Image 11	9.1947	9.1947	0.00%
Image 12	9.6366	9.6366	0.00%
Image 13	11.7421	12.4174	5.75%
Image 14	9.4524	9.5002	0.51%
Image 15	10.6424	10.6736	0.29%

4. Discussion

The comparative evaluations demonstrated in Section 3 reveal the effectiveness of the proposed method for micro-droplet detection. With the precise micro-droplet detection, the AP-labeled nanoparticle concentration for the experimental analysis can be calculated accurately. However, it should be noted that the AP-labeled nanoparticle concentration measurement is sensitive to the results of micro-droplet detection. The results in Tables 2 to 4 show that a very slight micro-droplet detecting error may significantly increase the AP-labeled nanoparticle concentration measurement error. Therefore, there is certainly room for further improvement of the proposed method.

5. Conclusions

AP-labeled nanoparticle concentration measurement is of great importance for quantitative biomolecular analysis and measurement. Because the micro-droplet can encapsulate a single AP-labeled nanoparticle and be imaged in fluorescence microscope, the AP-labeled nanoparticle concentration measurement is usually calculated by accurately counting the fluorescent micro-droplets and the overall micro-droplets. This work proposes a micro-droplet detection method for high accuracy AP-labeled nanoparticle concentration measurement by precisely and robustly detecting the weakly luminescent empty micro-droplets that are closely clustered in the complex background noises. The comparative evaluations using the state-of-the-art methods have demonstrated that the proposed method has the best accuracy for micro-droplet detection and AP-labeled nanoparticle concentration measurement.

Acknowledgments: This work was supported by the National Natural Science Foundation of China (21075082 and 61271320) and Medical Engineering Cross Fund of Shanghai Jiao Tong University (YG2014MS29). Baowei Fei was partially supported by NIH Grants CA156775, CA176684 and CA204254 and the Georgia Research Alliance Distinguished Scientists Award. The authors would like to thank all authors for opening source codes used in the experimental comparison in this work. We are thankful to the anonymous reviewers for their valuable comments that greatly helped to improve this paper.

Author Contributions: Rufeng Li and Binjie Qin conceived of and designed the experiments. Rufeng Li and Yibei Wang performed the experiments. Yibei Wang and Hong Xu analyzed the data. Rufeng Li, Baowei Fei and Binjie Qin wrote the paper. Hong Xu and Binjie Qin supervised the experiments.

References

1. Nketia, T.; Sailem, H.; Rohde, G.; Machiraju, R.; Rittscher, J. Analysis of live cell images: Methods, tools and opportunities. *Methods* **2017**, *115*, 65–79.
2. Specht, E.A.; Braselmann, E.; Palmer, A.E. A Critical and Comparative Review of Fluorescent Tools for Live-Cell Imaging. *Annu. Rev. Physiol.* **2017**, *79*, 93–117.
3. Qiang, Y.; Lee, J.Y.; Bartenschlager, R.; Rohr, K. Colocalization analysis and particle tracking in multi-channel fluorescence microscopy images. In Proceedings of the 2017 IEEE 14th International Symposium on Biomedical Imaging (ISBI 2017), Melbourne, Australia, 18–21 April 2017; pp. 646–649.
4. Rissin, D.M.; Kan, C.W.; Campbell, T.G.; Howes, S.C.; Fournier, D.R.; Song, L.; Piech, T.; Patel, P.P.; Chang, L.; Rivnak, A.J.; et al. Single-molecule enzyme-linked immunosorbent assay detects serum proteins at subfemtomolar concentrations. *Nat. Biotechnol.* **2010**, *28*, 595–599.
5. Basova, E.Y.; Foret, F. Droplet microfluidics in (bio)chemical analysis. *Analyst* **2015**, *140*, 22–38.
6. Joensson, H.N.; Andersson Svahn, H. Droplet Microfluidics—A Tool for Single-Cell Analysis. *Angew. Chem. Int. Ed.* **2012**, *51*, 12176–12192.
7. Rissin, D.M.; Walt, D.R. Digital concentration readout of single enzyme molecules using femtoliter arrays and Poisson statistics. *Nano Lett.* **2006**, *6*, 520–523.
8. Thompson, R.E.; Larson, D.R.; Webb, W.W. Precise nanometer localization analysis for individual fluorescent probes. *Biophys. J.* **2002**, *82*, 2775–2783.
9. Kervrann, C.; Sorzano, C.o.S.; Acton, S.T.; Olivo-Marin, J.C.; Unser, M. A guided tour of selected image processing and analysis methods for fluorescence and electron microscopy. *IEEE J. Sel. Top. Signal Process.* **2016**, *10*, 6–30.
10. Wiesmann, V.; Franz, D.; Held, C.; Munzenmayer, C.; Palmisano, R.; Wittenberg, T. Review of free software tools for image analysis of fluorescence cell micrographs. *J. Microsc.* **2015**, *257*, 39–53.
11. Arena, E.T.; Rueden, C.T.; Hiner, M.C.; Wang, S.; Yuan, M.; Eliceiri, K.W. Quantitating the cell: Turning images into numbers with ImageJ. *Wiley Interdiscip. Rev.: Dev. Biol.* **2017**, *6*, doi:10.1002/wdev.260.
12. Smal, I.; Loog, M.; Niessen, W.; Meijering, E. Quantitative comparison of spot detection methods in fluorescence microscopy. *IEEE Trans. Med. Imaging* **2010**, *29*, 282–301.

13. Zhang, B.; Fadili, M.J.; Starck, J.L.; Olivo-Marin, J.C. Multiscale variance-stabilizing transform for mixed-Poisson-Gaussian processes and its applications in bioimaging. In Proceedings of the 2007 14th IEEE International Conference on Image Processing (ICIP 2007), San Antonio, TX, USA, 16–19 September 2007; Volume 6, p. VI-233.

14. Smal, I.; Niessen, W.; Meijering, E. A new detection scheme for multiple object tracking in fluorescence microscopy by joint probabilistic data association filtering. In Proceedings of the 2008 5th IEEE International Symposium on Biomedical Imaging: From Nano to Macro (ISBI 2008), Paris, France, 14–17 May 2008; pp. 264–267.

15. Mallat, S.G. A theory for multiresolution signal decomposition: The wavelet representation. *IEEE Trans. Pattern Anal. Mach. Intell.* **1989**, *11*, 674–693.

16. Rezatofighi, S.H.; Hartley, R.; Hughes, W.E. A new approach for spot detection in total internal reflection fluorescence microscopy. In Proceedings of the 2012 9th IEEE International Symposium on Biomedical Imaging (ISBI 2012), Barcelona, Spain, 2–5 May 2012; pp. 860–863.

17. Jaiswal, A.; Godinez, W.J.; Eils, R.; Lehmann, M.J.; Rohr, K. Tracking virus particles in fluorescence microscopy images using multi-scale detection and multi-frame association. *IEEE Trans. Image Process.* **2015**, *24*, 4122–4136.

18. Basset, A.; Boulanger, J.; Bouthemy, P.; Kervrann, C.; Salamero, J. SLT-LoG: A vesicle segmentation method with automatic scale selection and local thresholding applied to TIRF microscopy. In Proceedings of the 2014 IEEE 11th International Symposium on Biomedical Imaging(ISBI), Beijing, China, 29 April–2 May 2014; pp. 533–536.

19. Basset, A.; Boulanger, J.; Salamero, J.; Bouthemy, P.; Kervrann, C. Adaptive spot detection with optimal scale selection in fluorescence microscopy images. *IEEE Trans. Image Process.* **2015**, *24*, 4512–4527.

20. Acosta, B.M.T.; Basset, A.; Bouthemy, P.; Kervrann, C. Multi-scale spot segmentation with selection of image scales. In Proceedings of the 2017 IEEE International Conference on Acoustics, Speech and Signal Processing (ICASSP), New Orleans, LA, USA, 5–9 March 2017; pp. 1912–1916.

21. Traore, D.; Rietdorf, K.; Al-Jawad, N.; Al-Assam, H. Automatic Hotspots Detection for Intracellular Calcium Analysis in Fluorescence Microscopic Videos. In *Annual Conference on Medical Image Understanding and Analysis*; Springer: Cham, The Netherlands, 2017; pp. 862–873.

22. Zuiderveld, K. Contrast limited adaptive histogram equalization. In *Graphics Gems IV*; Academic Press Professional, Inc.: New York, NY, USA, 1994; pp. 474–485.

23. Otsu, N. A threshold selection method from gray-level histograms. *IEEE Trans. Syst. Man Cybern.* **1979**, *9*, 62–66.

24. Ghaye, J.; Kamat, M.A.; Corbino-Giunta, L.; Silacci, P.; Vergeres, G.; Micheli, G.; Carrara, S. Image thresholding techniques for localization of sub-resolution fluorescent biomarkers. *Cytom. Part A* **2013**, *83*, 1001–1016.

25. Bartell, L.R.; Bonassar, L.J.; Cohen, I. A watershed-based algorithm to segment and classify cells in fluorescence microscopy images. *arXiv* **2017**, arXiv:1706.00815.

26. Acharya, V.; Kumar, P. Identification and Red Blood Cell Automated Counting from Blood Smear Images using Computer Aided System. *Med. Biol. Eng. Comput.* **2017**, doi:10.1007/s11517-017-1708-9.

27. Jain, R.; Kasturi, R.; Schunck, B.G. *Machine Vision*; McGraw-Hill: New York, NY, USA, 1995; Volume 5.

28. Zhu, F.; Qin, B.; Feng, W.; Wang, H.; Huang, S.; Lv, Y.; Chen, Y. Reducing Poisson noise and baseline drift in X-ray spectral images with bootstrap Poisson regression and robust nonparametric regression. *Phys. Med. Biol.* **2013**, *58*, 1739.

6

Identification of Human Ovarian Adenocarcinoma Cells with Cisplatin-Resistance by Feature Extraction of Gray Level Co-Occurrence Matrix Using Optical Images

Chih-Ling Huang [1],*, Meng-Jia Lian [2], Yi-Hsuan Wu [3], Wei-Ming Chen [2] and Wen-Tai Chiu [4]

[1]   Center for Fundamental Science, Kaohsiung Medical University, Kaohsiung 807, Taiwan

[2]   School of Dentistry, College of Dental Medicine, Kaohsiung Medical University, Kaohsiung 807, Taiwan; sy2es93103@gmail.com (M.-J.L.); bill321cm1@gmail.com (W.-M.C.)

[3]   Department of Medicinal and Applied Chemistry, College of Life Science, Kaohsiung Medical University, Kaohsiung 807, Taiwan; qoo860724@gmail.com

[4]   Department of Biomedical Engineering, National Cheng Kung University, Tainan 701, Taiwan; wtchiu@mail.ncku.edu.tw

*   Correspondence: chihling@kmu.edu.tw

Abstract: Ovarian cancer is the most malignant of all gynecological cancers. A challenge that deteriorates with ovarian adenocarcinoma in neoplastic disease patients has been associated with the chemoresistance of cancer cells. Cisplatin (CP) belongs to the first-line chemotherapeutic agents and it would be beneficial to identify chemoresistance for ovarian adenocarcinoma cells, especially CP-resistance. Gray level co-occurrence matrix (GLCM) was characterized imaging from a numeric matrix and find its texture features. Serous type (OVCAR-4 and A2780), and clear cell type (IGROV1) ovarian carcinoma cell lines with CP-resistance were used to demonstrate GLCM texture feature extraction of images. Cells were cultured with cell density of 6×10^5 in a glass-bottom dish to form a uniform coverage of the glass slide to get the optical images by microscope and DVC camera. CP-resistant cells included OVCAR-4, A2780 and IGROV and had the higher contrast and entropy, lower energy, and homogeneity. Signal to noise ratio was used to evaluate the degree for chemoresistance of cell images based on GLCM texture feature extraction. The difference between wile type and CP-resistant cells was statistically significant in every case ($p < 0.001$). It is a promising model to achieve a rapid method with a more reliable diagnostic performance for identification of ovarian adenocarcinoma cells with CP-resistance by feature extraction of GLCM in vitro or ex vivo.

Keywords: chemoresistance; cisplatin; gray-level co-occurrence matrix; ovarian adenocarcinoma

1. Introduction

Ovarian cancer is the most malignant of all gynecological cancers [1]. A challenge that deteriorates with ovarian adenocarcinoma in neoplastic disease patients has been associated with the chemoresistance of cancer cells. Cisplatin (CP) is a platinum-containing compound, which belongs to the first-line chemotherapeutic agents for the treatment of human ovarian cancer [2]. Therefore, it would be beneficial for cancer therapy to identify various chemoresistance for human ovarian adenocarcinoma cells, especially CP-resistance.

Ovarian carcinomas consist of at least five distinct diseases: high-grade serous, low-grade serous, clear cell, endometrioid, and mucinous [3]. High-grade serous ovarian cancer is responsible for approximately 80% of ovarian cancer cases and two-thirds of ovarian cancer deaths. OVCAR-4 ranked as one of the highest matches to high-grade serous ovarian cancer, a cell-line collected from a 42-year-old ovarian cancer patient and found to be resistant to combination chemotherapy [4]. A2780 is serous carcinoma cell line with platinum sensitivity [5]. IGROV1 is human clear cell type ovarian carcinoma cell line. It has the propensity to float as clusters isolated from tumor tissue and ascites [6].

Gray level co-occurrence matrix (GLCM) characterizes the texture of images by calculating from a numeric matrix [7], which was defined by Haralick et al. [8]. It can be used to analyze the medical imaging from magnetic resonance imaging or ultrasonography and find the potential relationship with tumor malignancies [9], such as brain tumor detection [10], liver tumors [11], and histopathological images [12].

In general, it is not easy to take images of ovarian cancer, but ovarian cancer cells can be extracted from ascites of patients. The cells can be cultured mono-layered to dissolve the problem for the image taken. In our previous study, detection of various characteristics of cancer cells by feature extraction of GLCM can be applied in real clinical cases for metastatic cancer cells [13] or biopsy [14] images which were successfully taken from camera.

In search of novel mechanisms that may lead to CP chemoresistance, scientists used a lot of cells and subtractive hybridization to identify differentially expressed genes [15]. However, chemoresistance happens in cells where equivalent effects of various expressed genes is expressed outside of cell imaging. In this study, we proposed a promising method based on GLCM image processing model to achieve a rapid method with a more reliable diagnostic performance for various chemoresistance for CP of human ovarian adenocarcinoma cells by feature extraction of GLCM.

2. Materials and Methods

The optical image system used in this study comprised a microscope (BX-53 OLYMPUS, Tokyo, Japan) and DVC camera (Model: 1500M-T1-GE S/N 3797) with an image capture software (DVC View™). The different images (1392×1040 pixels) of the samples were obtained. The diameter of a cell was approximately 10–20 pixels in obtained images and the processing image was 150×150 pixels with 256 gray level for extracting the characteristic texture feature of cells [13].

GLCM was used to calculate contrast, energy, entropy, and homogeneity to analyze the images texture features. The variable C (i, j) expressed in Equations (1)–(4) refer to the value at the (i, j) position in a GLCM. These four indexes corresponded to the disorder in cell images and indicate the surface characteristic of cancer cells. For example, contrast displayed the edges and three-dimensional (3D) structures of cell; energy represented the orderliness; homogeneity represented the smoothness of the distribution for gray level and entropy showed the disorder degree.

$$\text{Contrast}: \sum_{ij=1}^{G} C_{ij}(i-j)^2 \tag{1}$$

$$\text{Energy}: \sum_{ij=1}^{G} C_{ij}^2 \tag{2}$$

$$\text{Homogeneity}: \sum_{ij=1}^{G} \frac{1}{1+|i-j|} C_{ij} \tag{3}$$

$$\text{Entropy}: -\sum_{ij=1}^{G} C_{ij} \log C_{ij} \tag{4}$$

Due to ovarian cancer being the most malignant of all gynecological cancers its chemoresistance was challenging the first-line chemotherapeutic agents for the treatments. High-grade serous ovarian cancer is responsible for approximately 80% of ovarian cancer cases so we selected human serous type ovarian adenocarcinoma cell lines (OVCAR-4 and A2780), and human clear cell type ovarian carcinoma cell line (IGROV1) to demonstrate the GLCM texture feature extraction and analysis of images. Furthermore, wild type (WT) human ovarian adenocarcinoma cell lines and that with chemoresistance for CP were used. All cells were maintained in RPMI1640 medium solution (Gibco) containing 10% fetal calf serum and incubated at 37 °C with 5% CO_2. A2780 were cultured in PMI1640 medium with non-essential amino acids, glutamine, and 0.5 units insulin.

Before acquiring the images, cells were cultured with cell density of 6×10^5 in a glass-bottom dish. A silicone separator (Culture-Insert 2 Well, iBidi, Martinsried, Germany) was placed to trap cells to form a uniform coverage of the glass slide and create a clear region as the blank. Samples were incubated for 48 h and then washed twice in a phosphate buffered saline solution (PBS, 0.1 M, pH = 7.4).

To evaluate the reliability of the detection method, the statistical differences were evaluated using a one-way analysis of variance (ANOVA) technique. In evaluating the test results, a * p value of <0.05 was statistically significant, a ** p value of <0.01 was very statistically significant, and a *** p value of <0.001 was highly statistically significant.

3. Results and Discussion

Figure 1 shows cell images for serous cell type of OVCAR-4, A2780, and clear cell type IGROV1 of WT and CP-resistantance of ovarian adenocarcinoma cells. Under the optical microscope, little morphological differences could be observed between the WT ovarian adenocarcinoma cells (Figure 1a–c) and its CP-resistant counterpart (Figure 1d–f). However, chemoresistance is a very complex phenomenon, and it involves multiple interconnected mechanisms [16]. CP is localizing to the nucleus and binding to DNA, and then it gives rise to intrastrain DNA adducts. Subsequently, cancer cells apoptosis was caused by triggering G2 cell cycle arrest [17]. In a previous study, ovarian adenocarcinoma cells with CP-resistance recovered a normal proliferation state after a treatment with 5 µg/mL CP for 41 days. At confluence, the cell layer displayed some morphological differences and cells were becoming able to pile and to form three dimensional spherical structures [18]. It means that the cells with chemoresistance were tending to form stereoscopic structures and this characteristic can be analyzed by GLCM texture feature extracting of images. It will be promising and potentially detect chemoresistance before the new therapeutics.

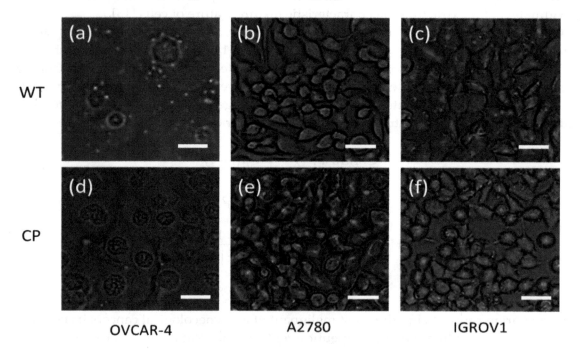

Figure 1. Cell images for serous cell type (**a**) OVCAR-4, (**b**) A2780, and (**c**) clear cell type IGROV1 of wild type (WT) ovarian adenocarcinoma cells and (**d–f**) which were cisplatin-resistant (CP). (Scale bar: 20 µm)

Figure 2 shows GLCM texture features of energy, contrast, homogeneity, and entropy for serous type (OVCAR-4) of ovarian adenocarcinoma cells with various interpixel distance with chemoresistance for CP and WT cells. The inflection points of texture feature can be found in Figure 2 around interpixel distances of 10–20 pixels. The size of the image used for processing is 150×150 pixels and the diameter of ovarian adenocarcinoma cells is approximately 10–20 pixels, which implies that the characteristic texture feature commonly occurs in the boundary of cells, and that we can set up the interpixel distance as a specific value (e.g., 10 pixels) around the cell diameter to obtain the typical texture features. The ovarian adenocarcinoma cells with CP-resistance exhibit more 3D structures with characteristic rough surfaces. These structures enhance the optical scattering effect and it is difficult to observe the cells in the same focus plane and enhance the margins of cells. These characteristics indicate that the images of ovarian adenocarcinoma cells with CP-resistance have lower energy and homogeneity but higher contrast and entropy due to the morphologies. These four texture features can be used to predict the ability for CP-resistance of ovarian adenocarcinoma cells.

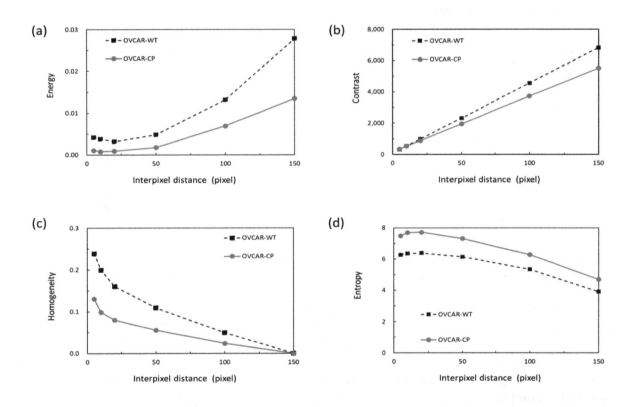

Figure 2. Gray level co-occurrence matrix (GLCM) texture feature: **(a)** energy, **(b)** contrast, **(c)** homogeneity, and **(d)** entropy for serous type (OVCAR-4) of ovarian adenocarcinoma cells with various interpixel distance with wild type (WT) and chemoresistance for cisplatin (CP).

Texture feature of GLCM extracting for WT and CP-resistant ovarian adenocarcinoma cell images are shown in Table 1. The texture features of WT ovarian adenocarcinoma cells were used as the benchmark and statistically compared with those of the CP-resistant cells for OVCAR-4, A2780, and IGROV-1, respectively. In general, the results show that for each of the cell lines, the CP-resistant ovarian adenocarcinoma cells have a higher contrast and entropy than the WT. Figure 3 shows GLCM texture features of WT and CP-resistant ovarian adenocarcinoma cells for OVCAR-4, A2780, and IGROV1. Table 1 and Figure 3 show that almost the differences in these four GLCM texture features of CP-resistant and WT cells were statistically significant in every case ($p < 0.01$ or $p < 0.001$). In other words, it provides the means to reliably differentiate between WT and CP-resistant cells for all three cell lines.

Table 1. Gray level co-occurrence matrix (GLCM) texture features for wild type (WT) and cisplatin-resistant (CP) of ovarian adenocarcinoma cells.

Cell	Feature	WT	CP	p-Value
OVCAR-4	Contrast ($\times 10^3$)	0.54 ± 0.08	0.53 ± 0.07	0.86
	Entropy ($\times 10^0$)	6.36 ± 0.22	7.70 ± 0.26	***
	Energy ($\times 10^{-3}$)	3.80 ± 0.84	0.83 ± 0.32	***
	Homogeneity ($\times 10^{-1}$)	1.99 ± 0.18	0.99 ± 0.10	***
A2780	Contrast ($\times 10^3$)	0.91 ± 0.13	1.35 ± 0.19	**
	Entropy ($\times 10^0$)	8.23 ± 0.21	8.85 ± 0.11	***
	Energy ($\times 10^{-3}$)	0.45 ± 0.11	0.20 ± 0.03	***
	Homogeneity ($\times 10^{-1}$)	0.60 ± 0.08	0.40 ± 0.03	**
IGROV1	Contrast ($\times 10^3$)	0.74 ± 0.15	1.32 ± 0.09	***
	Entropy ($\times 10^0$)	7.92 ± 0.21	9.41 ± 0.06	***
	Energy ($\times 10^{-3}$)	0.61 ± 0.12	0.18 ± 0.01	***
	Homogeneity ($\times 10^{-1}$)	0.71 ± 0.09	0.33 ± 0.01	***

Note: GLCM sampling offset was (10.0) and compare to WT and * $p < 0.05$, ** $p < 0.01$, and *** $p < 0.001$.

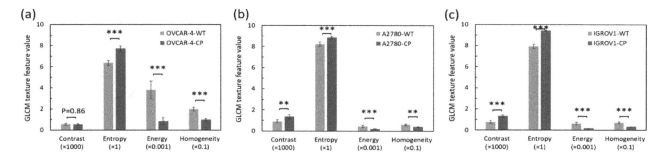

Figure 3. Gray level co-occurrence matrix (GLCM) texture feature of wild type (WT) and cisplatin (CP)-resistant ovarian adenocarcinoma cells for (**a**) OVCAR-4, (**b**) A2780, and (**c**) IGROV1.

Due to the multi-factor analysis being complex, signal-to-noise (S/N) ratios of these four GLCM texture features for WT and CP-resistant ovarian adenocarcinoma cells were calculated and shown in Table 2. The basic concept was according to Taguchi method [19]. In this study, S/N ratio was meaning the degree of the images influenced by the various factors. It was calculated by equations from the Taguchi method. Taguchi method was used to improve the qualities of products efficiently with parameters designed in engineering fields. S/N ratio was meaning the degree of the product influenced by the various factors. In this study, the various GLCM texture features can be the parameter of cell images. For CP-resistant type cells, two of the four GLCM texture features were for smaller-is-better (i.e., energy and homogeneity) and two for larger-is-better (i.e., contrast and entropy). It was same as the basic concept of Taguchi method, so we used it for multi-factor calculation. S/N ratio was calculated by Equations (5) and (6) [20]:

$$\text{Smaller-is-better}: \text{ S/N ratio} = -10 \log\left(\frac{1}{n} \sum y_i^2\right) \tag{5}$$

$$\text{Larger-is-better}: \text{ S/N ratio} = -10 \log\left(\frac{1}{n} \sum \frac{1}{y_i^2}\right) \tag{6}$$

S/N ratio can be referred to the degree for chemoresistance of cells based on GLCM texture feature extraction. The higher S/N ratio means the cell images were more like CP-resistant type. In Table 2, the S/N ratio of WT of ovarian adenocarcinoma cells were 17.93 ± 0.59, 23.37 ± 0.42, and 22.81 ± 0.43 for OVCAR-4, A2780 and IGROV1, respectively. The S/N ratio of CP-resistant ovarian adenocarcinoma cells were 21.76 ± 0.50, 24.44 ± 0.17, and 25.09 ± 0.07 for OVCAR-4, A2780 and IGROV1, respectively.

The differences in these cells were statistically significant in every case ($p < 0.001$). Compared to Table 1, the results of false positive CP were eliminated using multi-factor calculation. In this study, S/N ratio was meaning the degree of the images influenced by the various factors. Moreover, multi-factors included the tumor heterogeneity caused by different cell types in vivo.

Table 2. Signal-to-noise (S/N) ratio of gray level co-occurrence matrix (GLCM) texture feature for wild type (WT) and cisplatin-resistant (CP) ovarian adenocarcinoma cells.

Cells	WT	CP	p-Value
OVCAR-4	17.93 ± 0.59	21.76 ± 0.50	***
A2780	23.37 ± 0.42	24.44 ± 0.17	***
IGROV1	22.81 ± 0.43	25.09 ± 0.07	***

Note: GLCM sampling offset was (10.0) and compare to WT and * $p < 0.05$, ** $p < 0.01$, and *** $p < 0.001$.

The main factors which limit treatment efficiency are recurrence and progressive acquisition of chemoresistance. Chemoresistance is a complex process involving many stages. As a result, there is an urgent requirement for low-cost, high-throughput methods for assessing the risk of chemoresistance in a timely and quantitative manner. Accordingly, this study has proposed an optical method for chemoresistance detection based on GLCM texture features extraction. The feasibility of the proposed approach has been demonstrated using three pairs of ovarian adenocarcinoma cells, namely OVCAR-4, A2780, and IGROV1. Notably, the proposed method enables physical characterization of ovarian adenocarcinoma cells even in the case where the size and morphologies of the CP-resistant cells are very similar to those of WT.

Optical images could be used to study biophysical processes in living systems and to monitor morphological and physiological changes such as precancerous or cancerous conditions [21]. In a previous study, it has been indicated that epithelial-mesenchymal transition (EMT) contributes to chemoresistance acquisition [22] and indeed CP-resistant cell images result in the formation of dense 3D structures with characteristic rough surfaces compared to wild type cells. These cell structures enhance the higher contrast and entropy, and lower energy and homogeneity in GLCM texture feature of images.

The proposed method in this study has many advantages over in vitro tests, including a faster optical detection, a lower cost, a larger sample size, and a greater throughput. Most importantly, it provides the means to obtain a quantitative evaluation of the chemoresistance risk and therefore reduces the reliance on the practical skill and experience of the practitioner. Figure 4 shows the sketch of this promising model to achieve a rapid method with a more reliable diagnostic performance for identification of ovarian adenocarcinoma cells with cisplatin-resistance by feature extraction of GLCM in vitro or ex vivo. In the same time, machine learning was rapidly developing as the artificial intelligence technique [23]. The proposed method in this study was based on computer aided diagnosis [24] and it can be combined with the support vector machine [25] to train the model for proceeding the mass identification of chemoresistance risk for cancer cells. According to our previous study [13,14], more than ten cancer species were selected for feature extraction using optical images and we get positive results for various identification. It has potential for other cancer cells due to their equivalent effect for epithelial-mesenchymal transition expressed in cell imaging. However, it was required for the high throughput platform and combined with machine learning to train the model for proceeding the mass identification of chemoresistance risk for more cancer species. It provides a highly promising solution for physical characterization of ovarian adenocarcinoma cells with chemoresistance in vitro. Even for clinical practice, multiple invasive biopsies also can be used to analyze for feature extraction using optical images, but it was required to use scanned laser pico-projection system (SLPP) which has the narrower bandwidth compared to traditional white light to enhance the contrast and entropy of images for analysis [14].

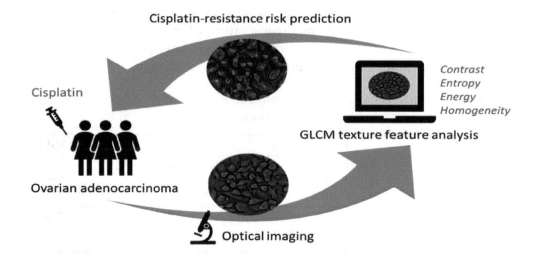

Figure 4. Sketch of the proposed promising model to achieve a rapid method with a more reliable diagnostic performance for identification of ovarian adenocarcinoma cells with cisplatin-resistance by feature extraction of GLCM in vitro or ex vivo.

4. Conclusions

Serous type ovarian adenocarcinoma cells with chemoresistance have more obvious edges and 3D structures, and the images were respected to have the higher contrast and entropy, lower energy and homogeneity. This provides the means to obtain a quantitative evaluation of the chemoresistance risk. It is a promising model to achieve a rapid method with a more reliable diagnostic performance for identification of ovarian adenocarcinoma cells with cisplatin-resistance by feature extraction of GLCM in vitro or ex vivo. In the future, the cells of the same patient could be taken from various stages of treatments to monitor morphological and physiological changes for cancerous conditions. It provides a quantitative evaluation of chemoresistance risk for chemotherapeutic agents in the next treatments. It can help to detect chemoresistance of cancer cells before the new therapeutics.

Author Contributions: Conceptualization, C.-L.H. and W.-T.C.; investigation, M.-J.L., Y.-H.W. and W.-M.C.; supervision, C.-L.H. All authors have read and agreed to the published version of the manuscript.

Acknowledgments: The authors would like to thank the financial support provided to this study by College Student Research Scholarship of Ministry of Science and Technology (MOST) in Taiwan under grant no. (107-2813-C-006-179-B) and sponsored by the Ministry of Education in Taiwan.

References

1. Janda, M.; McGrath, S.; Obermair, A. Challenges and controversies in the conservative management of uterine and ovarian cancer. *Best Pract. Res. Clin. Obstet. Gynaecol.* **2019**, *55*, 93–108. [CrossRef] [PubMed]
2. Jendželovský, R.; Jendželovská, Z.; Hiľovská, L.; Kovaľ, J.; Mikeš, J.; Fedoročko, P. Proadifen sensitizes resistant ovarian adenocarcinoma cells to cisplatin. *Toxicol. Lett.* **2016**, *243*, 56–66. [CrossRef] [PubMed]
3. Anglesio, M.S.; Wiegand, K.C.; Melnyk, N.; Chow, C.; Salamanca, C.; Prentice, L.M.; Senz, J.; Yang, W.; Spillman, M.A.; Cochrane, D.R.; et al. Type-specific cell line models for type-specific ovarian cancer research. *PLoS ONE* **2013**, *8*, e72162. [CrossRef] [PubMed]
4. Shaw, S.K.; Schreiber, C.L.; Roland, F.M.; Battles, P.M.; Brennan, S.P.; Padanilam, S.J.; Smith, B.D. High expression of integrin $\alpha v \beta 3$ enables uptake of targeted fluorescent probes into ovarian cancer cells and tumors. *Bioorg. Med. Chem.* **2018**, *26*, 2085–2091. [CrossRef] [PubMed]
5. Rivard, C.; Geller, M.; Schnettler, E.; Saluja, M.; Vogel, R.I.; Saluja, A.; Ramakrishnan, S. Inhibition of epithelial ovarian cancer by Minnelide, a water-soluble pro-drug. *Gynecol. Oncol.* **2014**, *135*, 318–324. [CrossRef] [PubMed]

6.	Carduner, L.; Picot, C.R.; Leroy-Dudal, J.; Blay, L.; Kellouche, S.; Carreiras, F. Cell cycle arrest or survival signaling through αv integrins, activation of PKC and ERK1/2 lead to anoikis resistance of ovarian cancer spheroids. *Exp. Cell Res.* **2014**, *320*, 329–342. [CrossRef] [PubMed]

7.	Lloyd, K.; Rosin, P.L.; Marshall, D.; Moore, S.C. Detecting violent and abnormal crowd activity using temporal analysis of grey level co-occurrence matrix (GLCM)-based texture measures. *Mach. Vis. Appl.* **2017**, *28*, 361–371. [CrossRef]

8.	Haralick, R.; Shanmugam, K.; Dinstein, I.H. Textural features for image classif. *IEEE Trans. Ind. Electron.* **1973**, *3*, 610–621. [CrossRef]

9.	Molina, D.; Pérez-Beteta, J.; Martínez-González, A.; Martino, J.; Velásquez, C.; Arana, E.; Pérez-García, V.M. Influence of gray level and space discretization on brain tumor heterogeneity measures obtained from magnetic resonance images. *Comput. Biol. Med.* **2016**, *78*, 49–57. [CrossRef] [PubMed]

10.	Vallabhaneni, R.B.; Rajesh, V. Brain tumour detection using mean shift clustering and GLCM features with edge adaptive total variation denoising technique. *Alex. Eng. J.* **2018**, *57*, 2387–2392. [CrossRef]

11.	Xian, G.-M. An identification method of malignant and benign liver tumors from ultrasonography based on GLCM texture features and fuzzy SVM. *Expert Syst. Appl.* **2010**, *37*, 6737–6741. [CrossRef]

12.	Öztürk, Ş.; Akdemir, B. Application of Feature Extraction and Classification Methods for Histopathological Image using GLCM, LBP, LBGLCM, GLRLM and SFTA. *Procedia Comput. Sci.* **2018**, *132*, 40–46. [CrossRef]

13.	Lian, M.-J.; Huang, C.-L. Texture feature extraction of gray-level co-occurrence matrix for metastatic cancer cells using scanned laser pico-projection images. *Lasers Med. Sci.* **2019**, *34*, 1503–1508. [CrossRef] [PubMed]

14.	Lian, M.-J.; Huang, C.-L.; Lee, T.-M. Automation Characterization for Oral Cancer by Pathological Image Processing with Gray-Level Co-occurrence Matrix. *J. Image Graph.* **2018**, *6*, 80–83. [CrossRef]

15.	Solár, P.; Sytkowski, A.J. Differentially expressed genes associated with cisplatin resistance in human ovarian adenocarcinoma cell line A2780. *Cancer lett.* **2011**, *309*, 11–18. [CrossRef] [PubMed]

16.	Ji, X.; Lu, Y.; Tian, H.; Meng, X.; Wei, M.; Cho, W.C. Chemoresistance mechanisms of breast cancer and their countermeasures. *Biomed. Pharmacother.* **2019**, *114*, 108800. [CrossRef] [PubMed]

17.	Kawahara, B.; Ramadoss, S.; Chaudhuri, G.; Janzen, C.; Sen, S.; Mascharak, P.K. Carbon monoxide sensitizes cisplatin-resistant ovarian cancer cell lines toward cisplatin via attenuation of levels of glutathione and nuclear metallothionein. *J. Inorg. Biochem.* **2019**, *191*, 29–39. [CrossRef] [PubMed]

18.	Villedieu, M.; Deslandes, E.; Duval, M.; Héron, J.F.; Gauduchon, P.; Poulain, L. Acquisition of chemoresistance following discontinuous exposures to cisplatin is associated in ovarian carcinoma cells with progressive alteration of FAK, ERK and p38 activation in response to treatment. *Gynecol. Oncol.* **2006**, *101*, 507–519. [CrossRef] [PubMed]

19.	Rezania, A.; Atouei, S.A.; Rosendahl, L. Critical parameters in integration of thermoelectric generators and phase change materials by numerical and Taguchi methods. *Mater. Today Energy* **2020**, *16*, 100376. [CrossRef]

20.	Avikal, S.; Nithin Kumar, K.C.; Singh, A.R.; Jain, R. Grey based Taguchi optimization for multi-lobe bearing. *Mater. Today Proc.* **2020**. [CrossRef]

21.	Duran-Sierra, E.; Cheng, S.; Cuenca-Martinez, R.; Malik, B.; Maitland, K.C.; Lisa Cheng, Y.S.; Wright, J.; Ahmed, B.; Ji, J.; Martinez, M.; et al. Clinical label-free biochemical and metabolic fluorescence lifetime endoscopic imaging of precancerous and cancerous oral lesions. *Oral Oncol.* **2020**, *105*. [CrossRef] [PubMed]

22.	Hoshiba, T. An extracellular matrix (ECM) model at high malignant colorectal tumor increases chondroitin sulfate chains to promote epithelial-mesenchymal transition and chemoresistance acquisition. *Exp. Cell Res.* **2018**, *370*, 571–578. [CrossRef] [PubMed]

23.	Waring, J.; Lindvall, C.; Umeton, R. Automated machine learning: Review of the state-of-the-art and opportunities for healthcare. *Artif. Intell. Med.* **2020**, *104*. [CrossRef] [PubMed]

24.	Raghavendra, U.; Gudigar, A.; Rao, T.N.; Ciaccio, E.J.; Ng, E.Y.K.; Rajendra Acharya, U. Computer-aided diagnosis for the identification of breast cancer using thermogram images: A comprehensive review. *Infrared Phys. Technol.* **2019**, *102*. [CrossRef]

25.	Wang, G.; Zhang, G.; Choi, K.-S.; Lam, K.-M.; Lu, J. Output based transfer learning with least squares support vector machine and its application in bladder cancer prognosis. *Neurocomputing* **2020**, *387*, 279–292. [CrossRef]

7

A Novel Laser Refractive Surgical Treatment for Presbyopia: Optics-Based Customization for Improved Clinical Outcome

Bojan Pajic [1,2,3,4], **Brigitte Pajic-Eggspuehler** [1], **Joerg Mueller** [1], **Zeljka Cvejic** [2] and **Harald Studer** [1,5,*]

[1] Eye Clinic Orasis, Swiss Eye Research Foundation, CH-5734 Reinach, Switzerland; bpajic@datacomm.ch (B.P.); brigitte.pajic@orasis.ch (B.P.-E.); joerg.mueller@nova-optik.ch (J.M.)
[2] Department of Physics, Faculty of Sciences, University of Novi Sad, Trg Dositeja Obradovica 4, 21000 Novi Sad, Serbia; zeljkac@uns.ac.rs
[3] Division of Ophthalmology, Department of Clinical Neurosciences, Geneva University Hospitals, CH-1205 Geneva, Switzerland
[4] Faculty of Medicine of the Military Medical academy, University of Defence, 11000 Belgrade, Serbia
[5] OCTlab, Department of Ophthalmology, University of Basel, CH-4001 Basel, Switzerland
* Correspondence: harald.studer@gmail.com

Academic Editor: Dragan Indjin

Abstract: Laser Assisted in Situ Keratomileusis (LASIK) is a proven treatment method for corneal refractive surgery. Surgically induced higher order optical aberrations were a major reason why the method was only rarely used to treat presbyopia, an age-related near-vision loss. In this study, a novel customization algorithm for designing multifocal ablation patterns, thereby minimizing induced optical aberrations, was used to treat 36 presbyopic subjects. Results showed that most candidates went from poor visual acuity to uncorrected 20/20 vision or better for near (78%), intermediate (92%), and for distance (86%) vision, six months after surgery. All subjects were at 20/25 or better for distance and intermediate vision, and a majority (94%) were also better for near vision. Even though further studies are necessary, our results suggest that the employed methodology is a safe, reliable, and predictable refractive surgical treatment for presbyopia.

Keywords: presbyopia; LASIK; presbyLASIK; uncorrected visual acuity

1. Introduction

Laser Assisted in Situ Keratomileusis (LASIK) is proven to be a safe, fast, and reliable procedure for corneal refractive surgery. The procedure comprises three steps: (i) cutting a thin flap on the outer corneal surface, (ii) ablating tissue underneath the flap with an excimer laser, and (iii) putting the flap back into place on the stromal bed. Only a relatively small number of side effects, such as dry-eye, halos, corneal ectasia, and epithelial ingrowth under the flap, have been reported. Modern excimer laser systems have demonstrated their ability and performance in treating various ametropic conditions, such as nearsightedness (myopia), farsightedness (hyperopia), and astigmatism. By 2009, more than 27 million eyes had successfully been treated with LASIK refractive surgery all around the world.

Even though various approaches—based on diverse technologies and methodologies—for the treatment of age-related far or nearsightedness have been proposed and documented in literature, effective presbyopia treatment remains a challenge in modern eye care. State-of-the-art treatment involves the implantation of multifocal intraocular lenses [1,2], which by nature is a highly invasive surgical procedure, and postoperative refraction planning remains highly complex. Other approaches such as mono-vision corneal procedures [3,4] use excimer lasers and LASIK to treat presbyopia, but these methods are unfortunately not well tolerated by many subjects. Corneal inlay implantation [5,6], intrastromal femtosecond laser corrections [7], or other excimer laser-based presbyopia treatments [8] have been used in clinics with some success over the last few years.

In any such procedure, besides restoring the patients' vision and ability to see far- as well as near-distance objects, the focus should always be that (i) the treatment is reversible and (ii) that postsurgical enhancement, or touch-up, is always possible. Generally speaking, corneal approaches are the least invasive, and are highly accurate and safe procedures. Furthermore, they omit risks that are inherent to the intraocular procedure. It has previously been reported that multifocal LASIK treatments, sometimes also called presbyLASIK treatments, in the cornea showed good refractive results for near, intermediate, and distance vision in hyperopic presbyopia patients [8–10]. The good results of those studies suggest that postoperative refraction was easily predictable, and that presbyLASIK was well tolerated by the study subjects. However, because LASIK ablation patterns for myopic eyes are fundamentally different from those of hyperopic treatments, this prospective study aimed to assess the performance of presbyLASIK customized multifocal procedures for myopic presbyopia patients.

2. Materials and Methods

This prospective, single-surgeon study of myopic presbyopia treatments with a multifocal presbyLASIK procedure included 72 eyes of 36 patients. All eyes underwent pre- and postoperative full clinical biomicroscopical examination, Orbscan IIz corneal topography (BAUSCH + LOMB, TECHNOLAS Perfect Vision GmbH, Munich, Germany) and Zywave II wavefront aberrometry analysis (BAUSCH + LOMB, Rochester, NY, USA). Additionally, monocular and binocular uncorrected near (UNVA), intermediate (UIVA), and distance (UDVA) visual acuity were assessed using a LogMAR chart. For all examinations, the eyes had undilated pupils, and were conducted preoperatively, as well as one week, one month, three months, and six months postoperatively.

All study subjects underwent Supracor refractive surgery, operated with a 217P Excimer laser (BAUSCH + LOMB, TECHNOLAS Perfect Vision GmbH, Munich, Germany). The dominant eye of each individual subject was targeted plano for far vision (0.0 diopters), while the respective non-dominant eye of the same subject was targeted at −0.5 diopters. All LASIK flaps were created with a Ziemer LDV femtosecond laser platform (Ziemer Ophthalmology, Port, Switzerland), and had a superior hinge and a thickness of 110 microns. All treatments were planned and executed in two main steps: first, the normal ablation pattern for the myopic condition of the subject's eyes were applied to the cornea, according to the surgeon's nomogram, and by targeting the mean refractive spherical equivalent (MRSE) to be optimal for distance vision. Second, the aforementioned 3-mm zone near the addition was applied (see Figure 1) to create the extra refractive power in the central cornea. The resulting multifocal shape allowed the patient to have clear vision over a wide range of depth of focus.

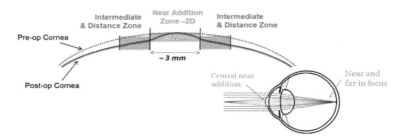

Figure 1. Schematic description of the Supracor treatment. The multifocal ablation pattern combines a regular ablation for the subjects' ametropic condition (shown in orange) with a 3-mm central zone near the vision add-on (shown in green). The add-on typically adds 2 diopters of refractive power to the central cornea.

The treatment planning software of a 217P laser system calculates a multifocal ablation pattern by combining the normal distance vision treatment plan for the ametropic condition of the subject, with a near vision addition in the 3-mm central zone of the treatment (see Figures 2 and 3). On one hand, the normal distance vision treatment thereby uses an adaptation of the original Munnerlyn formula [11] to flatten the overall cornea in the peripheral and paracentral zone. This flattening is customized to the individual eye, to reduce the cornea's refractive power and to bring the focus point of the eyes optical system right onto the retina. The near-vision addition, on the other hand, creates a small central region of higher curvature and hence a higher refractive power. The higher power is customized such that close-by targets are well focused on the retina. The hypothesis of multifocal ablations is that the brain is capable of blending the retinal images, and hence enables the subject to have good near, intermediate, and distance visual acuity. In order to prevent undesired optical side effects from the transition between the small area of high curvature and the flatter corneal region, a proprietary customization algorithm ensures that postoperative spherical aberrations are avoided.

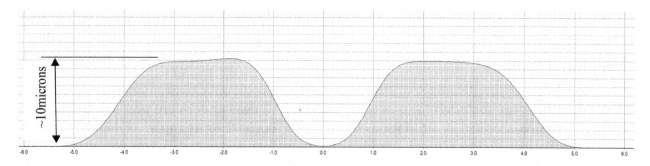

Figure 2. Typical multifocal ablation profile of a presbyopia-only treatment. The schematic indicates the amount of ablated tissue (blue area), with respect to the distance from the center of the cornea. Such a profile creates a steep central zone of 3 mm, providing extra refractive power for near-vision.

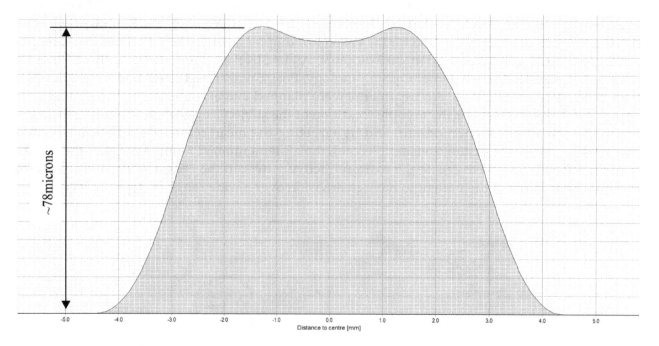

Figure 3. Typical multifocal ablation profile of a combined myopic and presbyopic treatment. The schematic indicates the amount of ablated tissue (blue area), with respect to the distance from the center of the cornea. Such a profile corrects the subjects' nearsightedness, as well as creates a steep central zone of 3 mm, providing extra refractive power for near-vision.

3. Results

All 72 surgical procedures were successfully executed, no side effects were detected, and not a single complication occurred during the study period. Measured on the LogMAR scale with respect to preoperative visual acuity (near: 0.29 ± 0.3, intermediate: 0.38 ± 0.36, distance: 0.75 ± 0.45), the visual acuity of subjects six months after surgery improved significantly, for near (-0.01 ± 0.11, $p = 5 \times 10^{-6}$), intermediate (-0.01 ± 0.07, $p = 2 \times 10^{-7}$), and distance vision (-0.09 ± 0.09, $p = 4 \times 10^{-12}$). Furthermore, the visual acuity of all eyes remained stable postoperatively after six months. The excimer laser system applied the planned ablation patterns at a very high precision, as the differences between the targeted and achieved spherical equivalent (SEQ), given in the unit of refractive power—diopters (D), at six months postoperative were -0.01 ± 0.14 D (standard deviation—SD) with an r-square of $R^2 = 0.997$ and -0.27 ± 0.30 D (SD) with $R^2 = 0.986$, for dominant and non-dominant eyes, respectively (see Figure 4). Moreover, 72% of the dominant eyes had an SEQ accuracy to the target of ± 0.13 D, 17% were between $+0.14$ D and $+0.50$ D, and 11% were between -0.14 D and -0.50 D. In the non-dominant eyes, 42% were within ± 0.13 D, 47% were within $+0.14$ D and $+0.50$ D, 8% were within -0.14 D and -0.50 D, and 3% were between $+0.51$ D and 1.00 D.

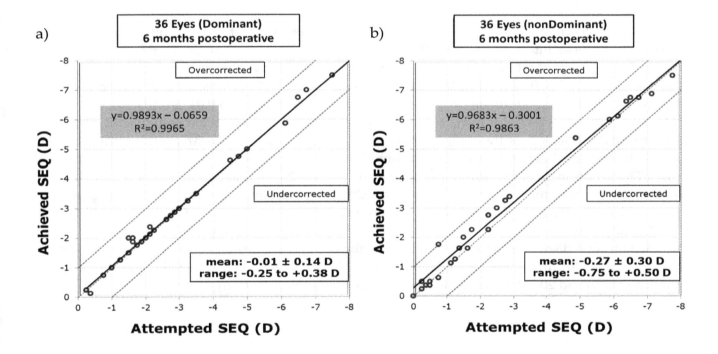

Figure 4. Attempted versus achieved spherical equivalent (SEQ) of (**a**) dominant and (**b**) non-dominant eyes, six months postoperatively. The regression lines in each graph indicate a small undercorrection for low values and a slight overcorrection for high values of spherical equivalent. SEQ: spherical equivalent; D: unit of refractive power, diopters.

The surgical treatment reduced spherical, and quadrafoil aberration in most eyes. Fifty-eight out of the 72 eyes had a decreased spherical aberration between 0.21 to 0.40 microns. Nine eyes had a decrease of quadrafoil aberration between 10 and 20 microns, and 62 eyes had a decrease of more than 20 microns of quadrafoil aberration (see Figure 5).

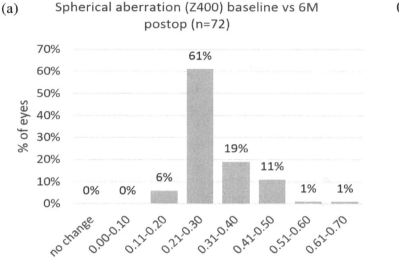
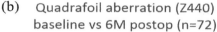
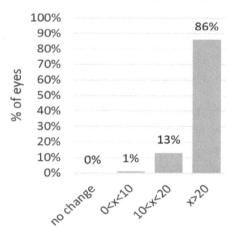

Figure 5. Surgically induced spherical (**a**) and quadrafoil (**b**) aberrations in micrometers, compared preoperatively (baseline) to postoperatively (postop). The treatment induced 0.21 to 0.40 microns of spherical aberration (Z400) and more than 20 microns of quadrafoil aberration (Z440) in most eyes.

Figure 6 presents the monocular mean and standard deviation of visual acuity before and after the surgery, for near, intermediate, and distance vision of all 36 subjects, in the LogMAR scale. At the six-month post-surgical follow-up for the dominant eyes, uncorrected near, intermediate, and distance visual acuity of 0.09 ± 0.11 (SD), 0.02 ± 0.04 (SD), and 0.02 ± 0.07 (SD) were observed, respectively. Meanwhile, for the non-dominant eyes, the six-month follow-up showed 0.04 ± 0.10 (SD), 0.01 ± 0.03 (SD), and 0.08 ± 0.08 (SD), for near, intermediate, and distance uncorrected visual acuity. Figure 7 indicates that while 36% of the dominant eyes had 20/20 uncorrected near visual acuity or better, six months after the intervention, 64% of the non-dominant were at 20/20 for uncorrected near visual acuity. The results in the figure further show that all eyes had 20/40 uncorrected visual acuity or better for distance and intermediate vision, while only 92% of the dominant and 97% of the non-dominant eyes had 20/40 uncorrected visual acuity for near vision. Figure 8 shows that the mean binocular visual acuity was at 0.03 ± 0.1 (SD), 0.01 ± 0.02 (SD), and 0.00 ± 0.05 (SD) for uncorrected near, intermediate, and distance vision, six months after the treatment. Further, the results show that 78% of the subjects had 20/20 uncorrected near visual acuity, 92% had 20/20 uncorrected intermediate visual acuity, and 86% had 20/20 distance visual acuity, at six months after surgery.

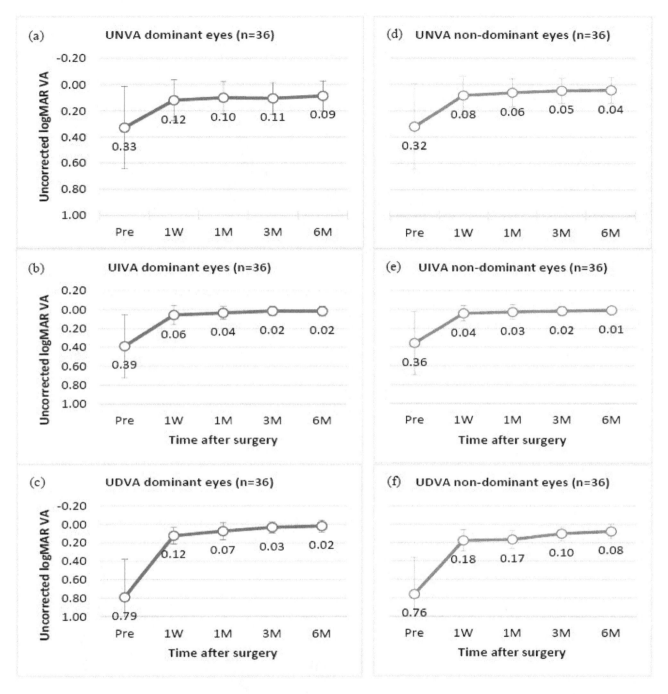

Figure 6. Mean and standard deviation of monocular uncorrected visual acuity for near (UNVA), intermediate (UIVA), and distance vision (UDVA) for 36 dominant (**a–c**) (shown in red), and 36 non-dominant (**d–f**) (shown in blue) eyes. Values are given preoperatively, and at one week (1 W), one month (1 M), three months (3 M), and six months (6 M) postsurgical follow-up.

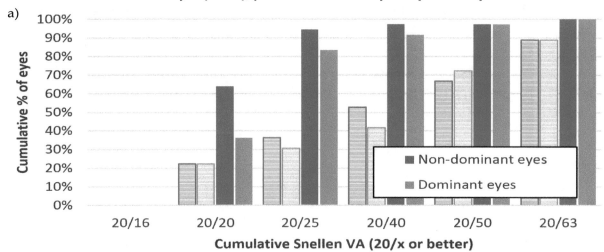

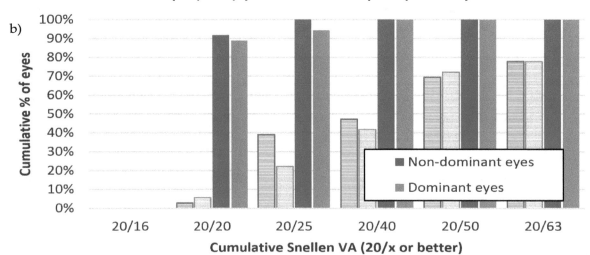

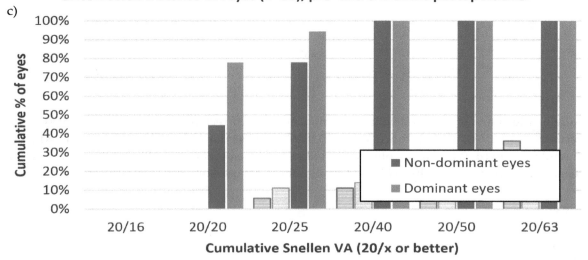

Figure 7. Cumulative percentage of subjects with 20/x dominant and non-dominant near (**a**), intermediate (**b**), and distance (**c**) visual acuity for 36 subjects. Dashed bars are preoperative, and solid bars are six-months postoperative data. Each percentage value is to be interpreted as 20/x vision or better.

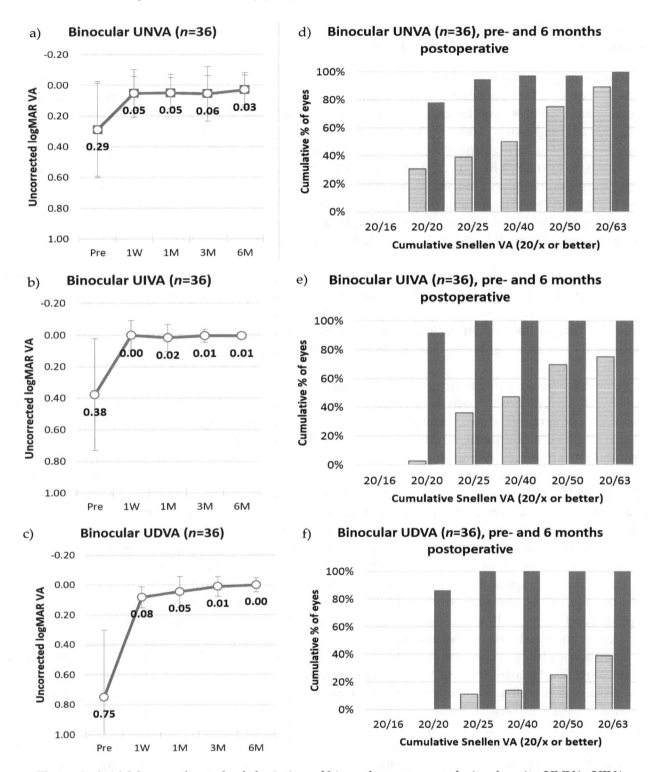

Figure 8. (a–c) Mean and standard deviation of binocular uncorrected visual acuity UNVA, UIVA, and UDVA vision for 36 subjects. Values are given preoperatively, and at one week (1 W), one month (1 M), three months (3 M), and six months (6 M) postsurgical follow-up. (d–f) Cumulative percentage of subjects with 20/x binocular near (UDVA), intermediate (UIVA), and distance (UDVA) vision for 36 subjects. Each percentage value is to be interpreted as 20/x vision or better.

4. Discussion

A prospective, single-center, single-surgeon clinical study on multifocal, myopic, presbyLASIK treatments, with an excimer laser, was carried out on 36 subjects. The applied treatment targeted the dominant eye to plano and the non-dominant eye to -0.5 diopters, while introducing a near addition of two diopters in the central cornea to increase the depth of focus.

Results suggest that the applied presbyLASIK procedure is an effective treatment for presbyopia. All study subjects had an uncorrected visual acuity of 20/40 or better for near, intermediate, and distance vision. Over 90% of the subjects were at 20/25 (LogMAR ≤ 0.10) or better, and about 80% were even at 20/20 (LogMAR ≤ 0.00) or better, again for the whole range of near, intermediate, and distance vision. In contrast to that, multifocal lens implantation results in the literature showed LogMAR 0.09 ± 0.08, LogMAR 0.10 ± 0.11, and LogMAR 0.07 ± 0.05, for near, intermediate, and distance vision [2], respectively, and in some cases even required spectacle correction for acceptable distance vision [1]. Mono vision treatments only showed 20/20 or better in 36.7% of the subjects for near, and in 31.1% of the subjects for distance visual acuity [3]. Results of intracorneal inlays were comparable for uncorrected near vision [6], and distance vision was not reported.

As expected, while the dominant eyes in this study generally had higher monocular visual acuity for distance vision, the non-dominant eyes performed better in monocular near vision. Presumably, the brains of the study candidates were capable of blending the two distinct monocular images into a binocular image, electively focusing on near, intermediate, and distant targets. This circumstance is supported by the thoroughly high satisfaction of all of the study patients.

Generally speaking, the excimer procedure employed in this study was less invasive compared to other presbyopia methods, such as refractive lens implantation. LASIK is a very well accepted and extensively proven procedure. It features high precision in positioning of the correction, in refractive outcome, as well as in predictability of the result. A key factor for this is the high precision and repeatability of flap quality and thickness [12]. A remaining problem with LASIK-based presbyopia treatments, however, is that the multifocal ablation may induce unwanted optical aberrations. Multifocal ablations usually are composed of a correction for distance vision (myopic or hyperopic), and a near addition. Lower order optical aberrations, specifically spherical aberrations, may be caused by the distance correction ablation. Additional higher order aberrations stemming from the transition between the distance treatment zone and the near addition might be induced, even though they may be outside of the region of the central addition, yet inside the optical zone of the distance vision correction. It seems apparent that the resulting refractive surface might evoke unfavourable optical aberrations [9,13,14]. Our wavefront results suggest that the customization algorithm for aberration reduction works very well. In almost all cases, spherical (Z400) as well as quadrafoil (Z440) aberrations were significantly reduced by the treatment.

The thoroughly positive results with the LASIK-based presbyopia treatment in this study can, at least partially, be attributed to the aspherical customization algorithm. The algorithm utilized the K-readings as well as the conic constant (Q) of the cornea to minimize the induction of adverse optical aberration effects [8,10,12]. In addition, using LASIK provides the option to re-touch the treatment with relative ease, and therefore has the potential to remove or enhance the presbyopic addition [9]. Even though further studies with more surgical cases are necessary to confirm these results, the presbyLASIK treatment employed in this study has great potential to become a gold standard for the treatment of presbyopia, as it safe and shows reliable, predictable, and satisfying outcomes.

Acknowledgments: The study was supported by the Swiss Commission for Technology and Innovation (CTI), through CTI project 13404.1.

Author Contributions: Bojan Pajic provided the treatment indication, developed the study design, acquired clinical data, and contributed to writing the paper. Brigitte Pajic-Eggspuehler performed data analysis and substantially contributed the study design. Joerg Mueller supplied surgical advices and substantially contribute to the design of the study. Zeljka Cvejic contributed substantially to the development of the study design. Harald Studer performed data analysis and contributed to writing the paper.

References

1. Chang, J.S.; Ng, J.C.; Lau, S.Y. Visual outcomes and patient satisfaction after presbyopic lens exchange with a diffractive multifocal intraocular lens. *J. Refract. Surg.* **2012**, *28*, 468–474. [CrossRef] [PubMed]

2. Tsaousis, K.T.; Plainis, S.; Dimitrakos, S.A.; Tsinopoulos, I.T. Binocularity anhances visual acuity of eyes implanted with multifocal intraocular lenses. *J. Refract. Surg.* **2013**, *29*, 246–250. [CrossRef] [PubMed]

3. Braun, E.H.; Lee, J.; Steinert, R.F. Monovision in LASIK. *Ophthalmology* **2008**, *115*, 1196–1202. [CrossRef] [PubMed]

4. Jain, S.; Ou, R.; Azar, D.T. Monovision outcomes in presbyopic individuals after refractive surgery. *Ophthalmology* **2001**, *108*, 1430–1433. [CrossRef]

5. Bouzoukis, D.I.; Kymionis, G.D.; Panagopoulos, S.I.; Diakonis, V.F.; Pallikaris, A.I.; Limnopoulou, A.N.; Portaliou, D.M.; Pallikaris, I.G. Visual outcomes and safety of small diameter intrastromal refractive inlay for the corneal compensation of presbyopia. *J. Refract. Surg.* **2012**, *28*, 168–173. [CrossRef] [PubMed]

6. Yilmaz, O.F.; Alagoz, N.; Pekel, G.; Azman, E.; Aksoy, E.F.; Cakır, H.; Bozkurt, E.; Demirok, A. Intracorneal inlay to correct presbyopia: Long-term results. *J. Cataract Refract. Surg.* **2011**, *37*, 1275–1281. [CrossRef] [PubMed]

7. Menassa, N.; Fitting, A.; Auffarth, G.U.; Holzer, M.P. Visual outcomes and corneal changes after intrastromal femtosecond correction of presbyopia. *J. Cataract Refract. Surg.* **2012**, *28*, 765–773. [CrossRef] [PubMed]

8. Saib, N.; Abrieu-Lacaille, M.; Berguiga, M.; Rambaud, C.; Froussart-Maille, F.; Rigal-Sastourne, J.C. Central PresbyLASIK for Hyperopia and Presbyopia Using Micro-monovision With the Technolas 217P Platform and SUPRACOR Algorithm. *J. Refract. Surg.* **2015**, *31*, 540–546. [CrossRef] [PubMed]

9. Vastardis, I.; Pajic-Eggspuehler, B.; Mueller, J.; Cvejic, Z.; Pajic, B. Femtosecond laser-assisted in situ keratomileusis multifocal ablation profile using a mini-monovision approach for presbyopic patients with hyperopia. *Clin. Ophthalmol.* **2016**, *10*, 1245–1256. [CrossRef] [PubMed]

10. Ryan, A.; O'Keefe, M. Corneal approach to hyperopic presbyopia treatment: Six-month outcomes of a new multifocal excimer laser in situ keratomileusis procedure. *J. Cataract Refract. Surg.* **2013**, *39*, 1226–1233. [CrossRef] [PubMed]

11. Munnerlyn, C.R.; Koons, S.J. Photorefractive keratectomy: A technique for laser refractive surgery. *J. Cataract Refract. Surg.* **1988**, *14*, 46–52. [CrossRef]

12. Pajic, B.; Vastardis, I.; Pajic-Eggspuehler, B.; Gatzioufas, Z.; Hafezi, F. Femtosecond laser versus mechanical microkeratome-assisted flap creation for LASIK: A prospective, randomized, paired-eye study. *Clin. Ophthalmol.* **2014**, *8*, 1883–1889. [CrossRef] [PubMed]

13. Alio, J.L.; Chaubard, J.J.; Caliz, A.; Sala, E.; Patel, S. Correction of Presbyopia by Technovision Central Multifocal LASIK (PresbyLASIK). *J. Refract. Surg.* **2006**, *22*, 453–460. [CrossRef] [PubMed]

14. Eppstein, R.L.; Gurgos, M.A. Presbyopia Treatment by Monocular Peripheral PresbyLASIK. *J. Refract. Surg.* **2009**, *25*, 516–523. [CrossRef]

8

New Approaches in the Study of the Pathogenesis of Urethral Pain Syndrome

Olga Streltsova [1], Anton Kuyarov [1], Muhhamad Shuaib Abdul Malik Molvi [1], Svetlana Zubova [2], Valery Lazukin [3], Ekaterina Tararova [4] and Elena Kiseleva [5,*]

[1] E.V. Shakhov Department of Urology, Privolzhsky Research Medical University, 10/1 Minin and Pozharsky Sq., 603950 Nizhny Novgorod, Russia; strelzova_uro@mail.ru (O.S.); kuyarov.anton@mail.ru (A.K.); msmolvi@mail.ru (M.S.A.M.M.)

[2] N.A. Semashko Nizhny Novgorod Regional Clinical Hospital, 190 Rodionova St., 603126 Nizhny Novgorod, Russia; zubova.svetlana.65@yandex.ru

[3] Department of Medical Physics and Informatics, Privolzhsky Research Medical University, 10/1 Minin and Pozharsky Sq., 603950 Nizhny Novgorod, Russia; valery-laz@yandex.ru

[4] Nizhny Novgorod Regional Oncology Dispensary, 190 Rodionova St., 603126 Nizhny Novgorod, Russia; tararova-ea@mail.ru

[5] Institute of Experimental Oncology and Biomedical Technologies, Privolzhsky Research Medical University, 10/1 Minin and Pozharsky Sq., 603950 Nizhny Novgorod, Russia

* Correspondence: kiseleva84@gmail.com

Abstract: Introduction: Urethral pain syndrome (UPS) is still a pathology in which the diagnosis is formulated as a "diagnosis of exclusion". The exact pathogenetic mechanisms are not yet fully understood and clear recommendations for the prevention and treatment of UPS are absent. Methods and Participants: A clinical and laboratory evaluation of 55 patients with established UPS included history taking, basic laboratory tests (e.g., complete blood count and clinical urine test), physical examination, uroflowmetry, and cystourethroscopy. Additionally, transvaginal ultrasound (TVUS) with compression elastography and cross-polarization optical tomography (CP OCT) were performed in 24 and 33 patients with UPS, respectively. The control group consisted of 14 patients with no complaints from the urinary system. Results: TVUS showed an expansion in the diameter of the internal lumen of the urethra, especially in the proximal region compared with the norm. Compression elastography revealed areas with increased stiffness (presence of fibrosis) in urethral and surrounding tissues. The performed CP OCT study showed that in UPS, the structure of the tissues in most cases was changed: trophic alterations in the epithelium (hypertrophy or atrophy) and fibrosis of underlying connective tissue were observed. The proximal fragment of the urethra with UPS underwent changes identical to those of the bladder neck. Conclusion: This paper showed that the introduction of new technology—CP OCT—in conjunction with TVUS will allow verification of structural changes in tissues of the lower urinary tract at the level of their architectonics and will help doctors understand better the basics of the UPS pathogenesis.

Keywords: cross-polarization optical coherence tomography (CP OCT); ultrasound; urethral pain syndrome; epithelial atrophy; epithelial hyperplasia; inflammation; fibrosis; image evaluation

---

1. Introduction

The most common reason for women to seek medical attention is dysuria, and it is believed that in 40% of cases urethritis and/or urethral syndrome are involved [1]. According to the US National Institutes of Health, one third of women with chronic pelvic pain (CPP) have urethral pain syndrome (UPS) [2,3]. The European Association of Urology defines UPS as the occurrence of chronic or recurrent episodic pain lasting for more than 6 months, and felt in the urethra, in the absence of proven infection or other obvious local pathology. It is often associated with negative cognitive, behavioral, sexual or emotional consequences [4], as well as with symptoms suggestive of lower urinary tract, sexual, intestinal, or gynecological dysfunction [5].

The problem of pain in the urethra with unchanged urinalysis, the absence of any other clinical manifestations, and the absence of somatically explainable causes, is complex and ultimately remains unresolved, since the exact pathogenetic mechanisms are not yet fully understood [6–9]. Neither are there any clear recommendations for the prevention and treatment of UPS, as a result of which the only effective form of medical care today is symptomatic therapy—involving the continuing intake of strong pain medications, antidepressants, and anticonvulsants [4,9]. In the methodological recommendations on CPP, published under the auspices of the the Moscow Department of Health (dated 14 July 2016), it is noted that there is no specific accepted treatment for UPS [10]. The approach should be interdisciplinary and the treatment should be multimodal, with the general principles of chronic pain syndrome management being applied [11–13].

The close embryological relationship between the urethra and the bladder makes it likely that there are causes similar to ones connected with the development of painful bladder syndrome [14]. According to the classification of the International Association for the Study of Pain (IASP, 2019) the mechanism of CPP and possible causes of its occurrence may include vascular lesions, persistent inflammatory processes, or violation of the innervation of organs due to mechanical compression in the pelvic region, but often the reason is not clear [15].

The connective tissue matrix of organs plays a key role in the occurrence and persistence of pain, as shown by the number of studies [16,17]. It is believed that connective tissue, as well as performing its supporting, protective and trophic functions, acts as a network-wide mechanosensitive signaling system—as a global unifying network [16,18].

Thus, it can be surmised that the above reasons for the development of CPP could be associated with factors that affect the state of the connective tissue matrix of the lower urinary tract. However, there are currently no methods for adequate, appropriate study of the structure of urethral tissues. According to the standards for examination of patients with CPP when using the UPOINT (Urinary, Psychosocial, Organ Specific, Infection, Neurologic/Systemic, Tenderness of Skeletal Muscles) classification [19] in the urology domain, the recommended list of examinations includes keeping a urination diary, cystoscopy, and the use of ultrasound (US) and uroflowmetry, while for complaints involving the urethra, urethroscopy is recommended. These methods allow only indirect assessment of the urethral tissues. Objective evaluation and accurate diagnosis of a disease that does not cause any visual changes, and results from a "diagnosis of exclusion" when using standard instrumental diagnostic methods, is important for understanding the pathogenetic aspects of the disease. In this work, we used traditional diagnostic methods, including US and uroflowmetry, and the non-traditional methods of ultrasound elastography (USE) and cross-polarization optical tomography (CP OCT) to study changes in the functioning of organs and their structure in UPS in comparison with the norm, and assessed the role of background diseases in the development of UPS.

The USE is a medical imaging modality that measures tissue mechanical properties by monitoring the response of tissue to acoustic energy [20,21]. In clinical settings, USE is emerging as a powerful tool for imaging and quantitatively monitoring cancer and fibrosis [22]. It provides a rapid visualization of the tissue elasticity using color-coding mode, even in organs deep within the body. Recently, USE is applied especially on the breast and liver, but the technique has been increasingly used for other tissues including the thyroid, prostate, lymph nodes, gastrointestinal tract, kidney, spleen, pancreas, and the musculoskeletal and vascular systems [22,23]. There are several USE techniques used in clinical practice, but USE with strain (compression) being the most common one allowing real-time visualization of the elastographic map on the screen [24]. With regard to the study of the urethra in UPS, the method can be useful for detecting fibrous changes in the urethral wall and adjacent tissues.

In general, OCT is similar to the ultrasonic technique, except for using light instead of sound and is centered on interferometry in the near-infrared range of wavelength (700–1300 nm) [25,26]. It measures the time delay and amplitude of backscattered light. The aim of the OCT technology is to perform a real-time, in vivo, optic biopsy, with direct label-free visualization of the histological structure of the human tissues at the level of the general architectonics to a depth of 1.5 mm [27]. High spatial resolution (5–15 µm) and performance simplicity with minimal expertise are the main advantages of OCT in contrast to US. The endoscopic nature of OCT probes not only enhances patient comfort and safety but also makes it especially suitable for assessing narrow tubular organs as well as for using standard guidewires for examining deeply located objects in the body [28].

CP OCT is a functional extension of OCT that enables the detection of changes in the state of polarization of light caused by birefringence and coupling between two polarization states due to scattering in the random media (cross-scattering) [29]. As a result, two types of images are obtained simultaneously: in the initial (co-) polarization and orthogonal (cross-) polarization, which allow assessing isotropic (cells) and anisotropic (collagen and elastic fibers of connective tissue) structures separately [30,31]. This is important in cases when precise observation of only connective tissue structures is needed.

The goal of the study was to assess the condition of the tissue in the female urethra in UPS, by using non-traditional methods for this pathology—compression US and CP OCT.

2. Materials and Methods

2.1. Patients

In total, 69 female patients were enrolled in this study: 55 with established UPS ("UPS" group, aged from 21 to 66 years) and 14 with a healthy urethra as a control group ("Norm" group, aged from 24 to 62 years). Patients with UPS received treatment in the urology department of the N.A. Semashko Nizhny Novgorod Regional Clinical Hospital between 2014 and 2019.

Inclusion criteria for the UPS group consisted of: age 18 years and older; presence of recurrent episodic pain localized in the urethra lasting more than 6 months; absence of infectious lesion or obvious organ pathology [32]. Exclusion criteria for UPS group were: age under 18; the presence of inflammatory processes in the lower urinary tract; the presence of tumors of the pelvic organs; radiation damage to the pelvic organs; pregnancy; lactation. The control group included women whose age was 18 years and older, with no detected pathology and complaints from the lower urinary tract. Otherwise, people were excluded from the study.

This study was approved by the review board of the Privolzhsky Research Medical University (Protocol #6 from 28 April 2020). The research was carried out within the framework of the RFBR project #19-07-00395, agreements 1236/19 from 11 April 2019 and #1365/20 from 30 March 2020. Informed consent to participate in the study was obtained from the participants. All conducted studies and the number of patients included are presented in Table 1.

Table 1. Clinical and laboratory methods for patient's examination and number of included patients.

Type of Study	Purpose of the Study	Number of Patients in the UPS Group	Number of Patients in the Norm Group
1. History taking	identification of the presence of any previously transferred concomitant pathology	55	14
2. Laboratory tests of blood and urine	identification of inflammatory processes	55	14
3. Physical examination and palpation of the urethra and the walls of the vagina (on a gynecological chair)	assessment of the state of the external opening of the urethra, detection of the presence of any myofascial aspect in the disease	55	-
4. Uroflowmetry	assessment of the condition of the sphincters of the urethra and bladder	55	-
5. Transvaginal US/compression US	assessment of the size, shape, structure of the urethra and bladder neck/mapping of the urethral wall and surrounding tissues stiffness	24	6

Table 1. *Cont.*

Type of Study	Purpose of the Study	Number of Patients in the UPS Group	Number of Patients in the Norm Group
6. Cystoscopy	examination the inside of the bladder in detail; identification and recording of abnormal findings	33 *	14 [0]
7. CP OCT [#]	visualization of the internal structure of the bladder neck and urethral wall, evaluation the condition of epithelium and connective tissue layers	33	14

* carried out to exclude the presence of interstitial cystitis; [0] patients with stones of the upper urinary tract but without pyelonephritis who have been assigned cystoscopy; [#] performed in conjunction with cystoscopy.

2.2. Transvaginal US

Transvaginal US (TVUS) was performed using a Philips Epiq5 system (Philips Ultrasound., Inc., 22100 Bothell-Everett Highway, Bothell, Washington, 98021-8431, USA). The sensor was inserted directly into the vagina, allowing visualization of the state of the bladder neck and urethra (assessment of their structure, the condition of their walls, and the width of the internal lumen) and detecting abnormalities in the structure of the urethra compared with the norm. This was also the first study in which patients with UPS underwent compression elastography of the adjacent urethral tissues. Compression elastography is a technique that displays the relative deformation of tissues in the form of their color mapping in real time [33]. When the tissue is subjected to an external force (deformation), the harder/denser areas of the tissue exhibit relatively less compression than the softer areas [24]. In our study, on the USE images, the adjustment scale was set to display the harder areas in blue, with the softer areas appearing in red [34].

2.3. CP OCT Study and Image Analysis

Time-domain device "Polarization-sensitive optical coherence tomograph OCT-1300U" (BioMedTech LLC, Nizhny Novgorod, Russia) (Figure 1a), that provides two image acquisition in co- and cross-polarizations was used in the study [29,35]. The device is approved for clinical use (product license №FCP 2012/13479 of 30 May 2012) and is equipped with replaceable endoscopic probe (Figure 1b,c). It has the following characteristics: the radiation source is a superluminescent diode, of operating wavelength 1310 nm, spectrum width 100 nm, axial resolution 15 μm, lateral resolution 25 μm, and radiation power at the object 3 mW. OCT image size in each polarization is 1.8 × 1.3 mm (width × height), image acquisition time is 2 s. Due to the presence of a flexible endoscopic probe with an outer diameter of 2.7 mm, the examination of the urethral tissue could be carried out simultaneously with cystoscopy through a standard endoscope. Our group's application of the CP OCT method to the study of the female urethral wall in patients with UPS, is a global "first" [36].

From 4 to 13 images were obtained from each patient: of the bladder neck and three regions of the urethra (Figure 1d) at the 6 o'clock position corresponding to a conventional clockface, and, if possible, with other additional images of the urethra in the three directions (9, 12, and 3 h of the clockface).

In the "UPS"/"N" groups, 169/58 CP OCT images were obtained, which included 43/16 CP OCT images of the bladder neck, as the section closest to the urethra and therefore potentially involved in processes occurring in the proximal urethra and 126/42 CP OCT images of the urethra (its proximal 41/14, middle 40/12, and distal 45/16 regions) (Table 2).

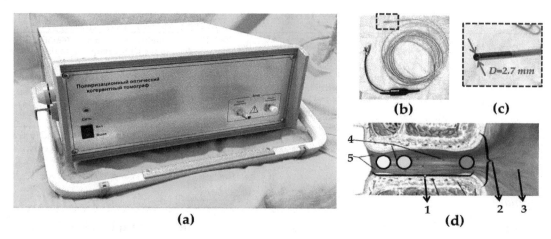

Figure 1. Cross-polarization optical tomography (CP OCT) device and areas under study shown on a diagram of the female urethra. (**a**) CP OCT device; (**b**) Flexible endoscopic forward-looking CP OCT probe; (**c**) Enlarged tip of the probe from (**b**). (**d**) Drawing of the urethra where it transitions to the bladder. Here, the circles indicate the locations from which CP OCT images were obtained in the proximal (blue), middle (green), and distal parts of the urethra (yellow) [37]. 1—urethra, 2—neck of urinary bladder, 3—triangle of urinary bladder, 4—lacunae and openings of urethral ducts, 5—openings of paraurethral Skene's ducts.

Table 2. Distribution of the CP OCT images by patient's groups and parts of the urethra.

Group	Number of Patients	Number of CP OCT Images	Average Number of CP OCT Images Created from 1 Patient	Number of CP OCT Images of Each Location			
				Bladder Neck	Distal Urethra	Medium Urethra	Proximal Urethra
UPS	33	169	5.12	43	41	40	45
Norm	14	58	4.14	16	14	12	16
Total	47	227	4.63	59	55	52	61

A visual assessment of the CP OCT images of the bladder neck and urethra was performed by two readers. The objects of interest were the epithelium and the state of the connective tissue structures of the urethra in patients with UPS, relative to the normal state of these structures. In the epithelium, the thickness was assessed as: normal, thickening (hyperplasia), or thinning (atrophy); in the connective tissue stroma, attention was paid to the presence of any element in the images corresponding to an inflammatory process or fibrosis. The CP OCT features of inflammation were: (1) lack of clarity of the border between the first (epithelial) and the second (connective tissue) layers, (2) the absence of horizontal ordering of the structures that are representative of the norm, and (3) the presence of any indistinctness in their images, which would correspond to cellular tissue infiltration. Significant thickening of the connective tissue layer, up to the lower border of the image with maintaining a high signal level was considered a sign of fibrosis [36,38]. Before qualitative evaluation of CP OCT images readers were trained by training test. After an independent blind visual assessment of the CP OCT images, the «UPS» group was divided into 2 age subgroups: patients under 50 and those over 50.

2.4. Statistical Analysis

The statistical analysis was performed using IBM SPSS Statistics software, V20 (IBM Corporation, Somers, NY, USA). The inter-reader reliability was calculated using the Fleiss' kappa (κ) coefficient: $\kappa > 0.8$—perfect agreement; $0.7 \leq \kappa < 0.8$—substantial agreement; $\kappa < 0.7$—poor agreement.

3. Results

3.1. The Role of Background Diseases in the Development of UPS

An analysis of concomitant pathology in patients with UPS, identified by their history is presented in Table 3. From Table 3 it follows that the predominant area of comorbidity was gynecological (70.9%). Hormonal abnormalities (94.8%) were found in 24 sexually active women in the pre-menopausal period, as well as in 13 women of the menopausal period; inflammatory diseases of the female genital area of bacterial and viral etiology were also present (76.9%).

Table 3. Concomitant pathology and the source of its occurrence in the group of patients with urethral pain syndrome (UPS) ($n = 55$).

Organ System with Pathology	n-Abs. (%)	Genesis of Pathology	n-Abs. (%)
1. Gynecological	39 (70.9)	Hormonal	37 (94.8)
		Inflammatory	30 (76.9)
		Surgical interventions on the pelvic organs	12 (30.7)
2. Respiratory	37 (67.2)	Upper (nose, nasal cavity, pharynx, larynx)	32 (86.4)
		Lower (trachea, bronchi, lungs)	5 (13.5)
		Psycho-emotional sphere	23 (41.8)
3. Neurological	35 (63.6)	Central nervous system	10 (18.2)
		Peripheral nervous system	42 (76.4)
		Psycho-emotional sphere	23 (41.8)
4. Urological	24 (43.6)	Inflammatory	10 (41.6)
		Non-inflammatory	17 (70.8)
5. Gastroenterological	18 (32.7)	Inflammatory diseases of the stomach, duodenum, biliary tract	38 (69.0)
		Bowel disease	21 (38.2)
6. Cardiovascular	9 (16.3)	Arterial hypertension	5 (55.5)
		Other	4 (44.5)
Total cases of pathology	162		

Anamnesis of upper respiratory tract pathology, more common in adolescence, was recorded in 67.2% of women, of whom the bulk of patients (64.9%) reported frequent viral diseases or herpes infection. The premorbid background in patients with UPS was neurological pathology (63.6%), and these are diseases associated with the involvement of the peripheral nervous system and as is important, with the state of the psycho-emotional sphere.

Each patient suffering from UPS had 2.94 (162/55) cases of comorbidity. Thus, the role of other factors in the presence of foci of chronic infection in the body, and a decrease in immune defense factors, as a comorbid background for the development of UPS, cannot be denied, since the presence in the patients' history of inflammatory diseases of the respiratory tract, gastrointestinal tract, urological and gynecological organs was revealed.

3.2. Results of Cystoscopic Examination

In 32.7% of cases (18 out of 55), clinical manifestations of UPS were combined with urinary pain syndrome. Low-volume (less than 300 mL) urination was reordered. The number of urinations exceeded 12 per day. Pains over the womb were present. During cystoscopy in patients of the "UPS" group, the bladder mucosa was unchanged—shiny, pale pink, while, in 16 cases (29.0%), there was a slight hyperemia in the bladder neck. A picture corresponding to interstitial cystitis—the presence of glomerulations in the mucous membrane of the bladder after the hydrodistension procedure, was found in 23.6% ($n = 13$).

3.3. Uroflowmetry Results

In 72.7% of cases (40 out of 55), there was a decrease in the urination rate to 13.7 ± 3.2 mL/s in combination with low-volume urination while the normal values of the urination rate for women are 23–32 mL/s [39]. The average volume of excreted urine was 172 ± 33 mL.

3.4. Results of TVUS Research

The results of TVUS studies showed that in the norm group in women, the urethra looks like a tube with a uniform lumen diameter without dilatations and contractions, which was 4.6 ± 0.6 mm, wall thickness 4.8 ± 1.1 mm. According to research by a group of authors [40], normally, the outer diameter of the urethra is 10.0 mm, the inner lumen of the urethra is closed during TVUS or 0.3 mm (Figure 2a,b). According to the authors [41], who conducted a study with an intraurethral sensor, the thickness of the urethra in the proximal section was normally 3.7 mm.

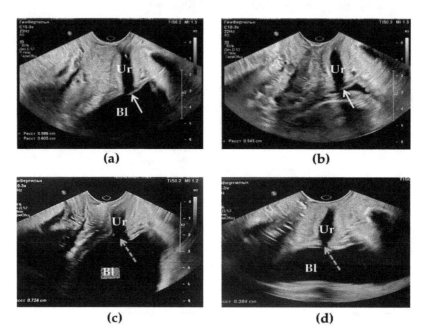

Figure 2. Transvaginal ultrasound (TVUS) of the urethra and adjacent tissues in normal conditions and with UPS. (**a,b**) A healthy woman 30 years of age before (**a**) and after (**b**) urination. The urethral tongue closes the opening to the urethra, as indicated by the yellow arrow; (**c**) Patient K., 30 years old, with a UPS disease duration of more than 10 years; (**d**) Patient Z., 38 years old, over 13 years of illness. In both cases, with UPS, the urethral tongue is indistinguishable and the gaping opening at the transition of the bladder into the urethra is indicated by the blue dashed arrows. Bl—bladder, Ur—urethra.

In women with UPS (*n* = 24), the structural features of the urethra were revealed: the urethra was funnel-shaped (Figure 2d), opening to the bladder. The internal lumen of the urethra in the proximal segment was expanded to 5.9 ± 2.1 mm. At the same time, 44% of patients had an expansion up to 7.5 ± 0.5 mm, in 56% up to 5.5 ± 0.5 mm. The thickness of the urethral walls in our study averaged 3.6 mm (from 2.4 to 6.0 mm). Thus, in all patients with UPS, an increase in the diameter of the internal lumen of the urethra, especially in the proximal region, was recorded.

In 7 (29.1%) cases, pathological changes were recorded in the urethral tongue, a cavernous structure that, as the bladder fills, normally increases in volume due to becoming engorged with blood and, together with the sphincter trigonalis, closes the exit from the bladder into the urethra. With the contraction of the urethra the posterior semicircle of the bladder neck is pressed against the anterior wall of the urethra and this closes its internal opening [42]. In patients with UPS, an absence of urethral tongue visualization (Figure 2c,d), or the absence of its adherence to the entrance to the urethra, was revealed. No residual urine was found in patients with UPS.

Compression US of the urethra and adjacent tissues of patients with UPS in the proximal and middle regions showed a significant predominance of areas colored blue, indicating tissue stiffness and rigidity (Figure 3b) compared to the norm, where no blue color was observed (Figure 3a). Thus, our studies confirm the presence of fibrosis of the tissues surrounding the urethra in UPS.

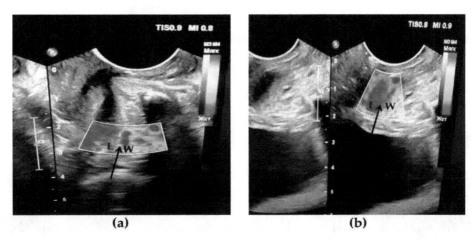

Figure 3. Compression ultrasound (US) in the normal condition (**a**) and in UPS (**b**). (**a**) Normally, the urethral wall is softer (red color) than in UPS (**b**) (predominance of green and blue colors). L—lumen of the urethra, W—urethral wall. The black arrow indicates the border between the lumen of the urethra and its wall.

3.5. Results of CP OCT Study

CP OCT images of all sections of the female urethra in the norm are structural. In co-polarization images (Figure 4a1–d1), the epithelium is clearly visualized in all areas of interest, its border contrasting with the underlying mucous layer. The epithelial layer and its thickness are marked in Figure 4a–d with dark blue rectangle. The signal from the connective tissue in the cross-polarization images (Figure 4a2–d2) is of medium intensity, has a horizontal orientation; in the middle and distal segments of the urethra, single, gland-like lacunas with clear contours can be determined. In cross-polarization, the OCT signal is determined mainly by the collagen fibers of the connective tissue layer, therefore, only this layer of the urethral wall is clearly visible in such images, and the epithelium and muscles are not visualized.

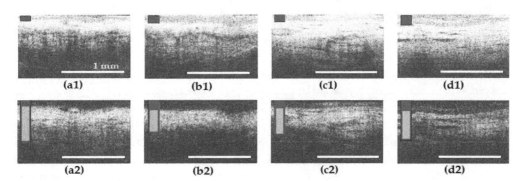

Figure 4. CP OCT images of the bladder neck (**a**) and three segments of normal urethra (**b**–**d**): (**b**) proximal; (**c**) middle; and (**d**) distal. The first row shows co-polarization images, the second row shows corresponding cross-polarization images. The first (epithelial) layer and its thickness are marked in all images with a dark blue rectangle. The second layer (connective tissue of lamina propria) in (**a2**–**d2**) is indicated by a vertical rectangle in light blue color: its height shows the average height of the layer and the blue color inside the frame indicates its normal condition.

In the normal group, there were no changes in the visible thickness in the zones of interest (Figure 4a1–d1). However, in women over 50 years old, a tendency of the epithelium to atrophy was revealed, which can be explained by the influence of hormonal changes. The connective tissue stroma generated approximately the same signal level in the cross-channel, without any extensive dark or bright areas and occupied 40–50% of the entire image height (Figure 4a2–d2), connective tissue is marked by vertical rectangle in light blue color: its height shows an average height of the layer and the light blue color inside the frame indicates its normal condition).

Visual analysis of CP OCT in the UPS group revealed that, in terms of the characteristics of the epithelium and connective tissue, the proximal part of the urethra was more similar to the bladder neck than to the middle and distal parts of itself. Examples are shown in Figures 5 and 6.

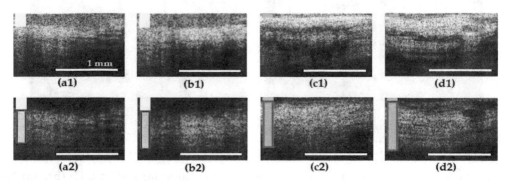

Figure 5. CP OCT images of the bladder neck (**a**) and three segments of the urethra (**b–d**) in patient I., 22 years old with UPS lasting 5 years. (**b**) Proximal; (**c**) middle; and (**d**) distal parts of the urethra. The first row shows co-polarization images, the second row shows corresponding cross-polarization images. (**a,b**) Epithelium hyperplasia is marked with yellow rectangle. Connective tissue in (**a2,b2**) have normal thickness (dark blue frame of vertical rectangle), but signs of inflammation (yellow color inside the rectangle); (**c,d**) Epithelial atrophy is marked with green rectangle. Connective tissue in (**c2,d2**) has increased thickness (red frame of vertical rectangle) and signs of fibrosis (pink color inside the rectangle).

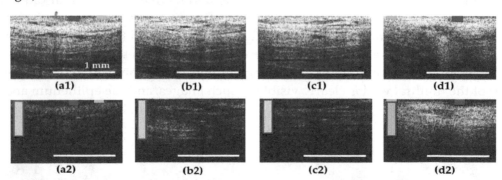

Figure 6. CP OCT images of the bladder neck (**a**) and three segments of the urethra (**b–d**) in patient E., 60 years old with UPS lasting 5 years. (**b**) proximal; (**c**) middle; and (**d**) distal parts of the urethra. The first row shows co-polarization images, the second row shows corresponding cross-polarization images. (**a,d**) Epithelium has signs of norm (blue rectangle), but mostly atrophic (green rectangle); (**b,c**) total epithelial atrophy is observed. (**a–c**) Connective tissue have normal thickness (dark blue frame of vertical rectangle), but signs of active inflammation (yellow color of vertical rectangle); (**d**) connective tissue has normal thickness (dark blue frame of vertical rectangle), but signs of fibrosis (pink color of vertical rectangle).

Figure 5 shows an example of patient I., 22 years old with UPS lasting 5 years. Epithelial hyperplasia is visible in the bladder neck and the proximal urethra (Figure 5a1,b1), the yellow rectangle), the border of the epithelium with the underlying connective tissue layer is blurred, indicating the presence of inflammatory processes in these tissues (Figure 5a1,b1). The signal from the connective tissue structures in cross-polarization has a noticeable local decrease in intensity caused by the shadows of dilated blood vessels and by tissue edema (Figure 5a2,b2), the vertical rectangle in yellow color shows tissue inflammation, dark blue frame indicates normal thickness of the layer). In the middle and distal parts of the urethra, by contrast, thinning of the epithelium is noticeable (Figure 5c1,d1), green rectangle), while in the middle part, the border with the underlying connective tissue layer is clear (Figure 5c1)).

The connective tissue layer is thickened (Figure 5c2,d2), the red frame of vertical rectangle indicates increased thickness of the layer, pink color indicates signs of tissue fibrosis and looks more homogeneous in structure (Figure 5c2) than in the non-pathogenic case (Figure 4c2,d2). In this subgroup of patients, a thickening of the connective tissue layer in cross-polarization to occupy over 60% of the image height was observed in 44.4% (32 CP OCT images out of 72). In this case, an increase in the OCT signal was observed in all the images.

Figure 6 shows an example of patient E., 60 years old with UPS lasting 5 years. In the bladder neck and proximal urethra (Figure 6a1,b1), as well as in the rest of the urethra (Figure 6c1,d1), the epithelium is atrophic, and in places where it is partially preserved (Figure 6a,d, blue and green rectangle), the border of the epithelium with the underlying connective tissue layer is blurred (Figure 6a1,d1)). The signal from connective tissue structures in cross-polarization is weak, presumably due to severe tissue edema (Figure 6a2–c2), vertical rectangle in yellow color shows tissue inflammation, dark blue frame indicates normal thickness of the layer). In the distal urethra, on the other hand, the connective tissue layer exhibits cross-scattering, but appears homogeneous in structure (Figure 6d2), pink color of vertical rectangle indicates fibrosis) compared to normal (Figure 4d2). In this subgroup of patients, thickening of the connective tissue layer in cross-polarization to over 60% of the image height was observed in 46.7% (28 CP OCT images out of 60); 71.4% of them with an increase in the OCT signal (20 of 28), while 28.6% (8 out of 28) showed a weakening of the signal.

The inter-reader reliability in qualitative evaluation of CP OCT images was 0.93 that indicates high concordance between the two readers. Disagreements were observed in cases of focal epithelial atrophy (an example, Figure 6a,d): one of the readers rated the epithelium as atrophic, the other as normal. In other cases, the answers were completely the same.

The results of the incidence of the bladder neck + proximal conditions are presented in Table 4. 132 CP OCT images obtained at the '6 o'clock position' from 33 patients were analyzed.

Table 4. State of the epithelium of the bladder neck and the proximal region of the urethra compared with the epithelium of the middle and distal regions at the '6 o'clock position' in patients with UPS, depending on age.

Subgroup of Patients by Age, Years	Number of Patients	Number of CP OCT Images	Hyperplasia of the Bladder Neck + Proximal Urethra	Atrophy of the Bladder Neck + Proximal Urethra	Total Matches	% of Changes in the Bladder Neck + Proximal Urethra of the Total Number of Patients
≤49	18	72	4	4	8	44.4% (8/18)
50≥	15	60	7	7	14	93.3% (14/15)
Total (n = 33)	33	132	11	11	22	68.8% (22/33)

It was revealed that changes in the epithelium of the bladder neck and proximal urethra—hyperplasia or atrophy, which differed from the middle and distal segments of the urethra—coincided in 22 cases out of 33, representing 68.8%. Hyperplasia was identified in 34.4% of cases (n = 11) as well as atrophy in 34.4% of cases (n = 11). It is noteworthy that in women over 50 years of age (n = 15), changes in the analyzed area were more common—93.3%, compared with women of reproductive age (n = 18)—44.4%. It can be surmised that hormonal levels undoubtedly play a role in changing the state of the tissues of the bladder neck and urethra.

Of the 11 cases of hyperplasia detected in the proximal urethra, only in the case of the epithelium was there also thickening in the middle and distal urethra. In other situations, atrophy was recorded—our cases, while, in six the epithelium was of normal thickness. In the presence of atrophy in the proximal urethra (n = 11), atrophy was recorded in the underlying regions—five cases, while the epithelium was of normal thickness in six cases.

Thus, the CP OCT method allowed us non-invasively to determine the state of the epithelium and connective tissue structures of the bladder neck and urethra in vivo. It was shown that with UPS, the structure of the tissues in most cases is changed. In this case, the proximal fragment of the urethra with UPS undergoes changes identical to those of the bladder neck.

4. Discussion

UPS is still a pathology in which the diagnosis is formulated as a "diagnosis of exclusion". It is not specific for women, as it can also occur in men [43], but in this case, it is customary to speak about prostatic, scrotal, or penile chronic pelvic pain [8]. A large number of studies have been devoted to the study of UPS and chronic pelvic pain in men [44–48], while UPS in women has been studied significantly less [3,6]. Therefore, one of the motivations was to conduct research on the female urethra. In any case, the problems of correct and quick diagnosis and the appointment of effective treatment for UPS in men there remain the same [5]. An idea to diagnose male UPS by using ultrasound and CP OCT devices seems to be reasonable and appropriate.

Despite significant global use of OCT in many fields of medicine [49–53], in urology, our study demonstrated the first use of this technique for examining the urethra [36]. This paper shows that the introduction of new technology—CP OCT—in conjunction with TVUS allows verification of tissue changes and assessment of the structures of the connective tissue matrix of the lower urinary tract at the level of their architectonics.

According to TVUS, in our study, women with UPS had an enlarged internal lumen of the urethra in the proximal segment—on average of 5.9 ± 2.1 mm. According to the literature, with an intraurethral ultrasound study performed on sectioned material, the inner diameter of the proximal segment of the urethra at distances of 10, 15, and 20 mm from the neck was 3.73, 4.18, and 2.64 mm, respectively [41]. In another study, when measuring the internal diameter of the urethra using TVUS in women with urinary incontinence [54], the diameter in the middle third of the urethra in the control (healthy) group of patients was 4.7 ± 1.1 mm. Thus, we have recorded an increase in the diameter of the internal lumen of the proximal urethral segment in all patients with UPS. Normally, upon initiation of urination, the mechanism for opening the funnel-shaped depression in the bladder neck is associated with contraction of the muscles of the deep triangle and of muscles located anterior to the internal opening of the urethra, as well as with the simultaneous contraction of the longitudinal muscle fibers of the urethra [42]. This means, we can assume the presence of insufficiency of these muscle groups in UPS.

Trophic disorders recorded by CP OCT in the epithelium of the urethral neck and the proximal segment of the urethra were more common in women over 50 years of age—in 93.3%, indicating their dependence on the patient's hormonal background. The hormonal dependence of a number of urinary disorders is explained in [55,56]. In these works, it was shown that in the deep layers of the mucous membrane of the urethra there is a powerful venous plexus, and that this has a large number of anastomoses with the venous uterovaginal plexus. At the same time, the work of Petros et al. [57] indicated that the epithelium of the urinary system (urothelium) acts as a mechanoreceptor, using its sensitive nerve endings, and that it controls the activity of the afferent nerves, so this may contribute a pathogenetic component of chronic pelvic pain, and of urethral syndrome in particular.

Using the CP OCT method, we have previously shown that the thickness of the tissue of the urethral membrane in women is dependent on age [58]. The work reported that, with UPS, there are corresponding tendencies towards thinning of the epithelium and an increase in the thickness of the connective tissue matrix of the bladder neck, as occurs in women without pathology of the urological sphere, but that these processes proceed at a higher rate.

The recorded changes in the thickness of the epithelium are undoubtedly associated with the state of the connective tissue matrix of the subepithelium of the structural components. The compaction of the walls of the urethra and surrounding tissues that we have revealed using elastometry data, as well as in our earlier CP OCT data on the state of the connective tissue matrix of the urethra during UPS [36], indicate the presence of fibrosis processes both within the wall of the urethra and around it, the cause of which, at present, is not clear. Our studies have previously shown that the state of the urethral tissues in UPS is not normal, with changes in the urethral tissues occupying an intermediate place between the norm and the changes seen in chronic bacterial inflammatory processes [36].

Changes in the state of the connective tissue can lead to a decrease in the sensitivity of the stretch receptors at the base of the bladder, affecting the functionality results [57], in particular, influencing the uroflowmetry data that we obtained. The results of the uroflowmetry allow us to assume the presence of functional disorders of the urethra in women with UPS. Considering the indices of the normal values of the urination rate for women, which are 23–32 mL/s [40], our results of uroflowmetry showing 13.7 ± 3.2 mL/s are likely to be associated with anatomical changes that are not detected in standard clinical studies, or with dysfunctional and/or obstructive urination due to an overactive urethra. However, it is known that the presence of symptoms of urinary disorders is not a reliable marker of pathological processes [40]. We are continuing our research in this direction.

There is reason to believe that the cause of the development of chronic inflammatory processes in UPS is located in the tissues of the urethra and, accordingly, this serves as an additional stimulus for the occurrence of disorders of the microcirculation, innervation, and functioning of the urethra, indirectly influencing the appearance of pain. Our anamnestic data on the presence of a prevailing gynecological pathology of inflammatory genesis suggest that the cause of such changes in the tissues of the bladder and urethra may be viral-bacterial associations in the tissues of the organs of the gynecological sphere. This aspect requires more detailed study. At present, the effect of the translocation of microorganisms in the tissues of the urinary system, vagina, and intestines has been proven in cases of upper urinary tract infection [59], although research in this area is ongoing. Analyses of the composition of the microflora of urine and of the large intestine in cases of infection of the lower urinary tract have also indirectly confirmed the presence of a translocation mechanism in microorganisms [59].

It is known that the close anatomical connection of the bladder, urethra, and vagina provides associated functional mechanisms for the urination process. A component of this mechanism is illustrated by the fact that in the distal urethra the circular fibers of the striated sphincter are transformed into loop structures, the ends of which are woven into the framework of the anterior vaginal wall [55]. According to the anamnesis, hormonal disorders, inflammatory diseases, and surgical interventions on the pelvic organs, which could result in dysfunction of the muscles of the urethra and vagina, were found in 70.9% of patients with UPS who were interviewed. At the same time, it is known that functional disorders, on their own, can generate pain [60]. The results of our study indicated that a reason for the development of pain and chronic dysuria in patients with UPS may be failure of the structures of the internal urethral sphincter. This sphincter is formed by the muscles of the external muscular layer of the bladder that pass into the urethra in the bladder neck region, forming spiral structures, occupying about 20% of its length. In the present study on TVUS, 29.1% of women were found to have an insufficiency of structures, namely the urethral tongue, in the area of this sphincter. This fact requires further research.

Thus, it has been shown that there are many factors that cause persistent long-term pain in the urethral region, or that contribute to the intensification of pain, some of which have yet to be studied. Given the non-obviousness of the causes of UPS, new research protocols and additional imaging and diagnostic methods are required for a comprehensive examination of such patients, without focusing only on their pathologies in the urological field.

The main shortcoming of our study was its retrospective nature and moderate patient number in the norm group. Therefore, our results are not definitive and require confirmation on a larger number of patients. However, we identified certain new patterns in patients with UPS compared with healthy women. We can suggest including our approach—the combined study of patients with UPS by TVUS/compression US and CP OCT—in the daily practice of urologists in order to undergo validation and prospective–comparative clinical trials.

Another drawback of our study was the lack of histological verification of CP OCT data. We proceeded from the results of our previous study [36], where the morphology of the female urethra was analyzed on cadaveric material and compared with CP OCT images. This fact and numerous studies on CP OCT visualization of mucous membranes in health and pathology [30,31,52,61,62] afford ground for confidence in the interpretation of CP OCT features, such as changes in the epithelium thickness and the state of connective tissue.

As soon as the limitations of the used methods are concerned, it is necessary to compare their imaging depth and resolution. With a fairly low resolution of TVUS, the advantage of the method is a sufficient imaging depth. The technique allows observing the entire urethra, estimating its size and shape, identifying concomitant pathologies in adjacent organs, and conducting a functional study (compare the state of the urethra and bladder before and after miction). In addition to the USE mode, which is used in this paper, the method also makes it possible to study the blood supply to the pelvic organs, which is an important part in the pathogenesis of UPS.

One of the limitations of the CP OCT method is the small depth of tissue visualization, namely, the inability to fully assess the muscle layer located deeper than the connective tissue. On the other hand, tissue imaging to a depth of 1–1.5 mm is an advantage over urethroscopy, which allows the assessment of the urethral mucosa only from the surface. The forward-looking CP OCT probe used in this study allows visualizing the urethral wall in a certain place, while it would be optimal to study the urethral mucosa along its entire length, for example, when using rotary or needle OCT probes with manual scanning [28]. Despite this, the advantage of CP OCT is the rapid assessment of the urethral wall structure at the tissue level: the high resolution of the method (5–15 μm) is sufficient for the rapid assessment of epithelium and connective tissue—structures that play a key role in the emergence of UPS [63].

As a prospect, we intend to continue research on the pathogenesis of UPS by adding neurophysiological methods for diagnosing lesions of the pudendal nerve and sacral pathways, assessing the hormonal status of women, and studying the microflora of the tissues of the urethra and the bladder neck.

5. Conclusions

For the first time in the case of UPS, the layered structure of the urethral wall was investigated in vivo using CP OCT to assess some of the pathogenetic aspects of the development and progression of this disease. The CP OCT method covers the range of possibilities of traditional cystoscopy and allows information to be obtained about the state of the urethral tissues that cannot be adequately assessed during cystoscopic examination alone. The predominant changes in the tissues of the urethra are fibrosis of the subepithelial structures and trophic changes in the epithelial layer. In 68.8% of cases, the "behavior" of the tissues of the proximal segment of the urethra coincided with changes in the bladder neck. The importance of the in vivo acquisition and operative analysis possible with CP OCT in combination with TVUS/compression US data in patients with UPS is beyond doubt.

Deep objective analysis of tissues can reveal the basis of pathogenesis. Real-time visualization of structural changes in the tissues of the urethra (epithelium, connective tissue, muscle layer, vasculature, and paraurethral glands) is important because it influences the final diagnosis, understanding of the pathogenesis of the disease and treatment tactics. An analysis of the comorbidities of patients with UPS showed that inflammatory gynecological diseases can become a premorbid background/one of the triggering mechanisms for the development of UPS.

Author Contributions: Conceptualization, O.S. and E.K.; methodology, E.T.; software, M.S.A.M.M. and V.L.; investigation, O.S., A.K., M.S.A.M.M., S.Z., and E.T.; data curation, V.L.; writing—original draft preparation, O.S., A.K., E.K., and S.Z.; writing—review and editing, O.S., A.K., and E.K.; funding acquisition, O.S. All authors have read and agreed to the published version of the manuscript.

Acknowledgments: The authors would like to thank Grigory V. Gelikonov and Valentin M. Gelikonov (Institute of Applied Physics of the RAS, Russia) for the provision of the CP OCT device and its technical support during the research.

References

1. Rothberg, M.B.; Wong, J.B. All dysuria is local a cost-effectiveness model for designing site-specific management algorithms. *J. Gen. Intern. Med.* **2004**, *19*, 433–443. [CrossRef] [PubMed]
2. Cho, S.T. Urethral pain syndrome really part of bladder pain syndrome? *Urogenit. Tract Infect.* **2017**, *12*, 22–27. [CrossRef]
3. Phillip, H.; Okewole, I.; Chilaka, V. Enigma of urethral pain syndrome: Why are there so many ascribed etiologies and therapeutic approaches? *Int. J. Urol.* **2014**, *21*, 544–548. [CrossRef] [PubMed]
4. Piontek, K.; Ketels, G.; Albrecht, R.; Schnurr, U.; Dybowski, C.; Brünahl, C.A.; Riegel, B.; Löwe, B. Somatic and psychosocial determinants of symptom severity and quality of life in male and female patients with chronic pelvic pain syndrome. *J. Psychosom. Res.* **2019**, *120*, 1–7. [CrossRef] [PubMed]
5. Passavanti, M.B.; Pota, V.; Sansone, P.; Aurilio, C.; De Nardis, L.; Pace, M.C. Chronic pelvic pain: Assessment, evaluation, and objectivation. *Pain Res. Treat.* **2017**, *2017*, 9472925. [CrossRef] [PubMed]
6. Kaur, H.; Arunkalaivanan, A.S. Urethral pain syndrome and its management. *Obstet. Gynecol. Surv.* **2007**, *62*, 348–351. [CrossRef]
7. Elsenbruch, S.; Häuser, W.; Jänig, W. Visceral pain. *Schmerz* **2015**, *29*, 496–502.
8. Fall, M.; Baranowski, A.P.; Elneil, S.; Engeler, D.; Hughes, J.; Messelink, E.J.; Williams, A.D.C. EAU guidelines on chronic pelvic pain syndrome. *Europ. Urol.* **2010**, *57*, 35–48. [CrossRef]
9. Dreger, N.; Degener, S.; Roth, S.; Brandt, A.S.; Lazica, D. Urethral pain syndrome: Fact or fiction—An update. *Urol. A* **2015**, *54*, 1248–1255. [CrossRef]
10. Zaitsev, A.V.; Sharov, M.N.; Pushkar, D.Y.; Khodyreva, L.A.; Dudareva, A.A. *Chronic Pelvic Pain Methodical Recommendations № 20*; LLC Publishing House ABV-Press: Moscow, Russia, 2006; p. 46.
11. Flor, H.; Fydrich, T.; Turk, D.C. Efficacy of multidisciplinary pain treatment centers: A meta-analytic review. *Pain* **1992**, *49*, 221–230. [CrossRef]
12. Jarrell, J.F.; Vilos, G.A.; Allaire, C.; Burgess, S.; Fortin, C.; Gerwin, R.; Lapensée, L.; Lea, R.H.; Leyland, N.A.; Martyn, P.; et al. Chronic pelvic pain working group; society of obstetricians and gynaecologists of canada. consensus guidelines for the management of chronic pelvic pain. *J. Obstet. Gynaecol. Can.* **2005**, *27*, 869–910. [PubMed]
13. Grinberg, K.; Sela, Y.; Nissanholtz-Gannot, R. New insights about chronic pelvic pain syndrome (CPPS). *Int. J. Environ. Res. Public Health* **2020**, *17*, 3005. [CrossRef] [PubMed]
14. Persu, C.; Cauni, V.; Gutue, S.; Blaj, I.; Jinga, V.; Geavlete, P. From interstitial cystitis to chronic pelvic pain. *J. Med. Life* **2010**, *3*, 167–174.
15. Aziz, Q.; Giamberardino, M.A.; Barke, A.; Korwisi, B.; Baranowski, A.P.; Wesselmann, U.; Treede, R.D. The IASP Classification of Chronic Pain for ICD-11: Chronic secondary visceral pain. *Pain* **2019**, *160*, 69–76. [CrossRef] [PubMed]
16. Stecco, C. *Functional Atlas of the Human Fascial System*, 1st ed.; Elsevier Health Sciences: London, UK, 2014; p. 384.
17. Muiznieks, L.D.; Keeley, F.W. Molecular assembly and mechanical properties of the extracellular matrix: A fibrous protein perspective. *Biochim. Biophys. Acta.* **2013**, *1832*, 866–875. [CrossRef]
18. Langevin, H.M. Connective tissue: A body-wide signaling network? *Med. Hypotheses* **2006**, *66*, 1074–1077. [CrossRef]
19. Shoskes, D.A.; Nickel, J.C.; Kattan, M.W. Phenotypically directed multimodal therapy for chronic prostatitis/chronic pelvic pain syndrome: A prospective study using UPOINT. *Urology* **2010**, *75*, 1249–1253. [CrossRef]
20. Wells, P.N.; Liang, H.D. Medical ultrasound: Imaging of soft tissue strain and elasticity. *J. R. Soc. Interface* **2011**, *8*, 1521–1549. [CrossRef]
21. Bamber, J.; Cosgrove, D.; Dietrich, C.F.; Fromageau, J.; Bojunga, J.; Calliada, F.; Cantisani, V.; Correas, J.M.; D'Onofrio, M.; Drakonaki, E.E.; et al. EFSUMB guidelines and recommendations on the clinical use of ultrasound elastography. Part 1: Basic principles and technology. *Ultraschall Med.* **2013**, *34*, 169–184. [CrossRef]
22. Cosgrove, D.; Piscaglia, F.; Bamber, J.; Bojunga, J.; Correas, J.M.; Gilja, O.H.; Klauser, A.S.; Sporea, I.; Calliada, F.; Cantisani, V.; et al. EFSUMB guidelines and recommendations on the clinical use of ultrasound elastography. Part 2: Clinical applications. *Ultraschall Med.* **2013**, *34*, 238–253.

23. Lupsor-Platon, M. *Ultrasound Elastography*; IntechOpen: London, UK, 2020; p. 146.

24. Sigrist, R.; Liau, J.; Kaffas, A.E.; Chammas, M.C.; Willmann, J.K. Ultrasound elastography: Review of techniques and clinical applications. *Theranostics* **2017**, *7*, 1303–1329. [CrossRef] [PubMed]

25. Huang, D.; Swanson, E.A.; Lin, C.P.; Schuman, J.S.; Stinson, W.G.; Chang, W.; Hee, M.R.; Flotte, T.; Gregory, K.; Puliafito, C.A.; et al. Optical coherence tomography. *Science* **1991**, *254*, 1178–1181. [CrossRef] [PubMed]

26. Drexler, W.; Liu, M.; Kumar, A.; Kamali, T.; Unterhuber, A.; Leitgeb, R.A. Optical coherence tomography today: Speed, contrast, and multimodality. *J. Biomed. Opt.* **2014**, *19*, 071412. [CrossRef] [PubMed]

27. Lamirel, C. Optical Coherence Tomography. In *Encyclopedia of the Neurological Sciences*, 2nd ed.; Aminoff, M.J., Daroff, R.B., Eds.; Academic Press: Waltham, MA, USA, 2014; pp. 660–668.

28. Gora, M.J.; Suter, M.J.; Tearney, G.J.; Li, X. Endoscopic optical coherence tomography: Technologies and clinical applications [Invited]. *Biomed. Opt. Express* **2017**, *8*, 2405–2444. [CrossRef] [PubMed]

29. Gelikonov, V.M.; Gelikonov, G.V. New approach to cross-polarized optical coherence tomography based on orthogonal arbitrarily polarized modes. *Laser Phys. Let.* **2006**, *3*, 445–451. [CrossRef]

30. Gladkova, N.; Kiseleva, E.; Robakidze, N.; Balalaeva, I.; Karabut, M.; Gubarkova, E.; Feldchtein, F. Evaluation of oral mucosa collagen condition with cross-polarization optical coherence tomography. *J. Biophotonics* **2013**, *6*, 321–329. [CrossRef]

31. Kiseleva, E.; Kirillin, M.; Feldchtein, F.; Vitkin, A.; Sergeeva, E.; Zagaynova, E.; Gladkova, N. Differential diagnosis of human bladder mucosa pathologies in vivo with cross-polarization optical coherence tomography. *Biomed. Optic. Express* **2015**, *6*, 1464–1476. [CrossRef]

32. Abrams, P.; Cardozo, L.; Fall, M.; Griffiths, D.; Rosier, P.; Ulmsten, U.; van Kerrebroeck, P.; Victor, A.; Wein, A. Standardisation Sub-Committee of the International Continence Society. The standardisation of terminology in lower urinary tract function: Report from the standardisation sub-committee of the International Continence Society. *Urology* **2003**, *61*, 37–49. [CrossRef]

33. Prado-Costa, R.; Rebelo, J.; Monteiro-Barroso, J.; Preto, A.S. Ultrasound elastography: Compression elastography and shear-wave elastography in the assessment of tendon injury. *Insights Imaging* **2018**, *9*, 791–814. [CrossRef]

34. Zahran, M.H.; El-Shafei, M.M.; Emara, D.M.; Eshiba, S.M. Ultrasound elastography: How can it help in differentiating breast lesions? *Egypt. J. Radiol. Nucl. Med.* **2018**, *49*, 249–258. [CrossRef]

35. Gelikonov, V.M.; Gelikonov, G.V. Fibreoptic methods of cross-polarisation optical coherence tomography for endoscopic studies. *IEEE J. Quantum Electron.* **2008**, *38*, 634–640.

36. Kiseleva, E.B.; Moiseev, A.A.; Kuyarov, A.S.; Molvi, M.A.; Gelikonov, G.V.; Maslennikova, A.V.; Streltsova, O.S. In vivo assessment of structural changes of the urethra in lower urinary tract disease using cross-polarization optical coherence tomography. *J. Innov. Opt. Health Sci.* **2020**, *13*, 2050024-1-16.

37. Netter, F.H. *Atlas of Human Anatomy*, 6th ed.; Elsevier Inc.: Philadelphia, PA, USA, 2014; pp. 339–400.

38. Kiseleva, E.; Gladkova, N.; Streltzova, O.; Kirillin, M.; Maslennikova, A.; Dudenkova, V.; Sergeeva, E. Cross-polarization OCT for in vivo diagnostics and prediction of bladder cancer. In *Bladder Cancer—Management of NMI and Muscle-Invasive Cancer*; Ather, M., Ed.; InTech: Rijeka, Croatia, 2017; pp. 43–61.

39. Afraa, T.A.; Mahfouz, W.; Campeau, L.; Corcos, J. Normal lower urinary tract assessment in women: I. Uroflowmetry and post-void residual, pad tests, and bladder diaries. *Int. Urogynecol. J.* **2012**, *23*, 681–685.

40. Makrushina, N.V.; Fastykovskaya, E.D. Ultrasound diagnosis of pelvic floor muscle insufficiency in women. *Sib. Med. J. Tomsk* **2012**, *27*, 91–96.

41. Schaer, G.N.; Schmid, T.; Peschers, U.; Delancey, J.O. Intraurethral ultrasound correlated with urethral histology. *Obstet. Gynecol.* **1998**, *91*, 60–64. [PubMed]

42. Jung, J.; Ahn, H.K.; Huh, Y. Clinical and functional anatomy of the urethral sphincter. *Int. Neurourol. J.* **2012**, *16*, 102–106.

43. Cakici, Ö.U.; Hamidi, N.; Ürer, E.; Okulu, E.; Kayigil, O. Efficacy of sertraline and gabapentin in the treatment of urethral pain syndrome: Retrospective results of a single institutional cohort. *Cent. European J. Urol.* **2018**, *71*, 78–83. [PubMed]

44. Nickel, J.C. Clinical evaluation of the man with chronic prostatitis/chronic pelvic pain syndrome. *Urology* **2002**, *60*, 20–22.

45. Trinchieri, A.; Magri, V.; Cariani, L.; Bonamore, R.; Restelli, A.; Garlaschi, M.C.; Perletti, G. Prevalence of sexual dysfunction in men with chronic prostatitis/chronic pelvic pain syndrome. *Arch. Ital. Urol. Androl.* **2007**, *79*, 67.
46. Juan, Y.-S.; Shen, J.-T.; Jang, M.-Y.; Huang, C.-H.; Li, C.-C.; Wu, W.-J. Current Management of Male Chronic Pelvic Pain Syndromes. *Urol. Sci.* **2010**, *21*, 157–162.
47. Smith, C.P. Male chronic pelvic pain: An update. *Indian J. Urol.* **2016**, *32*, 34–39. [CrossRef] [PubMed]
48. Archambault-Ezenwa, L.; Markowski, A.; Barral, J.-P. A comprehensive physical therapy evaluation for Male Chronic Pelvic Pain Syndrome: A case series exploring common findings. *J. Bodyw. Mov. Ther.* **2019**, *23*, 825–834. [CrossRef]
49. Wang, Y.; Liu, S.; Lou, S.; Zhang, W.; Cai, H.; Chen, X. Application of optical coherence tomography in clinical diagnosis. *J. X-ray Sci. Technol.* **2019**, *27*, 995–1006. [CrossRef]
50. Carrasco-Zevallos, O.M.; Viehland, C.; Keller, B.; Draelos, M.; Kuo, A.N.; Toth, C.A.; Izatt, J.A. Review of intraoperative optical coherence tomography: Technology and applications. *Biomed. Opt. Express* **2017**, *8*, 1607–1637. [CrossRef]
51. Freund, J.E.; Buijs, M.; Savci-Heijink, C.D.; de Bruin, D.M.; de la Rosette, J.J.; van Leeuwen, T.G.; Laguna, M.P. Optical coherence tomography in urologic oncology: A comprehensive review. *SN Compr. Clin. Med.* **2019**, *1*, 67–84. [CrossRef]
52. Kirillin, M.Y.; Motovilova, T.; Shakhova, N.M. Optical coherence tomography in gynecology: A narrative review. *J. Biomed. Opt.* **2017**, *22*, 121709. [CrossRef]
53. Olsen, J.; Holmes, J.; Jemec, G.B.E. Advances in optical coherence tomography in dermatology—A review. *J. Biomed. Opt.* **2018**, *23*, 040901. [CrossRef]
54. Oliveira, F.R.; Ramos, J.G.L.; Martins-Costa, S. Translabial ultrasonography in the assessment of urethral diameter and intrinsic urethral sphincter deficiency. *J. Ultrasound Med.* **2006**, *25*, 1153–1158. [CrossRef] [PubMed]
55. Petros, P.P.E.; Ulmsten, U.I. An integral theory and its method for the diagnosis and management of female urinary incontinence. *Scand. J. Urol. Nephrol. Suppl.* **1993**, *153*, 1–93. [PubMed]
56. Petros, P.E.P.; Ulmsten, U.I. An integral theory of female urinary incontinence: Experimental and clinical considerations. *Acta Obstet. Gynecol. Scand. Suppl.* **1990**, *153*, 7–31. [CrossRef]
57. Petros, P. *The Female Pelvic Floor. Functions, Dysfunctions and Their Treatment in Accordance with the Integral Theory*, 3rd ed.; Springer: Berlin/Heidelberg, Germany, 2010; p. 352.
58. Streltsova, O.S.; Kiseleva, E.B.; Molvi, M.A.; Lazukin, V.F. Structural features of the urethra in patients with urethral pain syndrome. *Exper. Clin. Urol.* **2019**, *3*, 170–177. [CrossRef]
59. Naboka, Y.L.; Gudima, I.A.; Dzhalagoniya, K.T.; Chernitskaya, M.L.; Ivanov, S.N. Urine and colon microbiota in patients with recurrent uncomplicated lower urinary tract infection. *Urol. Herald.* **2019**, *7*, 59–65. [CrossRef]
60. Crofford, L.J. Chronic pain: Where the body meets the brain. *Trans. Am. Clin. Climatol. Assoc.* **2015**, *126*, 167–183.
61. Bibas, A.G.; Podoleanu, A.G.; Cucu, R.G.; Bonmarin, M.; Dobre, G.M.; Ward, V.M.M.; Odell, E.; Boxer, A.; Gleeson, M.J.; Jackson, D.A. 3-D optical coherence tomography of the laryngeal mucosa. *Clin. Otolaryngol.* **2004**, *29*, 713–720. [CrossRef] [PubMed]
62. Di Stasio, D.; Lauritano, D.; Iquebal, H.; Romano, A.; Gentile, E.; Lucchese, A. Measurement of oral epithelial thickness by optical coherence tomography. *Diagnostics* **2019**, *9*, 90. [CrossRef]
63. Parsons, C.L. The role of a leaky epithelium and potassium in the generation of bladder symptoms in interstitial cystitis/overactive bladder, urethral syndrome, prostatitis and gynecological chronic pelvic pain. *BJU Int.* **2011**, *107*, 370–375. [CrossRef]

9

Image-Guided Laparoscopic Surgical Tool (IGLaST) Based on the Optical Frequency Domain Imaging (OFDI) to Prevent Bleeding

Byung Jun Park [1,†], Seung Rag Lee [1,†], Hyun Jin Bang [1], Byung Yeon Kim [1], Jeong Hun Park [1], Dong Guk Kim [1], Sung Soo Park [2,*] and Young Jae Won [1,*]

[1] Medical Device Development Center, Osong Medical Innovation Foundation, Cheongju, Chungbuk 361-951, Korea; yachon.park@gmail.com (B.J.P.); naviman78@gmail.com (S.R.L.); crisenc@kbiohealth.kr (H.J.B.); nick.kimby@gmail.com (B.Y.K.); pjh8311@kbiohealth.kr (J.H.P.); dgkim@kbiohealth.kr (D.G.K.)

[2] Department of Surgery, Korea University College of Medicine, Seoul 02841, Korea

* Correspondence: sungsoo.park.md@gmail.com (S.S.P.); yjwon000@gmail.com (Y.J.W.)

† These authors contributed equally to this work.

Academic Editors: Dragan Indjin, Željka Cvejić and Małgorzata Jędrzejewska-Szczerska

Abstract: We present an image-guided laparoscopic surgical tool (IGLaST) to prevent bleeding. By applying optical frequency domain imaging (OFDI) to a specially designed laparoscopic surgical tool, the inside of fatty tissue can be observed before a resection, and the presence and size of blood vessels can be recognized. The optical sensing module on the IGLaST head has a diameter of less than 390 μm and is moved back and forth by a linear servo actuator in the IGLaST body. We proved the feasibility of IGLaST by in vivo imaging inside the fatty tissue of a porcine model. A blood vessel with a diameter of about 2.2 mm was clearly observed. Our proposed scheme can contribute to safe surgery without bleeding by monitoring vessels inside the tissue and can be further expanded to detect invisible nerves of the laparoscopic thyroid during prostate gland surgery.

Keywords: laser and laser optics; optical frequency domain imaging; optical coherence tomography; laparoscopic surgical tool; medical optics instrumentation

1. Introduction

Laparoscopic surgery, which is also called minimally invasive surgery (MIS) with laparoscopy, has become widely accepted as a part of general, gynecological, urological, and thoracic surgeries. Because laparoscopic surgery is performed with a laparoscope and thin rod-shaped surgical instruments through trocars settled on the body wall (the hole size is usually 0.5–1.5 cm), it provides many advantages to the patient compared with open surgery in terms of pain, incision size, and postoperative recovery [1].

While laparoscopic surgery is clearly advantageous in terms of patient outcomes, there are some drawbacks on the surgeon's side, such as a loss of dexterity, poor depth perception, the fulcrum effect, and a decreased sense of touch [2,3]. In particular, the loss of tactile sensation by depending on tools makes it difficult to avoid invisible blood vessels surrounded by the fatty tissues of the dissection area before resection. In open surgery, surgeons are not only able to feel pulsating blood vessels with their own hands but also use their comprehensive knowledge of gross human anatomy to trace specific local areas that need to be dissected. However, MIS takes away the surgeon's tactile senses of the tissue and applications of a wide anatomical map due to the magnified local camera view of the laparoscopic system. These inevitable drawbacks of MIS force surgeons to dissect tissues very meticulously to find vessels and expose them until they are nearly naked because they need to confirm them on the monitor and have no tactile sense. Even minor bleeding can make the laparoscopic surgical field very dirty and confusing. This situation sometimes lengthens the duration of MIS. To ensure perfect bleeding control from vessels, surgeons use more hemoclips than they actually need. Moreover, if a blood vessel is not fully captured within the sealing area of the advanced energy device, bleeding cannot be avoided.

The optical frequency domain imaging (OFDI) technique, which is also known as swept source optical coherence tomography (SS-OCT), is a high-sensitivity and high-resolution optical cross-sectional imaging technique based on optical frequency-domain interferometry with a wavelength sweeping laser [4]. Because the optical cross-sectional imaging technique is fast and minimally invasive compared to non-optical techniques such as MRI, CT, and X-rays, it has been extensively studied in a number of medical fields. Clinically, OFDI is used in ocular and cardiovascular applications and has been demonstrated to accurately image the normal eye and coronary artery in vivo as well as diseased states [5–9]. Typically, the penetration depth is about 1–3 mm in tissue, and the depth resolution is about 10–15 μm [10]. OFDI has also been applied to studying the structural features of skin, gynecological tissues, and gastrointestinal tract [11–14]. Most previous studies on medical devices using OFDI focused on discriminating between normal and diseased or cancerous tissues based on microstructural features. When the OFDI technique is applied in a laparoscopic surgical device such as a tissue dissector, safe surgery without unwanted bleeding can be realized by monitoring blood vessels inside a tissue before resection.

We developed an image-guided laparoscopic surgical tool (IGLaST) to observe blood vessels inside a tissue that uses a clinically qualified OFDI technique and the specially designed laparoscopic surgical tool. We demonstrated our proposed scheme in vivo by observing the blood vessels surrounded by the fatty tissues of a porcine model.

2. Materials and Methods

2.1. Design of IGLaST

Compared to previous medical devices using OFDI, IGLaST is for laparoscopic surgical devices that grasp a tissue or blood vessel for dissection or sealing. The proposed IGLaST comprises an optical imaging part based on the OFDI technique and a specially designed laparoscopic surgical part, as shown in Figure 1. We designed the laparoscopic surgical part to scan an optical sensing module with a linear actuator and operate the head with a handle. The optical imaging part consists of the OFDI system and an optical sensing module.

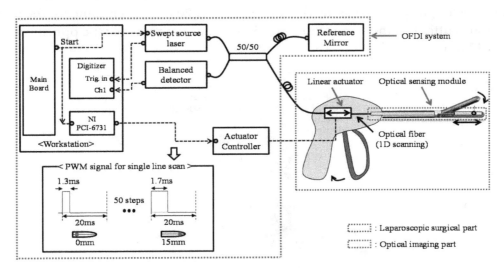

Figure 1. Schematic diagram of an image-guided laparoscopic surgical tool (IGLaST) based on the optical frequency domain imaging (OFDI) technique.

Because laparoscopic surgery is minimally invasive, the head size for the surgical instruments is restricted to a diameter of 5–10 mm. The optical sensing module can be simply realized by an optical fiber with a diameter of less than 0.35 mm. Such an optical fiber is inexpensive and easily separated and combined by an optical connector. Thus, OFDI can be an effective technique for realizing an image-guided disposable laparoscopic surgical tool.

2.2. OFDI for IGLaST

A swept sourced laser with a center wavelength λ_0 of 1300 nm and a spectral bandwidth λ_{full} of 100 nm at a cutoff point of -20 dB (SL1310V1-10048, Thorlabs, Sterling, VA, USA) was used as the light source. The swept source is separated by a 3 dB fiber coupler. One of two beams after the 3 dB fiber coupler goes to a reference mirror, and the other goes to the sample. The two reflected beams from the reference mirror and sample pass through the same root in opposite directions and are interfered with. The interference optical signal is detected by a balanced detector and acquired by a digitizer with a sampling rate of up to 500 MS/s at a 12 bit resolution.

In an experiment, the mechanical movement of the optical sensing module was performed by using a linear servo actuator (PLS-5030, POTENIT, Seoul, Korea) for 15 mm transverse line scanning within 1 s. Generally, OFDI imaging requires a high-speed line scanning system (HSLS) for biomedical applications [5–9]. However, HSLS-based OFDI is not required for laparoscopic surgical applications because the sample is tightly fixed by the IGLaST head. Our proposed line scanning scheme with a linear servo actuator provides a low-cost and miniaturized device for practical use in laparoscopic surgical applications. To control the linear servo actuator, an NI PCI-6731 board (National Instruments, Austin, TX, USA) was equipped with a workstation, and pulse-width modulation (PWM) signals were generated as described in Figure 1.

To facilitate clear imaging, the swept source laser, digitizer, and linear servo actuator were synchronized, as represented in Figure 1.

The repetition rate of the light source was 100 kHz, and 100,000 interference signals were generated in a single scan. For a higher signal-to-noise ratio (SNR), the 20 adjacent interference signals were averaged after fast Fourier transform (FFT). Finally, a 5000 × 701 pixel OFDI image was acquired.

2.3. Realization of IGLaST

To apply the proposed method to a laparoscopic tissue dissector, we developed the IGLaST head with an optical sensing module and tissue cutter. The IGLaST head with biocompatible material (SUS304) contains two routes for the optical sensing module and tissue cutter, as shown in Figure 2. The size of the area for grasping the tissue is about 5.3 mm × 20 mm. Each route for the optical sensing module and tissue cutter has the same width of 0.5 mm, and the route for the optical sensing module has a length of 17 mm.

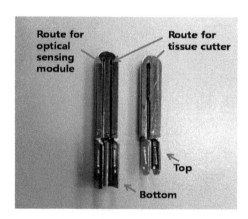

Figure 2. IGLaST head with the route for the optical sensing module.

In order to transmit the laser beam into a sample, a ball-lens fiber functioning as a reflective mirror at the end of a fiber was manufactured, as shown in Figure 3a. This was predetermined by using a simulation tool (Light Tools, Synopsys, Mountain View, CA, USA) to satisfy a spot size (Full width at half maximum) of 27 μm at a working distance of 1.6 mm, as shown in Figure 3b. A coreless fiber (FG125LA, Thorlabs, Sterling, VA, USA) was fusion-spliced to the SMF (SMF-28, Corning, Corning, NY, USA) and cleaved to a predetermined length. Then, the distal end of the coreless fiber was heated, while being translated in a tungsten filament furnace to form a ball lens. The translation length and speed, the temperature of the filament, and the duration of heating were empirically adjusted to form the optimal ball-lens fiber. The entire ball lens fabrication process was performed at a computer-controlled fusion splicing workstation (GPX-3000, Vytran, Morganville, NJ, USA). To perpendicularly reflect the beam into the tissue, the distal tip of the ball lens was polished with a fiber polishing machine (Ultrapol, Ultra Tech., Santa Ana, CA, USA). The angle between the fiber axis and polished surface was about 39°. We confirmed the spot size (FWHM) of the beam was about 22.8 μm at a working distance of 1.6 mm by using a beam profiler (SP620U, Spiricon, Jerusalem, Israel), as shown in Figure 3c. The distance between the SMF/coreless fiber interface and front of the ball lens was 302 μm, and the coronal diameter of the ball lens was 323 μm.

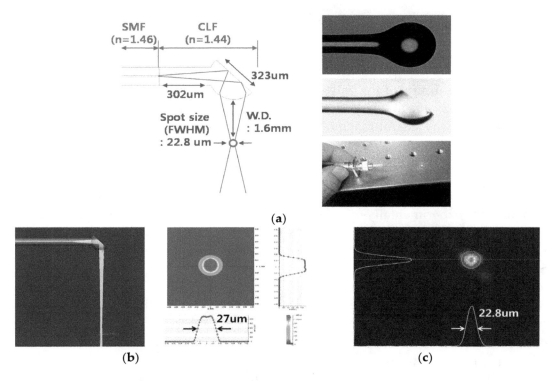

Figure 3. (a) Design and manufacture of the ball-lens fiber. (b) Simulation results for the ball-lens fiber. (c) Experimentally measured beam profile of the ball-lens fiber at a working distance of 1.6 mm.

Figure 4 shows the structure of proposed optical sensing module. To protect the ball-lens fiber, a polyimide with an inner diameter of 350 μm and outer diameter of 390 μm was used. The polyimide was inserted into the groove on the bottom of the IGLaST head and secured with epoxy, as shown at the bottom of Figure 4. The rest of the ball-lens fiber was guided by Shrinkable Tube 1. Between the polyimide and Tube 1, Shrinkable Tube 2 was used as a spacer and had a smaller inner diameter than Tube 1. The length of Tube 1 was about 500 mm, which is similar to the length of a laparoscopic surgical tool. After the end of Tube 1, a linear servomotor was used for one-dimensional scanning of the ball-lens fiber. To minimize twisting or bending of the ball-lens fiber, the linear servomotor was placed close to the end of Tube 1.

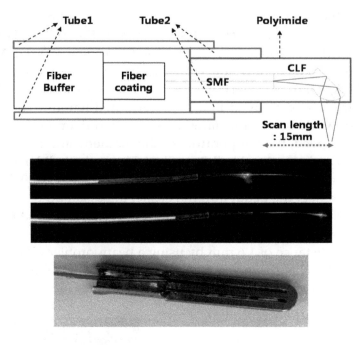

Figure 4. Optical sensing module for IGLaST.

One-dimensional scanning of the ball-lens fiber inside the optical sensing module was tested by using a laser diode with a central wavelength of 633 nm, as shown at the middle of Figure 4. After the optical sensing module was assembled, the head was attached to the IGLaST body.

3. Results

3.1. Optical Properties

Figure 5 plots the experimentally measured beam diameter (FWHM) of the optical sensing module of IGLaST. The beam shape was measured by using a microscope equipped with an IR camera [15]. The beam diameter plot started at 400 μm considering the air gap between the optical sensing module and IGLaST head surface. The beam profile was elliptically shaped after passing through the polyimide. The ratio of the x-axis/y-axis crossed at the focal plane. The measured x- and y-axis beam diameters were 29.3 and 31.8 μm, respectively. The lateral resolution expected by the FWHM beam width ranged from 20 to 65 μm in the first 2 mm after the IGLaST head.

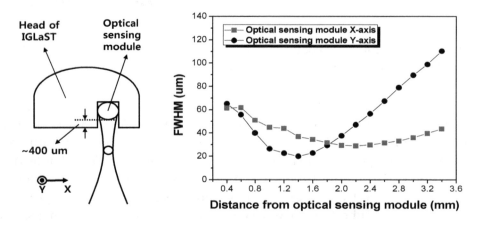

Figure 5. Beam diameter (FWHM) of the optical sensing module.

3.2. Imaging of a Vessel Inside the Fatty Tissues of a Porcine Model with IGLaST

As a demonstration, IGLaST was used to observe blood vessel inside fatty tissue during laparoscopic surgery. We prepared a 40 kg porcine model that was 3 months old. The pig underwent surgical procedures under general anesthesia. Three incisions with a length of 0.5–1 cm were made on the abdomen of the pig, and trocars were placed in the incisions. A laparoscope, laparoscopic dissection tool, and laparoscopic clamp were inserted inside the body through the trocars, and an operation was performed to find the region of interest. The animal experiment protocol was approved by the Institutional Animal Care and Use Committee (IACUC) of Korea University.

Figure 6 shows the in vivo imaging inside the fatty tissue of the pig with IGLaST. In laparoscopic surgery, tissues to be dissected should consist of adipose, lymphatics, and collagen, and blood vessels must be surrounded by the tissue complex. Therefore, the tissue complex that may cover major blood vessels of an artery or vein usually needs to be dissected to find them. In most cases, blood vessels inside the tissue are invisible, as shown in Figure 6a. We inserted our developed IGLaST inside the pig body through a trocar and grasped the tissue with the head of IGLaST to observe invisible blood vessels inside the tissue, as shown in Figure 6b. The red light is a guide source to inform the position of the head of the ball-lens fiber. The blood vessel inside the fatty tissue of the pig appeared with OFDI, as shown in Figure 6c. The yellow bar in Figure 6c represents a length of 0.5 mm. The size of the image was about 15×1.75 mm^2. After the tissue was grasped, the tissue was compressed, and the thickness of the tissue was reduced to about 0.5–0.6 mm. In this experiment, a blood vessel with a length of about 2.2 mm was clearly observed.

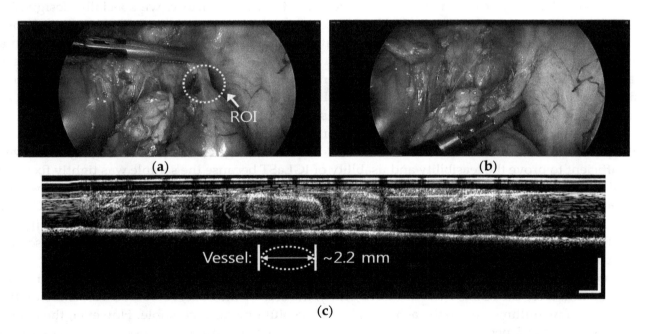

Figure 6. In vivo imaging inside the fatty tissue of a porcine model with IGLaST; the blood vessel inside the tissue is visible. (**a**) Laparoscopic image of the porcine model. (**b**) Laparoscopic image of the porcine model after the tissue is grasped with IGLaST. (**c**) OFDI image inside the fatty tissue.

When the IGLaST head grasping the tissue was slightly released, image blurring occurred at the vessel position because of blood flow, as shown in Figure 7a. If the morphological image processing technique to extract blurring pixels is applied, the contrast can be increased to improve awareness of the blood vessels inside the tissue, as shown in Figure 7b. This technique provides the functions of erosion, smooth filtering, simple threshold, and area sort to isolate the blurred part [16]. IGLaST can be further improved to discriminate arteries and veins by the application of Doppler and angiographic techniques [17–19]

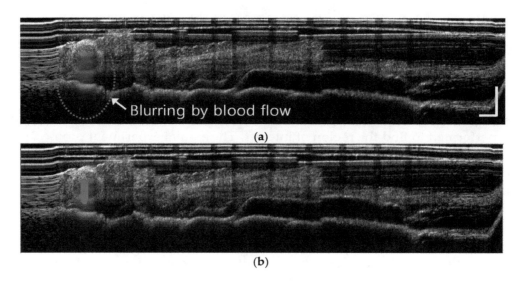

Figure 7. (a) In vivo imaging of the blood flow inside the fatty tissue of a porcine model with IGLaST. **(b)** Identification of blood flow with the morphological image processing technique.

4. Discussion and Conclusions

We proposed and developed IGLaST based on the OFDI technique to prevent bleeding. To observe within tissue that may cover invisible blood vessels of a vein or artery, we specially designed a laparoscopic surgical tool and applied the OFDI technique. We successfully demonstrated that our proposed scheme can be used to prevent unwanted bleeding by observing a blood vessel with a diameter of about 2.2 mm inside the fatty tissues of a porcine model during laparoscopic surgery. The experimental results suggest that IGLaST can be a useful tool for investigating blood vessels inside the tissue before resection. The utility of IGLaST may extend to other surgical devices such as laparoscopic surgical staplers, laparoscopic vessel sealing devices, and surgical scissors.

The use of a low-speed linear servo actuator may be unfamiliar for researchers interested in high-speed OFDI-based medical devices for cardiovascular imaging and ocular imaging. However, it is sufficient to prove the feasibility and usability of IGLaST because the sample was tightly fixed by the IGLaST head. The proposed line scanning scheme with a linear servo actuator provides a low-cost and miniaturized device for the practical use of laparoscopic surgical applications. In future IGLaST designs, we will apply the high-speed OFDI technique to the laparoscopic surgical tool to identify the blood flow of blood vessels inside the tissue so that arteries and veins can be discriminated based on Doppler and angiographic techniques.

For the optical sensing module, a beam diameter (FWHM) of less than 65 μm was obtained in the first 2 mm after the IGLaST head. In this study, the size of the observed blood vessel inside the tissue was a few millimeters, so the achieved lateral resolution was acceptable. However, the lateral resolution of IGLaST needs to be further improved to observe small blood vessels or nerves inside the tissue.

We believe that techniques using IGLaST can also be applied to identify invisible nerves or lymphatic vessels inside the tissue to avoid injuring them during minimally invasive surgery (MIS). Moreover, our proposed scheme has tremendous potential as a smart image-guided laparoscopic surgical tool for robot-assisted surgery.

Acknowledgments: This work was supported by the Industrial Strategic Technology Development Program (10051331) funded by the Ministry of Trade, Industry and Energy (MOTIE) of Korea.

Author Contributions: Young Jae Won and Sung Soo Park made the idea and designed the system; Byung Jun Park, Seung Rag Lee, and Byung Yeon Kim built the system; Hyun Jin Bang contributed to make optical head for IGLaST; Jung Hun Park and Dong Guk Kim contributed to make mechanical head for IGLaST; all authors performed the experiments; Byung Jun Park and Seung Rag Lee analyzed the data; Young Jae Won and Sung Soo Park wrote the paper.

References

1. Swanstrom, L.L.; Soper, N.J. *Mastery of Endoscopic and Laparoscopic Surgery*; Lippincott Williams & Wilkins: Philadelphia, PA, USA, 2013.
2. Der Putten, E.P.W.; Goossens, R.H.M.; Jakimowicz, J.J.; Dankelman, J. Haptics in minimally invasive surgery—A review. *Minim. Invasive Ther. Alied Technol.* **2008**, *17*, 3–16. [CrossRef] [PubMed]
3. Gallagher, A.G.; McClure, N.; McGuigan, J.; Ritchie, K.; Sheehy, N.P. An ergonomic analysis of the fulcrum effect in the acquisition of endoscopic skills. *Endoscopy* **1998**, *30*, 617–620. [CrossRef] [PubMed]
4. Fercher, A.F.; Drexler, W.; Hitzenberger, C.K.; Lasser, T. Optical coherence tomography—Principles and applications. *Rep. Prog. Phys.* **2003**, *66*, 239–303. [CrossRef]
5. Zysk, A.M.; Nguyen, F.T.; Oldenburg, A.L.; Marks, D.L.; Boppart, S.A. Optical coherence tomography: A review of clinical development from bench to bedside. *J. Biomed. Opt.* **2007**, *12*, 051403. [CrossRef] [PubMed]
6. Costa, R.A.; Skaf, M.; Melo, L.A.S.; Calucci, D.; Cardillo, J.A.; Castro, J.C.; Huang, D.; Wojtkowski, M. Retinal assessment using optical coherence tomography. *Prog. Retin. Eye Res.* **2006**, *25*, 325–353. [CrossRef] [PubMed]
7. Dogra, M.R.; Gupta, A.; Gupta, V. *Atlas of Optical Coherence Tomography of Macular Diseases*; Taylor & Francis: Boca Raton, FL, USA, 2004.
8. Brezinski, M.E.; Tearney, G.J.; Bouma, B.E.; Izatt, J.A.; Hee, M.R.; Swanson, E.A.; Southern, J.F.; Fujimoto, J.G. Optical coherence tomography for optical biopsy: Properties and demonstration of vascular pathology. *Circulation* **1996**, *93*, 1206–1213. [CrossRef] [PubMed]
9. Cho, H.S.; Jang, S.-J.; Kim, K.; Dan-Chin-Yu, A.V.; Shishkov, M.; Bouma, B.E.; Oh, W.-Y. High-frame-rate intravascular optical frequency-domain imaging in vivo. *Biomed. Opt. Exp.* **2014**, *5*, 223–232. [CrossRef] [PubMed]
10. Fujimoto, J.G.; Pitris, C.; Boppart, S.A.; Brezinski, M.E. Optical coherence tomography: An emerging technology for biomedical imaging and optical biopsy. *Neoplasia* **2000**, *2*, 9–25. [CrossRef] [PubMed]
11. Cogliati, A.; Canavesi, C.; Hayes, A.; Tankam, P.; Duma, V.-F.; Santhanam, A.; Thompson, K.P.; Rolland, J.P. MEMS—Based handheld scanning probe with pre-shaped input signals for distortion-free images in Gabor-domain optical coherence microscopy. *Opt. Express* **2016**, *24*, 13365–13374. [CrossRef] [PubMed]
12. Testoni, P.A.; Mangiavillano, B. Optical coherence tomography in detection of dysplasia and cancer of the gastrointestinal tract and bilio-pancreatic ductal system. *World J. Gastroenterol.* **2008**, *14*, 6444–6452. [CrossRef] [PubMed]
13. Suter, M.J.; Vakoc, B.J.; Yachimski, P.S.; Shishkov, M.; Lauwers, G.Y.; Mino-Kenudson, M.; Bouma, B.E.; Nishioka, N.S.; Tearney, G.J. Comprehensive microscopy of the esophagus in human patients with optical frequency domain imaging. *Gastrointest. Endosc.* **2008**, *68*, 745–753. [CrossRef] [PubMed]
14. Boppart, S.A.; Goodman, A.; Libus, J.; Pitris, C.; Jesser, C.A.; Brezinski, M.E.; Fusimoto, J.G. High resolution imaging of endometriosis and ovarian carcinoma with optical coherence tomography: Feasibility for laparoscopic-based imaging. *Br. J. Obstet. Gynaecol.* **1999**, *106*, 1071–1077. [CrossRef] [PubMed]
15. Lee, J.B.; Chae, Y.G.; Ahn, Y.C.; Moon, S.B. Ultra-thin and flexible endoscopy probe for optical coherence tomography based on stepwise transitional core fiber. *Biomed. Opt. Express* **2015**, *6*, 1782–1796. [CrossRef] [PubMed]
16. Dougherty, E.R.; Lotufo, R.A. *Hands-on Morphological Image Processing*; SPIE: Bellingham, WA, USA, 2003.
17. Rollins, A.M.; Yazdanfar, S.; Barton, J.K.; Izatt, J.A. Real-time in vivo color Doppler optical coherence tomography. *J. Biomed. Opt.* **2002**, *7*, 123–129. [CrossRef] [PubMed]
18. De Carlo, T.E.; Romano, A.; Waheed, N.K.; Duker, J.S. A review of optical coherence tomography angiography (OCTA). *Int. J. Retin. Vitr.* **2015**, *1*. [CrossRef] [PubMed]
19. Choi, W.J.; Li, Y.D.; Qin, W.; Wang, R.K. Cerebral capillary velocimetry based on temporal OCT speckle contrast. *Biomed. Opt. Express* **2016**, *7*, 4859–4873. [CrossRef] [PubMed]

10

Feasibility of Optical Coherence Tomography (OCT) for Intra-Operative Detection of Blood Flow during Gastric Tube Reconstruction

Sanne M. Jansen [1,2,*,†], Mitra Almasian [1,†], Leah S. Wilk [1], Daniel M. de Bruin [1], Mark I. van Berge Henegouwen [3], Simon D. Strackee [2], Paul R. Bloemen [1], Sybren L. Meijer [4], Suzanne S. Gisbertz [3] and Ton G. van Leeuwen [1]

[1] Department of Biomedical Engineering & Physics, Academic Medical Center, University of Amsterdam, 1105 AZ Amsterdam, The Netherlands; m.almasian@amc.uva.nl (M.A.); l.s.wilk@amc.uva.nl (L.S.W.); d.m.debruin@amc.uva.nl (D.M.d.B.); p.r.bloemen@amc.uva.nl (P.R.B.); t.g.vanleeuwen@amc.uva.nl (T.G.v.L.)

[2] Department of Plastic, Reconstructive & Hand Surgery, Academic Medical Center, University of Amsterdam, 1105 AZ Amsterdam, The Netherlands; s.d.strackee@amc.uva.nl

[3] Department of Surgery, Academic Medical Center, University of Amsterdam, 1105 AZ Amsterdam, The Netherlands; m.i.vanbergehenegouwen@amc.uva.nl (M.I.v.B.H.); s.s.gisbertz@amc.uva.nl (S.S.G.)

[4] Department of Pathology, Academic Medical Center, University of Amsterdam, 1105 AZ Amsterdam, The Netherlands; s.l.meijer@amc.uva.nl

* Correspondence: s.m.jansen@amc.uva.nl

† These authors contributed equally to this work.

Abstract: In this study; an OCT-based intra-operative imaging method for blood flow detection during esophagectomy with gastric tube reconstruction is investigated. Change in perfusion of the gastric tube tissue can lead to ischemia; with a high morbidity and mortality as a result. Anastomotic leakage (incidence 5–20%) is one of the most severe complications after esophagectomy with gastric tube reconstruction. Optical imaging techniques provide for minimal-invasive and real-time visualization tools that can be used in intraoperative settings. By implementing an optical technique for blood flow detection during surgery; perfusion can be imaged and quantified and; if needed; perfusion can be improved by either a surgical intervention or the administration of medication. The feasibility of imaging gastric microcirculation in vivo using optical coherence tomography (OCT) during surgery of patients with esophageal cancer by visualizing blood flow based on the speckle contrast from M-mode OCT images is studied. The percentage of pixels exhibiting a speckle contrast value indicative of flow was quantified to serve as an objective parameter to assess blood flow at 4 locations on the reconstructed gastric tube. Here; it was shown that OCT can be used for direct blood flow imaging during surgery and may therefore aid in improving surgical outcomes for patients.

Keywords: flow; monitoring; OCT; optical imaging; surgery; esophagectomy; gastric tube; perfusion; speckle

---

1. Introduction

The viability of cells and tissue mainly depends on blood flow as it transports oxygen and nutrients to the cells. Without oxygen and nutrients, ischemia occurs and tissue becomes necrotic [1]. An esophageal resection with ensuing gastric tube reconstruction is the cornerstone of treatment in patients with esophageal cancer. To be able to pull up the gastric tube, ligation of the left gastric artery, the left gastro-epiploic artery, the short gastric vessels and some branches of the right gastric artery is needed. As a result, perfusion of the tube's gastric tissue after reconstruction relies on the right gastroepiploic artery and some branches of the right gastric artery [2] leaving the future neo-esophageal anastomotic site depending only on collateral blood flow.

Anastomotic leakage (incidence 5–20%) and stricture (10–22%) are major complications following esophagectomy, and mortality is as high as 4% [2]. Perfusion deficiency of the gastric tube is seen as the major risk factor to develop these complications, which, in turn, correlate with high morbidity, IC-unit stay, high costs in healthcare and decreased quality of life [3]. Monitoring perfusion would allow surgeons to make different choices in their surgical design [4] and, if needed, involve anesthesiology interventions to optimize perfusion by the use of fluid or medication [5]. Consequently, intra-operative perfusion monitoring could potentially aid in achieving better patient outcomes after surgery and in decreasing complications and mortality.

Optical techniques are well-suited for intra-operative monitoring due to their minimal-invasive and real-time visualization capabilities [6]. Optical Coherence Tomography (OCT) allows high-resolution, non-invasive, real-time imaging of tissue [7]. It detects backscattered near-infrared light from tissue to obtain depth-resolved, in vivo images. As a result, this technique potentially allows visualization of vasculature in different tissue layers until a depth of approximately 2.5 mm [8]. Moreover, the underlying arteries will not influence the measured perfusion in the overlaying microvascular network, in contrast to other optical imaging techniques like fluorescence imaging, laser speckle contrast imaging or laser Doppler flowmetry [9–11]. Finally, a handheld OCT probe is easy to use in the operation room.

A large number of studies have investigated and established the link between OCT speckle and the flow of the imaged medium, ranging from qualitative detection of flow to quantitative analysis of the flow parameter in very controlled measurement settings [8,12–14]. By analyzing the speckle variance [15] or speckle decorrelation [12] of OCT data, flow can be discriminated from static tissue in order to visualize blood vessels and microcirculation. In previous studies we have shown that OCT speckle decorrelation can be used to obtain a quantitative blood flow parameter [8,14]. However, because of the needed fixation during imaging, these systems are not readily applicable in the operating room. Therefore, for the visualization of flow during surgery, in this study we use speckle contrast in the OCT M-mode scans to distinguish flow from static tissue.

The aim of this study is to research the feasibility of a commercially available OCT system to detect blood vessels in gastric tissue, in patients with esophageal cancer in a clinical setting during esophageal cancer surgery with gastric tube reconstruction. 3D OCT scans are obtained to image tissue layers in the reconstructed gastric tube and compared to histopathological slides, yielding information about tissue structure and blood vessel locations. In this paper, speckle contrast, the ratio of speckle variance over the mean, is calculated from OCT M-mode scans to distinguish areas with flow from static tissue. The percentage of pixels indicative of flow is used as an objective parameter to compare blood flow at different locations, ranging from normal perfusion, near the remaining right gastroepiploic artery and/or branches of the right gastric artery, to decreased perfusion, near the future anastomotic side.

2. Materials and Methods

This prospective, observational, in vivo pilot study of 26 patients with esophageal cancer who underwent an esophageal resection with gastric tube reconstruction was approved by the medical ethics committee (NL52377.018.15) of the Academic Medical Center of Amsterdam, and submitted at the clinicaltrials.gov database (NCT02902549) [16]. Patients were included in this study between October 2015 and June 2016 in the Academic Medical Center (Amsterdam, The Netherlands). Written informed consent was obtained at least one week before surgery. Surgery was performed by two experienced upper-gastrointestinal surgeons (MIvBH, SSG).

Usually, patients undergo a minimally invasive Ivor Lewis procedure (2-stage procedure with intra-thoracic anastomosis), however, in case of a mid- or proximal esophageal carcinoma, a minimally invasive McKeown procedure (3-stage procedure with cervical anastomosis) was performed. Mobilization and vascularization of the gastric conduit was the same in both procedures.

The procedures have been described in detail before [5]. In brief, during the abdominal phase a lymphadenectomy and mobilization of the stomach was performed, ligating the left gastric artery, some branches of the right gastric artery at the level of the angulus, the left gastro-epiploic artery and the short gastric vessels (Figure 1). During the thoracic phase a lymphadenectomy was performed, the esophagus was mobilized and after extraction of the specimen and gastric pull-up an intrathoracic or a cervical anastomosis was created. In all patients, a 3–4 cm wide gastric tube was reconstructed using a powered ECHOLON FLEX Stapler (Ethicon, Johnson & Johnson Health Care Systems, Piscataway, NJ, USA). Branches of the right gastric artery supply the remains of the lesser curvature. The right gastro-epiploic artery supplies the greater curvature until the watershed area with the left gastro-epiploic artery.

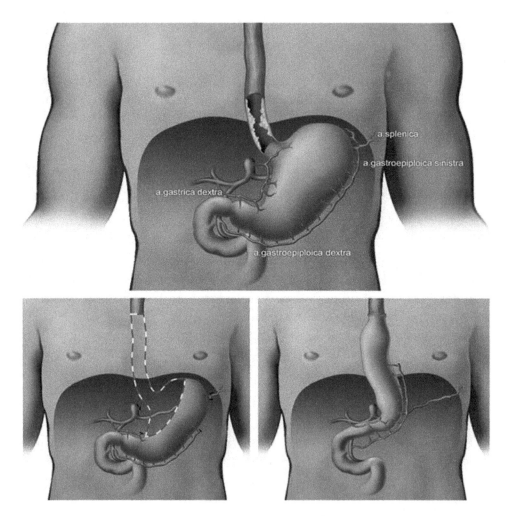

Figure 1. Esophageal cancer with gastric vascularization, esophagectomy and gastric tube reconstruction with only one artery left (gastroepiploic artery).

OCT data were recorded using a commercial 50 kHz IVS 2000 swept source OCT system (THORLABS, Newton, NJ, USA) operating at a center wavelength of ~1300 nm. The full width half maximum axial and lateral resolutions were measured to be ~14 μm and ~25 μm, respectively. Volumetric images (x, y, z) of 10 mm by 10 mm by 2.5 mm, containing 1024 by 1024 by 400 pixels, and M-mode scans (x, y, z) of 0 mm by 10 mm by 2.5 mm, containing 1024, 1024, 400 pixels were collected. The depth axis was corrected for the refractive index of tissue (n_{ref} = 1.4) (Figure 2).

A sterile sheet was placed around the probe for the intra-operative measurements on gastric tissue. Measurements were taken with a hand-held OCT probe directly after preparation of the gastric tube, at four perfusion areas: 3 cm proximal of the level of the watershed between the right and left gastro-epiploic arteries (location 1), at the level of the watershed between the right and left gastro-epiploic arteries (location 2), 3 cm distal to the watershed between the right and left gastro-epiploic arteries (location 3) and at the level of the gastric fundus (location 4), physiologically from normal perfusion to decreased perfusion. Time to obtain data was recorded in the CRF.

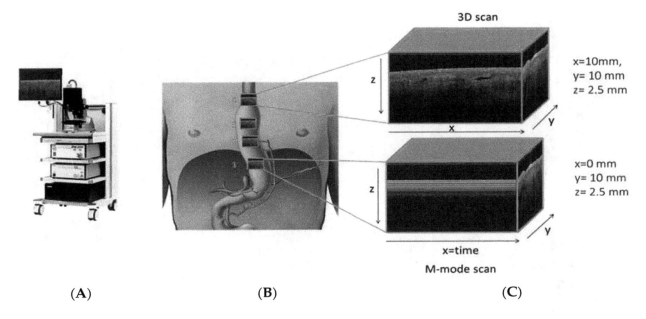

Figure 2. Santec OCT system (panel **A**), schematic figure (panel **B**) of gastric tube with ROI of 10 × 10 mm of OCT grayscale images at four perfusion areas, with shadowing of vessels in cross sectional OCT image (panel **C**).

Tissue from the fundus of the gastric tube was obtained for histology (n = 5) in 5 patients during surgery, with the aim to correlate these findings to the OCT scans. After routine processing of the tissue HE-stained, slides were digitized and evaluated by a pathologist (SLM) to define tissue layers and localize different structures, such as blood and lymph vessels. Different tissue layers (serosa, subserosa and muscularis propria) and blood and lymph vessels were annotated and compared to OCT scans.

All data analysis was performed using custom-made scripts written in MATLAB (Mathworks, Natick, MA, USA). Using the M-mode scans, the speckle contrast (C) as a function of time was quantified in order to differentiate regions of flow from regions of static tissue. To this end, the following processing steps were applied to the data (Figure 3). First, a dB mask (−2 dB) was applied to exclude noise from the OCT data, where after a region of interest (ROI) in the Y-Z image is chosen to exclude corrupted parts of the scan, if needed. Second, the pixel-specific speckle contrast is calculated along the time axis for all pixels selected. The speckle contrast is the ratio of the amplitude variance over the mean amplitude [17]. The amplitude of regions with flow on OCT M-mode scans are expected to be Rayleigh distributed and hence have a speckle contrast value of 0.52 [18]. Here, we have used a speckle contrast gate between 0.42 and 0.62 to detect areas with flow. Next, a median filter with a kernel of 7 by 3 pixels is applied to the speckle contrast images. The pixels remaining after filtering are labeled as flow. The boundaries of the speckle contrast gate and the size of the median filter kernel are optimized by comparing the resulting speckle contrast images with the original X-Z M-mode scans by eye in five randomly chosen scans. Finally, an overlay is created using a Y-Z plot of the gated and filtered speckle contrast and the Y-Z grayscale OCT image. The percentage of pixels labelled as flow relative to the total number of pixels is calculated as an objective parameter to indicate the amount of vessels in the analyzed area.

The ability of the proposed method to distinguish pixels with flow from static tissue based on a speckle contrast gate between 0.42 and 0.62 was validated on a tissue mimicking flow phantom [8]. To simulate human perfusion heparinized human whole blood was flown with a velocity of 5 mm/s through a channel with a 100 μm diameter embedded in scattering silicon. The details on the manufacturing of the flow phantom are described elsewhere [8]. Single M-mode OCT scans (400 × 400 pixels) were collected at a static and flow region of the phantom and the speckle contrast was calculated as a function of depth.

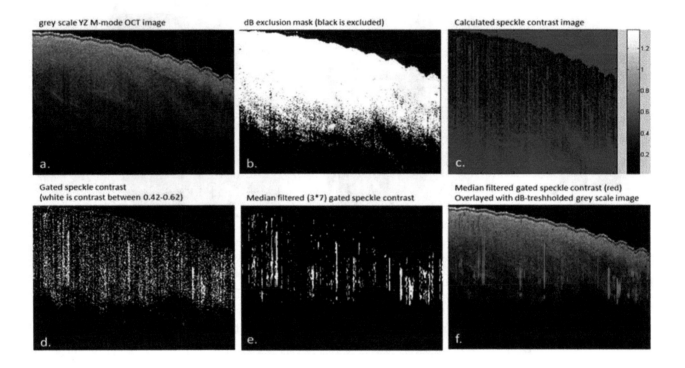

Figure 3. Data analysis steps of OCT M-mode scans, all images are shown from the y-z plane. (**a**) grayscale y-z M-mode scan; (**b**) applied dB mask to exclude noise from the data, the white areas on this image are included as data (**c**) over the time scale calculated speckle contrast values (of regions of included data after the dB threshold (**d**) speckle contrast within the 0.42–0.62 gate plotted in white (**e**) speckle contrast after applying a median filter with a 7 × 3 pixel kernel (**f**) gated and filtered speckle contrast (red) overlaid with the grayscale OCT image.

3. Results

3.1. Patients and Feasibility of Intra-Operative OCT Imaging

In total, 26 patients signed informed consent. Four patients were excluded based on delay in operation time (measurements interrupted the operation by ±20 min), which made imaging impossible considering patient safety. Therefore 22 patients were included for data acquisition (Figure 4). In all 22 patients, 3D OCT images were acquired at four locations of the gastric tube, from the base to the fundus, the future anastomotic site ($n = 88$). Furthermore, M-mode scans were acquired at the same four locations of the gastric tube, from physiologically expected normal to decreased perfusion ($n = 88$). Speckle contrast analysis was not possible for all acquired M-mode scans due to poor quality of the scans (e.g., specular reflections, out of focus, and crossing zero-delay). In most cases the quality of the scans was hampered by specular reflections from the sterile sheet on top of the tissue. In total 48 M-mode scans were excluded. In four patients ($n = 12$) OCT data acquisition and speckle contrast analysis yielding areas indicative of flow (%) was successful at all four locations.

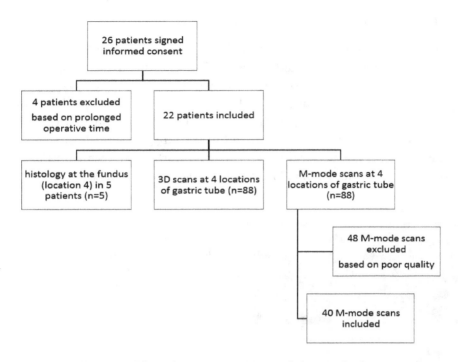

Figure 4. Flow diagram: patient and data inclusion.

3.2. 3D OCT Scans

3D images were obtained at four locations of the gastric tube (Figure 5). On the 3D scans, different tissue layers could be distinguished. By comparison with histopathology slides, these layers could be identified. Importantly, the localization of the blood vessels of the reconstructed gastric tube was similar in OCT images compared to histopathology (Figure 6). Furthermore, because lymph fluid is a low-scattering medium, lymph vessels could be identified in the OCT images as well.

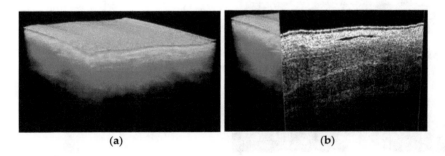

(a)   (b)

Figure 5. 3D OCT scan of the gastric tube, (**a**) volumetric representation (**b**) with cross section visualized.

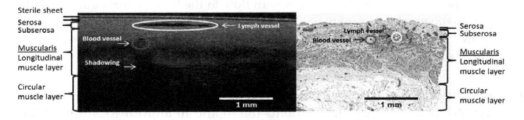

Figure 6. OCT B-scan of location 4, the fundus (at the left panel), and HE stained histology slide (the right panel) obtained at the end of the gastric tube. Blood and lymph vessels are indicated in red and yellow, respectively. The corresponding tissue layers, serosa, subserosa (purple/dark pink) and muscularis propria (light pink) are depicted in both panels. The scale bar depicts a length of 1 mm.

3.3. Speckle Contrast Analysis of M-Mode OCT Scans

Areas indicative of flow could be distinguished from static tissue by calculating the speckle contrast in the M-mode images. As depicted in Figure 7A, the contrast calculated for a single M-mode scan for static tissue was mostly below 0.4, unless the SNR was too low as observed at larger depths. When flow was present in the channel at 0.2 mm below the surface, the speckle contrast was between 0.42 and 0.62 (Figure 7B). Please note that an increase in the speckle contrast was observed below the flow channel as well. Similar effects were observed in the single M-mode scans of the reconstructed gastric tube, as depicted in Figure 7C for the less perfused part of the tissue and in Figure 7D in which a blood vessel was present at a depth of 0.2 mm below the tissue surface.

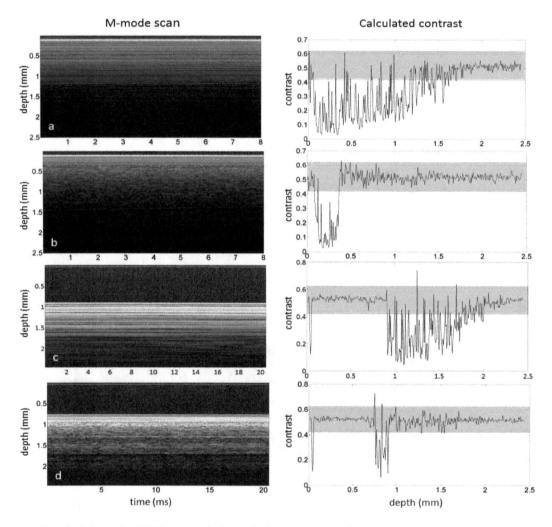

Figure 7. Single M-mode OCT scans (**left**) and the corresponding calculated contrast (**right**) of a. a static region of the flow phantom, b. a region with flow in the flow phantom in which the red line depicts the approximated location of the top of the flow channel, c. a static region of tissue and d. a region with flow in tissue by a blood vessel at approximately 0.2 mm below the tissue surface. The red bar depicts the speckle contrast threshold used in this manuscript.

Calculation of speckle contrast percentage (%) as a parameter for tissue areas with flow was possible in 13 ($n = 40$) of the 22 included patients (59%) and in all four locations in 4 ($n = 12$) of the 22 patients (14%) (for data inclusion and exclusion criteria, see first results section and Figure 4). We observed a decrease in speckle contrast percentage (%) from location 1 to location 4 in 6 of the 13 patients (46%) and an increase in 3 of the 13 patients (23%). The speckle contrast percentage data at location 1 or 4 was missing for 3 out of 13 patients.

The results, percentage pixels indicating flow relative to the total number of pixels, per patient and location are summarized in Table 1 and Figure 8. In 10 patients, data analysis was possible for location 4. In 80% of these patients, percentage of flow pixels was lower compared to location 1, 2 or 3.

Table 1. Percentage of pixels indicative of flow per patient per location obtained from the OCT M-mode scans. In red the flow in location 4 of the gastric tube.

Patient	pt2	pt3	pt4	pt5	pt6	pt9	pt12	pt14	pt16	pt17	pt18	pt19	pt20	pt21	pt22
location 1	5	8	18	22	x	24	x	16	x	13	20	8	12	11	15
location 2	x	x	x	x	x	28	2	17	8	10	6	9	4	8	8
location 3	14	8	x	x	x	23	5	14	x	24	x	2	x	x	3
location 4	11	1	14	17	18	16	x	13	x	21	x	0	1	x	x

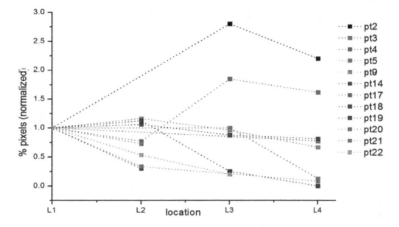

Figure 8. Normalized percentage of pixels per patient per location obtained from the OCT M-mode scans. The values are normalized relative to location 1, hence only the plots for patients with a value for location 1 are shown.

For patients 9, 14, 17 and 19 the speckle contrast analysis was possible on all four locations on the gastric tube. Figure 9 depicts the OCT M-mode scans of all four locations for patients 9, 14 17 and 19. A decrease of areas with speckle contrast indicative of flow (red) is visible towards the fundus in patients 9, 14 and 19. The expected shadowing due to multiple scattering [8] caused by the high scattering coefficient in blood is clearly observed in the images [18].

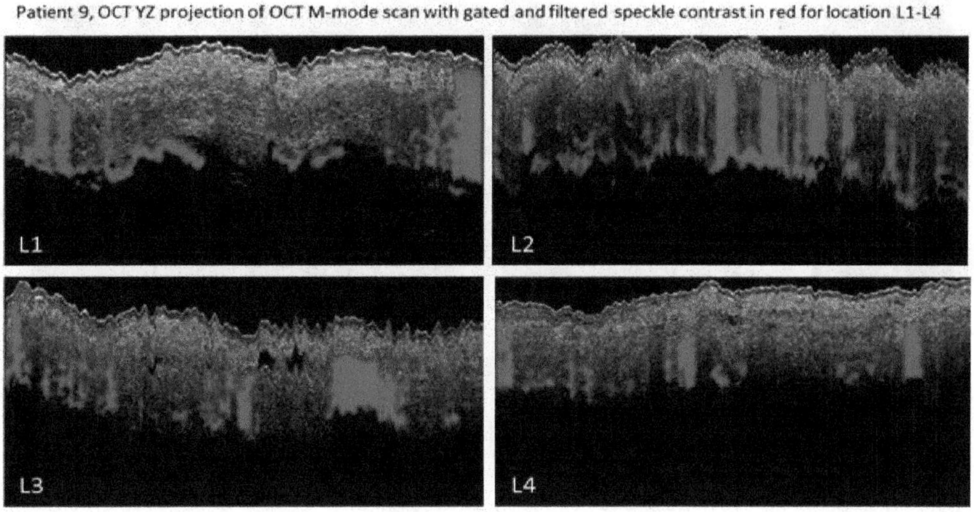

Patient 9, OCT YZ projection of OCT M-mode scan with gated and filtered speckle contrast in red for location L1-L4

Figure 9. *Cont.*

Patient 14, OCT YZ projection of OCT M-mode scan with gated and filtered speckle contrast in red for location L1-L4

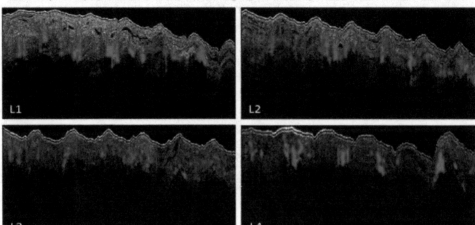

Patient 17, OCT YZ projection of OCT M-mode scan with gated and filtered speckle contrast in red for location L1-L4

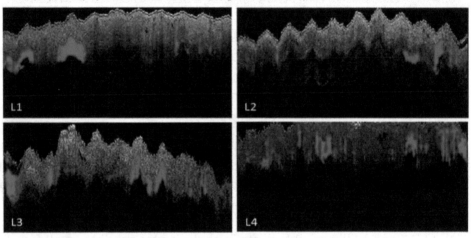

Patient 19, OCT YZ projection of OCT M-mode scan with gated and filtered speckle contrast in red for location L1-L4

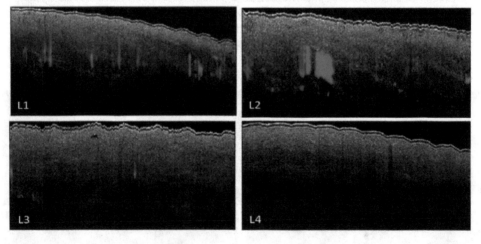

Figure 9. OCT speckle contrast indicative of flow overlaid with OCT grayscale (YZ) images from M-mode scans from location 1 (L1, 3 cm below the watershed), location 2 (L2, watershed), location 3 (L3, 3 cm above the watershed), location 4 (L4, fundus). In patient 9 high speckle contrast indicative of flow is seen in location 2 on the watershed area. In patient 14 and 19 a decreased speckle contrast indicative of flow is observed towards location 4. In patient 17 an increase in speckle contrast indicative of flow from location 1 to 4 is observed.

3.4. Histology Results

Histology of the fundus tissue was available for patients 14, 17 and 19. Figure 10 depicts the OCT M-mode scan of location 4 with speckle contrast in red and the histopathology slide also of location 4 with blood vessels in red and serosa, subserosa (purple/darkpink) and muscularis propria (light pink) tissue layers.

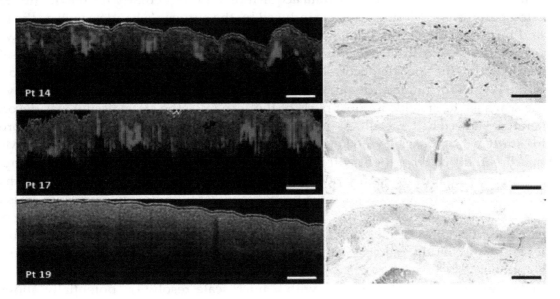

Figure 10. OCT scan of location 4 (fundus), the scale bar depicts a length of 1 mm, and histology slides HE-stained, of patient 14, 17 and 19 with blood vessels in red and tissue layers: serosa, subserosa (purple/dark pink), muscularis propria (light pink).

Although the OCT scan and the histology slide are not one to one correlated, the amount and location of the blood vessels tend to agree per patient. Histology of patient 14 demonstrates many blood vessels localized in the superficial subserosa, which is evidently visible in the OCT scan. Histology of patient 19, in contrary, shows no blood vessels, except for capillaries, which is demonstrated in the OCT scan as well.

4. Discussion

This study is the first that demonstrates OCT imaging of gastric tissue and detection of flow in vivo in patients with esophageal cancer during surgery. We show that intra-operative OCT imaging of gastric tissue and microcirculation is feasible. Moreover, regions of flow could be distinguished from static tissue by calculating speckle contrast in the M-mode scans. The percentage of pixels distinguished as flow was quantified as an objective parameter. This parameter can potentially be used to differentiate normal from decreased perfusion areas.

By comparing OCT data with HE-stained histopathology slides, it was possible to define tissue layers (serosal, subserosal, muscularis propria) and blood vessels. A network of blood vessels was observed in the subserosa. Similar blood vessels, in turn, were depicted in the OCT data exhibiting speckle contrast values between 0.42 and 0.62. Together, these findings substantiate our hypothesis that OCT speckle contrast in M-mode scans can be used to indicate regions of blood flow, while the tissue under study is moving due to the heart beat and respiration.

Lymph vessels were visible as well in the OCT images, assuming that the lymph fluid is a low-scattering medium [19]. Detection and segmentation of the lymphatic vessel, which is outside our scope in the presented work, could potentially add to the analysis of the reconstructed gastric tube OCT data. The clinical value of visualization of lymphatic vessels in the reconstructed gastric tube has yet to be studied.

A limitation of this study is the small number of patients with successful data analysis at all locations. Quality of the images was suboptimal as stabilization of the OCT probe was very difficult. Due to the intra-operative setting, a sterile operational field and hence a sterile drape over the OCT probe was required. This sterile drape introduced specular reflections, which hampered the automated image analysis. This problem could be solved by introducing a sterile probe. Mechanical stability is a general requirement for successful OCT data acquisition and particularly for the quantification of speckle-related parameters. Motion artefacts induced by the surgeon's hand as well as the patient's heartbeat and breathing diminished the quality of the OCT scans by introducing non-flow related speckle decorrelation. Next to visual information, we attempted to visualize blood vessel in the 3D OCT by calculating the speckle decorrelation in adjacent B-scans using the algorithm proposed by Gong et al. [12]. Unfortunately, due to external motion artefacts we were not able to visualize flow in these scans as the speckle in most parts of the scan (also the static tissue) was decorrelated. Previous literature showed better results of microvascular OCT imaging using fixation of the probe [20], which in this study was impossible due to the in vivo, intra-operative setting of this study. Moreover, heartbeat and breathing of the patient will be a problem in imaging intestinal organs, compared to extremities, since the organs are highly perfused and therefore connected to arteries with a large diameter. For future studies, we recommend a probe stabilizer with negative pressure, as is used in SDF imaging, to decrease motion artefacts [21]. Furthermore, optimization of the scanning protocol could increase feasibility of OCT imaging: by using a smaller scanning range, heartbeat and breathing will have less influence on the motions artefacts. Equally, a faster OCT system would decrease the influence of motion in the image and increase speckle stability.

OCT provides depth resolved images with a microscale resolution potentially allowing for visualization of the microvasculature. The visualization of blood vessels located directly underneath other blood vessels is hampered by the shadowing effect caused by multiply scattered photons in the vessels affecting both the OCT intensity and the speckle decorrelation. Red blood cells are highly forward scattering at common OCT wavelengths, which increases the probability of multiple scattering and therefore shadowing. This effect is clearly visible in Figure 7b, in which flow induces the speckle contrast of lower static parts to increase to values similarly to those of flowing blood.

The advantage of OCT over other optical modalities is the depth resolution provided in real-time. Previous research shows the potential benefit of different optical techniques in intra-operative perfusion imaging such as fluorescence imaging [4,22–26], thermography [27], laser speckle contrast imaging [28] and sidestream darkfield microscopy [8,29,30]. Fluorescence imaging creates a wide field overview of the vasculature of the tissue, enabling the surgeon to indicate the perfusion status of an organ or tissue by the intensity measurements of a fluorophore (e.g., indocyanine green, ICG). However, overlaying vessels cannot be distinguished. Therefore, microvascular tissue with impaired perfusion could look highly perfused because of the high flow in an underlying artery. Moreover, for the illumination of vessels with fluorescence imaging, a fluorophore is needed which makes this technique invasive. Thermography and laser speckle contrast imaging are both widely tested in vivo in patients. They both create an overview of the tissue perfusion in a color-coded scale, easily interpreted by clinicians. The disadvantage of thermography for intraoperative perfusion monitoring is the used parameter: temperature, is a parameter exhibiting a slow response to a change in tissue perfusion. Laser speckle contrast imaging, on the other hand, uses perfusion units to estimate the perfusion status, which is an arbitrary unit and therefore not easily interpreted as an absolute value to differentiate good from decreased perfusion. Sidestream darkfield microscopy provides tissue imaging, like OCT, on a millimeter scale. It is able to visualize single erythrocytes flowing through capillaries. However, it can only focus at one imaging depth up to 500 micrometer and surgeons need to focus the camera by hand, which is a challenge considering the motion artefacts discussed previously.

OCT could optimize surgery by improving the understanding of perfusion and intra-operative visualization of the microcirculation. Integration of the software is needed to create real-time evaluation of perfusion in tissue. The proposed speckle analysis algorithm is fast, automated and can be used unsupervised, and can be integrated in the image acquisition software to enable real-time visualization of blood flow during surgery. With this parameter, real-time intra-operative OCT data analysis will be possible. Future studies should focus on the speckle contrast percentage indicative of flow and patient outcome to study a possible correlation and define a threshold value to help the surgeon to decide whether to adjust the surgical plan or not. In the future, OCT-based quantitative perfusion imaging and -evaluation could potentially improve surgical outcome and decrease post-operative complications due to impaired perfusion.

5. Conclusions

This study shows the feasibility of intra-operative OCT-based imaging of gastric tissue and detection of flow in blood vessels in patients with esophageal cancer. Flow was detected by calculating off-line the speckle contrast in M-mode OCT images, from which the percentage of pixels indicative of flow was obtained. This objective parameter was obtained while the bulk tissue was moving and therefor it may be a useful for intra-operative perfusion evaluation. Potentially, surgeons could use a threshold value for quantitative assessment of the perfusion state of tissue and with that improve patient outcome.

Author Contributions: S.M.J., D.M.d.B., T.G.v.L., M.I.v.B.H., S.D.S. and S.S.G. conceived and designed the experiments; S.M.J., M.I.v.B.B., S.S.G. and P.R.B. performed the experiments; S.M.J. and M.A. analyzed the data; L.S.W. and S.L.M. contributed reagents/materials/analysis tools; S.M.J and M.A. wrote the paper with revisions of D.M.d.B., T.G.v.L., M.I.v.B.B., S.D.S., S.L.M. and S.S.G.

Acknowledgments: The authors would like to thank ZonMw for their financial support and Institute Quantivision for their support in trial conception, and I. Kos for her contribution in technical drawings.

References

1.   Futier, E.; Robin, E.; Jabaudon, M.; Guerin, R.; Petit, A.; Bazin, J.-E.; Constantin, J.-M.; Vallet, B. Central venous O_2 saturation and venous-to-arterial CO_2 difference as complementary tools for goal-directed therapy during high-risk surgery. *Crit. Care* **2010**, *14*, R193. [CrossRef] [PubMed]

2.   Biere, S.S.; van Berge Henegouwen, M.I.; Maas, K.W.; Bonavina, L.; Rosman, C.; Garcia, J.R.; Gisbertz, S.S.; Klinkenbijl, J.H.; Hollmann, M.W.; de Lange, E.S.; et al. Minimally invasive versus open oesophagectomy for patients with oesophageal cancer: A multicentre, open-label, randomised controlled trial. *Lancet* **2012**, *379*, 1887–1892. [CrossRef]

3.   Miyazaki, T.; Kuwano, H.; Kato, H.; Yoshikawa, M.; Ojima, H.; Tsukada, K. Predictive value of blood flow in the gastric tube in anastomotic insufficiency after thoracic esophagectomy. *World J. Surg.* **2002**, *26*, 1319–1323. [CrossRef] [PubMed]

4.   Zehetner, J.; DeMeester, S.R.; Alicuben, E.T.; Oh, D.S.; Lipham, J.C.; Hagen, J.A.; DeMeester, T.R. Intraoperative Assessment of Perfusion of the Gastric Graft and Correlation With Anastomotic Leaks After Esophagectomy. *Ann. Surg.* **2015**, *262*, 74–78. [CrossRef] [PubMed]

5.   Veelo, D.P.; Gisbertz, S.S.; Hannivoort, R.A.; Van Dieren, S.; Geerts, B.F.; Henegouwen, M.I.V.B.; Hollmann, M.W. The effect of on-demand vs deep neuromuscular relaxation on rating of surgical and anaesthesiologic conditions in patients undergoing thoracolaparoscopic esophagectomy (DEPTH trial): Study protocol for a randomized controlled trial. *Trials* **2015**, *331*. [CrossRef] [PubMed]

6.   Jansen, S.M.; de Bruin, D.M.; van Berge Henegouwen, M.I.; Strackee, S.D.; Veelo, D.P.; Van Leeuwen, T.G.; Gisbertz, S.S. Optical Techniques for Perfusion Monitoring of the Gastric Tube after Esophagectomy: A review of technologies & thresholds. *Dis. Esophagus* **2018**, in press.

7.   Huang, D.; Huang, D.; Swanson, E.A.; Lin, C.P.; Schuman, J.S.; Stinson, W.G.; Chang, W.; Hee, M.R.; Flotire, T.; Gregory, K.; et al. Optical Coherence Tomography. *Science* **1991**, *254*, 1178–1181. [CrossRef] [PubMed]

8.   Jansen, S.M.; de Bruin, D.M.; Faber, D.J.; Dobbe, I.J.G.G.; Heeg, E.; Milstein, D.M.J.; Strackee, S.D.; van Leeuwen, T.G. Applicability of quantitative optical imaging techniques for intraoperative perfusion diagnostics: A comparison of laser speckle contrast imaging, sidestream dark-field microscopy, and optical coherence tomography. *J. Biomed. Opt.* **2017**, *22*, 1–9. [CrossRef] [PubMed]

9. Alander, J.T.; Kaartinen, I.; Laakso, A.; Pätilä, T.; Spillmann, T.; Tuchin, V.V.; Venermo, M.; Välisuo, P. A Review of indocyanine green fluorescent imaging in surgery. *Int. J. Biomed. Imaging* **2012**, *2012*. [CrossRef] [PubMed]

10. Senarathna, J.; Member, S.; Rege, A.; Li, N.; Thakor, N.V. Laser Speckle Contrast Imaging: Theory, Instrumentation and Applications. *IEEE Rev. Biomed. Eng.* **2013**, *6*, 99–110. [CrossRef] [PubMed]

11. Rajan, V.; Varghese, B.; Van Leeuwen, T.G.; Steenbergen, W. Review of methodological developments in laser Doppler flowmetry. *Lasers Med. Sci.* **2009**, *24*, 269–283. [CrossRef] [PubMed]

12. Gong, P.; Es'haghian, S.; Harms, K.A.; Murray, A.; Rea, S.; Kennedy, B.F.; Wood, F.M.; Sampson, D.D.; Mclaughlin, R.A. Optical coherence tomography for longitudinal monitoring of vasculature in scars treated with laser fractionation. *J. Biophotonics* **2016**, *9*, 626–636. [CrossRef] [PubMed]

13. Mariampillai, A.; Leung, M.K.K.; Jarvi, M.; Standish, B.A.; Lee, K.; Wilson, B.C.; Vitkin, A.; Yang, V.X.D. Optimized speckle variance OCT imaging of microvasculature. *Opt. Lett.* **2010**, *35*, 1257–1259. [CrossRef] [PubMed]

14. Weiss, N.; Van Leeuwen, T.G.; Kalkman, J. Localized measurement of longitudinal and transverse flow velocities in colloidal suspensions using optical coherence tomography. *Phys. Rev. E Stat. Nonlinear Soft Matter Phys.* **2013**, *88*, 1–7. [CrossRef] [PubMed]

15. Liu, X.; Zhang, K.; Huang, Y.; Kang, J.U. Spectroscopic-speckle variance OCT for microvasculature detection and analysis. *Biomed. Opt. Express* **2011**, *2*, 2995–3009. [CrossRef] [PubMed]

16. Jansen, S.M.; de Bruin, D.M.; van Berge Henegouwen, M.I.; Strackee, S.D.; Veelo, D.P.; van Leeuwen, T.G.; Gisbertz, S.S. Can we predict necrosis intra-operatively? Real-time optical quantitative perfusion imaging in surgery: Study protocol for a prospective, observational, in vivo pilot study. *Pilot Feasibil. Stud.* **2017**, *3*, 65. [CrossRef] [PubMed]

17. Almasian, M.; van Leeuwen, T.G.; Faber, D.J. OCT Amplitude and Speckle Statistics of Discrete Random Media. *Sci. Rep.* **2017**, *7*, 14873. [CrossRef] [PubMed]

18. Mahmud, M.S.; Cadotte, D.W.; Vuong, B.; Sun, C.; Luk, T.W.H.; Mariampillai, A.; Yang, V.X.D. Review of speckle and phase variance optical coherence tomography to visualize microvascular networks. *J. Biomed. Opt.* **2013**, *18*, 50901. [CrossRef] [PubMed]

19. Gong, P.; Es'haghian, S.; Harms, K.-A.; Murray, A.; Rea, S.; Wood, F.M.; Sampson, D.D.; McLaughlin, R.A. In vivo label-free lymphangiography of cutaneous lymphatic vessels in human burn scars using optical coherence tomography. *Biomed. Opt. Express* **2016**, *7*, 4886. [CrossRef] [PubMed]

20. Liew, Y.M.; McLaughlin, R.A.; Gong, P.; Wood, F.M.; Sampson, D.D. In vivo assessment of human burn scars through automated quantification of vascularity using optical coherence tomography. *J. Biomed. Opt.* **2013**, *18*, 61213. [CrossRef] [PubMed]

21. Balestra, G.M.; Bezemer, R.; Boerma, E.C.; Yong, Z.-Y.; Sjauw, K.D.; Engstrom, A.E.; Koopmans, M.; Ince, C. Improvement of sidestream dark field imaging with an image acquisition stabilizer. *BMC Med. Imaging* **2010**, *10*, 15. [CrossRef] [PubMed]

22. Rino, Y.; Yukawa, N.; Sato, T.; Yamamoto, N.; Tamagawa, H.; Hasegawa, S.; Oshima, T.; Yoshikawa, T.; Masuda, M.; Imada, T. Visualization of blood supply route to the reconstructed stomach by indocyanine green fluorescence imaging during esophagectomy. *BMC Med. Imaging* **2014**, *14*, 14–18. [CrossRef] [PubMed]

23. Shimada, Y.; Okumura, T.; Nagata, T.; Sawada, S.; Matsui, K.; Hori, R.; Yoshioka, I.; Yoshida, T.; Osada, R.; Tsukada, K. Usefulness of blood supply visualization by indocyanine green fluorescence for reconstruction during esophagectomy. *Esophagus* **2011**, *8*, 259–266. [CrossRef] [PubMed]

24. Kubota, K.; Yoshida, M.; Kuroda, J.; Okada, A.; Ohta, K.; Kitajima, M. Application of the HyperEye Medical System for esophageal cancer surgery: A preliminary report. *Surg. Today* **2013**, *43*, 215–220. [CrossRef] [PubMed]

25. Kumagai, Y.; Ishiguro, T.; Sobajima, J.; Fukuchi, M.; Ishibashi, K.; Baba, H.; Mochiki, E.; Kawano, T.; Ishida, H. Indocyanine green fluorescence method for reconstructed gastric tube during esophagectomy. *Dis. Esophagus* **2014**, *27*, 106A. [CrossRef]

26. Yukaya, T.; Saeki, H.; Kasagi, Y.; Nakashima, Y.; Ando, K.; Imamura, Y.; Ohgaki, K.; Oki, E.; Morita, M.; Maehara, Y. Indocyanine Green Fluorescence Angiography for Quantitative Evaluation of Gastric Tube Perfusion in Patients Undergoing Esophagectomy. *J. Am. Coll. Surg.* **2015**, *221*, e37–e42. [CrossRef] [PubMed]

27. Pauling, J.D.; Shipley, J.A.; Raper, S.; Watson, M.L.; Ward, S.G.; Harris, N.D.; McHugh, N.J. Comparison of infrared thermography and laser speckle contrast imaging for the dynamic assessment of digital microvascular function. *Microvasc. Res.* **2012**, *83*, 162–167. [CrossRef] [PubMed]

28. Milstein, D.M.J.; Ince, C.; Gisbertz, S.S.; Boateng, K.B.; Geerts, B.F.; Hollmann, M.W.; Van Berge Henegouwen, M.I.; Veelo, D.P. Laser speckle contrast imaging identifies ischemic areas on gastric tube reconstructions following esophagectomy. *Medicine* **2016**, *95*. [CrossRef] [PubMed]

29. De Backer, D.; Hollenberg, S.; Boerma, C.; Goedhart, P.; Büchele, G.; Ospina-Tascon, G.; Dobbe, I.; Ince, C. How to evaluate the microcirculation: Report of a round table conference. *Crit. Care* **2007**, *11*, R101. [CrossRef] [PubMed]

30. De Bruin, A.F.J.; Kornmann, V.N.N.; van der Sloot, K.; van Vugt, J.L.; Gosselink, M.P.; Smits, A.; Van Ramshorst, B.; Boerma, E.C.; Noordzij, P.G.; Boerma, D.; et al. Sidestream dark field imaging of the serosal microcirculation during gastrointestinal surgery. *Color. Dis.* **2016**, *18*, O103–O110. [CrossRef] [PubMed]

11

Real-Time External Respiratory Motion Measuring Technique Using an RGB-D Camera and Principal Component Analysis [†]

Udaya Wijenayake and Soon-Yong Park *

School of Computer Science and Engineering, Kyungpook National University, 80 Daehakro, Bukgu, Daegu 41566, Korea; udaya@vision.knu.ac.kr
* Correspondence: sypark@knu.ac.kr

† This paper is an extended version of our paper published in the Wijenayake, U.; Park, S.Y. PCA based analysis of external respiratory motion using an RGB-D camera. In Proceedings of the IEEE International Symposium on Medical Measurements & Applications (MeMeA), Benevento, Italy, 15–18 May 2016.

Abstract: Accurate tracking and modeling of internal and external respiratory motion in the thoracic and abdominal regions of a human body is a highly discussed topic in external beam radiotherapy treatment. Errors in target/normal tissue delineation and dose calculation and the increment of the healthy tissues being exposed to high radiation doses are some of the unsolicited problems caused due to inaccurate tracking of the respiratory motion. Many related works have been introduced for respiratory motion modeling, but a majority of them highly depend on radiography/fluoroscopy imaging, wearable markers or surgical node implanting techniques. We, in this article, propose a new respiratory motion tracking approach by exploiting the advantages of an RGB-D camera. First, we create a patient-specific respiratory motion model using principal component analysis (PCA) removing the spatial and temporal noise of the input depth data. Then, this model is utilized for real-time external respiratory motion measurement with high accuracy. Additionally, we introduce a marker-based depth frame registration technique to limit the measuring area into an anatomically consistent region that helps to handle the patient movements during the treatment. We achieved a 0.97 correlation comparing to a spirometer and 0.53 mm average error considering a laser line scanning result as the ground truth. As future work, we will use this accurate measurement of external respiratory motion to generate a correlated motion model that describes the movements of internal tumors.

Keywords: respiratory motion; radiotherapy; RGB-D camera; principal component analysis (PCA)

1. Introduction

Radiotherapy is one of the highly-discussed topics in the modern medical field. It has been widely used in cancer treatments to remove tumors without causing any damages to the neighboring healthy tissues. However, inaccurate system setups, anatomical motion and deformation and tissue delineation errors lead to inconsistencies in radiotherapy approaches. Respiratory-based anatomical motion and deformation largely cause errors in both radiotherapy planning and delivery processes in thoracic and abdominal regions [1,2]. With respiration, tumors in abdominal and thoracic regions can move as much as 35 mm [3–6]. As a consequence, inaccurate respiratory motion estimations directly effect tissue delineation errors, dose miss-calculations, exposure of healthy tissues to high doses and erroneous dose coverage for the clinical target volume [7–11].

Motion encompassing, respiratory gating, breath holding and forced shallow berating with abdominal compression are some of the existing conventional respiratory motion estimation methods [1]. Difficulties in handling patient movements, longer treatment time, patient training and discomfort are some of the most common drawbacks of these methods. On the other hand, real-time tumor tracking techniques have started to gain much attention due to their ability in actively estimating respiratory motion and continuous synchronization of the beam with the motion of the tumor.

Apart from radiotherapy, measurement of the respiration is an important task in pulmonary function testing, which is crucial for early detection of potentially fatal illnesses. Spirometer and pneumotachography are two of the well-known methods of pulmonary function testing. These methods need a direct contact with the patient while measuring and may interfere with the natural respiration. Furthermore, they measure only the full respiratory volume and cannot assess the regional pulmonary function in different chest wall behaviors. Hence, there is a need for a non-contact respiratory measurement technique, which can evaluate not only the complete, but also regional respiration.

In this paper, we investigate the feasibility of using a commercial RGB-D camera as a non-contact, non-invasive and whole-field respiratory motion-measuring device, which will enhance the patient comfort. These low-cost RGB-D cameras can provide real-time depth information of a target surface. We can use this depth information for respiratory motion measurement, but cannot achieve higher accuracy due to a considerable amount of noise in the raw depth data. Therefore, we proposed a technique of making an accurate respiratory motion model using principal component analysis (PCA) and then using that model for real-time respiratory motion measurement. First, we apply hole-filling and bilateral filtering to the first 100 raw depth frames and use that filtered depth data to create a PCA-based motion model. In the real-time respiratory motion-measuring stage, we project each depth frame to the motion model (principal components) and reconstruct back, removing the spatial and temporal noise and holes in the depth data. We can achieve higher motion measurement accuracy by using these reconstructed depth data, instead of raw depth data. The initial result of our proposed method is published in [12].

The results of this study—accurate measurements of external surface motion—can be used to predict the internal tumor motion, which is an important task of radiotherapy systems. Correspondence models that make a relationship between respiratory surrogate signals, such as spirometry or external surface motion, and internal tumor/organ motion have been studied in the literature [13–16]. Neural networks, principal component analysis and b-spline are a few example models that have been used for predicting the internal motion.

This paper is organized as follows. First, a comprehensive review of related works is presented in Section 2. An overview of the proposed method that describes the key steps and how to handle the problems existing in related works is given in Section 3. A detailed description of all of the materials and methods followed in the proposed method is presented in Section 4. The results of the experiments we conducted to evaluate the accuracy of the proposed method are given in Section 5. Finally, Section 6 concludes the paper by discussing the results and issues of the proposed method.

2. Related Work

The Synchrony respiratory tracking system, a subsystem of CyberKnife, is the first technology that continuously synchronizes beam delivery to the motion of the tumor [17]. The external respiratory motion is tracked using three optical fiducial markers attached to a tightly-fitting vest. Small gold markers are implanted near the target area before treatment to ensure the continuous correspondence between internal and external motion. The Calypso, the prostate motion-tracking system integrated into Varian (Varian Medical Systems, Palo Alto, CA, USA), eliminates the need for internal-external motion modeling by implanting three tiny transponders with an associated wireless tracking [18]. The BrainLAB ExacTrac positioning system uses radiopaque fiducial markers, implanted near the target isocenter, with external infrared (IR) reflecting markers [19]. Internal markers are tracked by an X-ray localization system, while an IR stereo camera tracks the external markers. The Xsight Lung

Tracking system (an extension of the CyberKnife system) is a respiratory motion-tracking system of lung lesion that eliminates the need for implanted fiducial markers [20].

Another interesting respiratory motion modeling technique using 4D computed tomography (CT) images was introduced in [21], where PCA is used to reduce the motion artifacts appearing on the CT images and to synthesize the CT images in different respiratory phases. Mori et al. used cine CT images to measure the intrafractional respiratory movement of pancreatic tumors [22]. Yang et al. estimated and modeled the respiratory motion by applying an optical flow-based deformable image registration technique on 4D-CT images that were acquired in cine mode [23]. In contrast to CT, magnetic resonance imaging (MRI) provides lesser ionization and excellent soft tissue contrast that helps to achieve better characterization. Therefore, 4D and cine-MRI images have been widely used for measuring organ/tumor motion due to respiration [24–28]. Apart from that, researchers have been experimenting with ultrasound images for tracking organs that move with respiration [29,30].

Radiography and fluoroscopy imaging techniques such as X-ray, CT and MRI have the problems of higher cost, slow acquisition, low resolution, lower signal-to-noise ratio and especially exposure to an extra dose of radiation [2,21,31,32]. Additionally, some of these systems have the disadvantage of invasive fiducial marker implantation procedures that increase the patient preparation time and treatment time.

To avoid these problems, researchers have proposed optical methods, which mainly consist of cameras, light projectors and markers. With the advantage of non-contact measurement, optical methods have no interference with the natural respiration of the patient. Ferrigno et al. proposed a method to analyze the chest wall motion by using passive markers placed on the thorax and abdomen [33]. Motion measurement is carried out by computing the 3D coordinates of these markers with the help of specially-designed multiple cameras. In [34], the authors proposed a respiratory motion-estimation method based on coded visual markers. They also utilized a stereo camera to calculate the 3D coordinates of the markers and estimated the 3D motion of the chest wall according to the movements of the markers. Yan et al. investigated the correlation between the motion of external markers and an internal tumor target [35]. They placed four infrared reflective markers on different areas of the chest wall and used a stereo infrared camera to track the motion of the markers. Alnowami et al. employed the Codamotion infrared marker-based tracking system to acquire the chest wall motion and applied probability density estimation to predict the respiratory motion [36,37]. Some researchers have investigated respiratory motion evaluation by calculating curvature variance of the chest wall using a fiber optic sensor and fiber Bragg grating techniques [38,39]. Even though the marker-based methods provide higher data acquisition rates and accuracy, the marker attachment procedure is time consuming and results in inconveniences for the patient. Furthermore, a large number of markers is needed to achieve higher spatial resolution.

In contrast to marker-based methods, structured light techniques provide whole-field measurement with high spatial resolution. Structured light systems consist of a projector and camera and emit a light pattern onto the target surface, creating artificial correspondences. The 3D information of the target surface can be found by solving the correspondences on the captured image of the illuminated scene. Aoki et al. proposed a respiratory monitoring system using a near-infrared multiple slit-light projection [40]. Even though they were able to achieve a high correlated respiratory motion pattern to a spirometer, they could not measure the exact respiratory volume or motion due to the variable projection coverage on the chest wall, which is caused by patient movements. Chen et al. solved this problem by introducing active light markers to define the measuring boundary, offering a consistent region for volume evaluation [41]. They also used a projector to illuminate the chest wall with a structured light pattern of color stripes and a camera to capture the height-modulated images. Then, the 3D surface calculated by triangulation is used to derive the respiratory volume information. However, the long baseline and the restriction of the camera plane to be parallel to the reference frame limit the portability of this method. In [31], the authors adopted a depth sensor, which uses a near-UV structured light pattern, along with a state-of-the-art non-rigid registration algorithm to identified the 3D deformation of the chest wall and hence the tumor motion. Time of flight (ToF) is another well-known optical method that has been used by researchers for respiratory motion handling during radiotherapy [42–44].

With the recent advances in commercial RGB-D sensors such as the Microsoft Kinect and ASUS Xtion Pro, these have been used in a broad area of research work. Have a relatively low cost and the fact that these sensors can measure the motion without any markers or wearable devices encourage researchers to use them in respiratory motion analysis. However, the low depth resolution of these sensors, which is about 1 cm at a 2 m distance, restricts the usage mostly for evaluating respiratory functions such as respiratory rate [45–51], where highly accurate motion information is not needed. In the case of radiotherapy, respiratory motion induces tumor movements up to 2 cm in abdominal or thoracic regions and needs less than 1 mm accuracy in motion measurements [52]. Xia and Siochi overcome the low depth resolution of the Kinect sensor by using a translation surface, which magnifies the respiratory motion and reduces the noise of irregular surfaces [53]. A few other researchers utilized RGB-D sensors to acquire 3D surface data of the chest wall and applied PCA to capture 1D respiration curves of disjoint anatomical regions (thorax and abdomen), which is related to the principal axes [32,54]. However, the respiratory motion measurement accuracy of these methods is affected by the patient movements, as they have not provided a proper method for handling these.

3. Overview of the Proposed Method

In this study, we introduce a non-contact, non-invasive and real-time respiratory motion measurement technique using an RGB-D camera, which is small in size and more flexible for handling. Furthermore, we introduce a patient movement-handling method using four dot markers. These four markers define the measurement boundaries of the moving chest wall, providing a consistent region for respiratory motion estimation.

Using the RGB-D camera, we capture continuous depth images of the patient's chest wall at 6.7 fps covering the whole thoracic and abdominal area. Then, we create a respiratory motion model by applying PCA to the first 100 frames, decomposing the data into a set of motion bases that corresponded to principal components (PCs). Before applying PCA, we use an edge-preserving bilateral filter and a hole-filling method to remove the noise and the holes of the first 100 frames.

According to the experimental analysis, we found out that a respiratory motion model can be accurately obtained using the first three principal components. The remaining principal components represent the noise and motion artifact existing in the input data. We start the real-time respiratory motion measurement from the 101st frame, projecting each new depth frame onto the motion model to obtain the low-dimensional representation of the data. To evaluate the motion in metric space, depth images are reconstructed using the projection coefficient. Figure 1 shows the flowchart of the proposed respiratory motion measurement process.

Using an RGB-D camera for respiratory motion measurement has many advantages. First, compared to the CT/MRI techniques, the proposed method prevents patients from being exposed to an extra dose of radiation. The RGB-D camera is a non-contact optical method and has no interference with the natural breathing of the target. Moreover, this can give real-time depth information of the target surface. Therefore, we can provide a comfortable and efficient, but lesser duration, treatment to the patients. Compared to marker-based methods, the RGB-D camera has high spatial resolution and provides depth information of the entire target surface; hence, we can measure not only the entire chest wall motion, but also the regional motions. The RGB-D camera we use in our system provides depth data in 640 × 480 resolution, and we select a 200 × 350 ROI providing 70,000 data points for motion measurement, which is much higher than marker-based methods (as an example, [36] used a 4 × 4 marker grid providing only 16 data points). The smaller size and lower price of the RGB-D cameras facilitate building a more portable and inexpensive respiratory motion measurement system compared to some other optical methods.

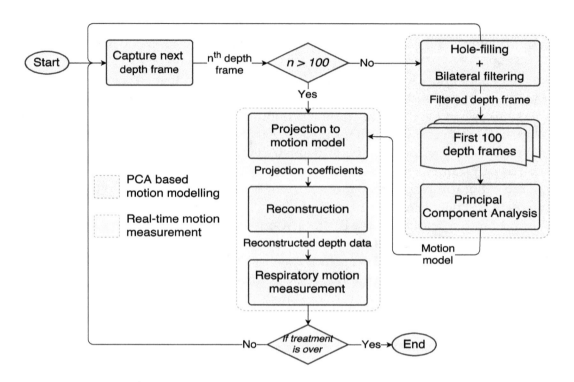

Figure 1. Flowchart of the proposed PCA-based respiratory motion-analyzing system. The first 100 depth frames are used to generate a PCA-based respiratory motion model. Then, that model (principal components) is used for real-time respiratory motion measurement starting from the 101st frame.

However, there is a known problem of low accuracy of the RGB-D cameras. Depth data acquired from low-cost RGB cameras has much noise and many holes that affect the accuracy of motion measurement. Alnowami et al. and Tahavori et al. used depth data acquired from an RGB-D camera for respiratory motion measurement, but could not achieve sub-millimeter level accuracy when it comes to experiments with real persons [55,56]. Using the PCA-based motion model, we increase the motion measurement accuracy by removing the spatial and temporal noise along with the holes in the depth data. When the filtered depth data are used as the input of the PCA-based motion model, we do not need to apply bilateral filtering or hole-filling for each depth frame during real-time motion measurement. Comparing with a laser line scanner, we prove that our method can achieve sub-millimeter accuracy in respiratory motion measurement using a low-cost RGB-D camera.

4. Materials and Methods

4.1. Data Acquisition

We use an Asus Xtion PRO RGB-D camera (consisting of an RGB camera, an infrared camera and a Class 1 laser projector that is safe under all conditions of normal use) to acquire real-time depth data and RGB images of the entire thoracic and abdominal region of the target subjects. The RGB-D camera provides both depth and RGB-D images in 640 × 480 resolution and 30 frames per second. However, due to the process of saving data to disk for later analysis, we could acquire only about 6.7 frames per second. The OpenNI library is used to grab the depth and RGB data from the camera and to convert them to matrix format for later usage. The depth camera covers not only the intended measuring area, but also the background regions. Moreover, the coverage of the chest wall is variable due to the surface motion and the patient movements. However, we should have an anatomically-consistent measuring area during the whole treatment time for delivering the radiation dose accurately.

To handle this problem, we attach four dot markers to define a measuring boundary on the chest wall covering the whole thoracic and abdominal area. Instead of using active LED markers or retroreflective markers, which can interfere with the RGB-D camera, we use small white color circles made of sticker paper.

After obtaining informed consent from all subjects following the institutional ethics, we collected respiratory motion data from ten healthy volunteers. All of the volunteers were advised to wear a skin-tight black color t-shirt and lay down in a supine position. The four markers are attached to the t-shirt, and the RGB-D camera is placed nearly 85 cm above the volunteer as shown in Figure 2. According to the specification of the RGB-D camera, it can provide depth information within an 80 cm to 350 cm range. However, [55] showed that the RGB-D camera gives the best accuracy within the 85 cm to 115 cm range. By keeping the camera closer to the volunteer, we can cover the measuring area with a higher number of pixels, which eventually provides more data points for motion analysis. Analyzing all of these facts, we place the RGB-D camera 85 cm above the patient. Along with the continuous depth frames, visual images are also captured using the built-in RGB camera nearly for a duration of one minute. The RGB images are used only for the purpose of detecting the markers to determine the measuring ROI.

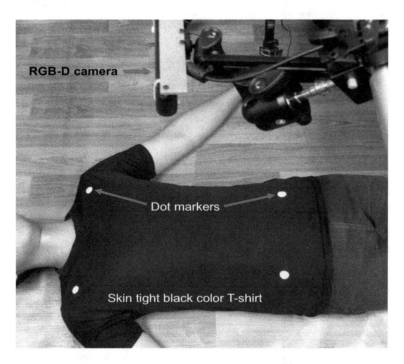

Figure 2. Experimental setup where the patient is laying down in the supine position wearing a skin-tight t-shirt with four white color dot markers. The RGB-D camera is placed nearly 85 cm above the patient.

4.2. Measuring Region

To define the measuring region, we detect the dot markers on the RGB image by applying few image processing techniques. Otsu's global binary thresholding method followed by contour detection and ellipse fitting [57] are applied to identify the center coordinates of each dot marker accurately. Using the intrinsic and extrinsic parameters of the depth and RGB cameras, which are acquired by a calibration process [58,59], depth images are precisely aligned (with sub-pixel accuracy) to the visual (RGB) images. Therefore, the marker coordinates found on visual images can be directly used on depth images to define the ROI, which marks the measuring area. The position, shape and size of the ROI are not consistent throughout all of the depth frames due to the motion of the chest wall and the movement of the patient. In order to make it consistent, the selected ROI on every depth frame is mapped into a predefined size of a rectangular shape using projective transformation [60]. Figure 3 shows the steps followed for detecting the dot markers and creating the rectangular ROI. We use this rectangular ROI for further processing of our proposed method.

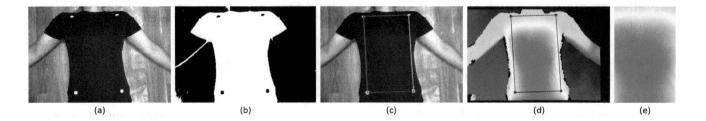

Figure 3. The process of rectangular ROI generation. (**a**) Captured visual image; (**b**) after binarization using Otsu's method; (**c**) defining the measuring area after finding the center coordinates of the four markers; (**d**) identified measuring area projected onto the aligned depth image; (**e**) generated rectangular ROI using perspective transformation.

4.3. Respiratory Motion Modeling Using PCA

4.3.1. Depth Data Pre-Processing

We use the first 100 depth frames to create a respiratory motion model using PCA. Since we use this model for real-time respiratory motion measurement, a precise model should be created using accurate input data. Due to the slight reflection of the t-shirt and device errors, holes can appear in the same spot of the chest wall area for a few continuous depth frames as depicted in Figure 4a. Moreover, there is much noise existing in the raw depth data provided by the sensor. If we directly use these data as the input for PCA without any pre-processing, we will encounter erroneous results as in Figure 4b, where most of the data variation is concentrated in the areas of holes.

To avoid this problem, we first apply a hole-filling technique on depth images using the zero-elimination mode filter. If there are enough non-zero neighbors, this filter replaces pixels with zero depth values with the statistical mode of its non-zero neighbors. Next, we remove noise from depth images using an edge-preserving bilateral filter [61]. Figure 4c shows the PCA result when we use filtered depth data as the input.

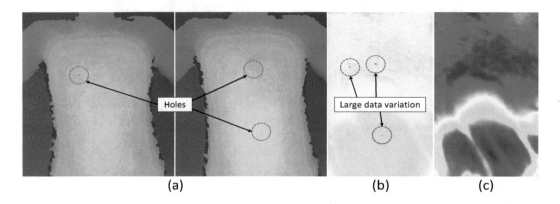

Figure 4. (**a**) Two example depth frames where holes appear in the chest wall region; (**b**) erroneous PCA result (eigenvector) where large data variations appear near the hole regions; (**c**) PCA result after applying hole-filling and bilateral filtering to input depth data.

4.3.2. Principal Component Analysis

After applying filtering to the first 100 depth frames, PCA [62] is applied to make a respiratory motion model that is integrated into the major principal components. By column-wise vectorization of the depth data (d_i) on the selected rectangular ROI, we create an input data matrix D of dimension $m \times n$:

$$D_{m \times n} = \left[\vec{d}_1, \vec{d}_2, \ldots, \vec{d}_n \right], \tag{1}$$

where n is the total number of depth frames ($n = 100$) and m is number of pixels in the rectangular ROI. First, we subtract the mean vector $\vec{d}$ calculated as:

$$\vec{d} = \frac{1}{n} \sum_{i=1}^{n} \vec{d}_i \tag{2}$$

from the input data matrix to create a normalized matrix $\hat{D}$:

$$\hat{D} = \left[\vec{d}_1 - \vec{d}, \vec{d}_2 - \vec{d}, \cdots, \vec{d}_n - \vec{d} \right]. \tag{3}$$

Since $m \gg n$, we use Equation (4) to calculate the $n \times n$ covariance matrix C, reducing the dimensionality of the input data.

$$C = \frac{1}{n-1} \hat{D}^T \hat{D} \tag{4}$$

The transformation, which maps the high-dimensional input depth data into a low-dimensional PC subspace, is obtained by solving the eigenvalues (λ_j) and eigenvectors ($\vec{\phi}_j$) of the covariance matrix using Equation (5).

$$C\vec{\phi}_j = \lambda_j \vec{\phi}_j \tag{5}$$

All of the eigenvectors, which correspond to principal components, are then arranged in descending order $\{\vec{\phi}_1, \vec{\phi}_2, \vec{\phi}_3, \cdots, \vec{\phi}_n\}$ according to the magnitude of the eigenvalues ($\lambda_1 \geq \lambda_2 \geq \lambda_3 \geq \cdots \geq \lambda_n$).

Using an experimental analysis, we found out that the first eigenvalue dominates the rest of the eigenvalues and accounts for over 98% of the data variation during regular respiration. However, when the respiration is irregular, three eigenvalues are required to cover 98% of the data variation. Figure 5 depicts the first ten eigenvalues of the covariance matrix calculated from five samples on regular breathing and three samples on irregular breathing. Figure 6 shows three graphs of projection coefficients (explained in Section 4.4.1) corresponding to the first three principal components calculated for regular breathing, while Figure 7 shows examples of irregular breathing. An apparent respiratory motion pattern is visible only on the first PC for regular breathing, while the first three PCs show a respiratory pattern in irregular breathing. Following this analysis, we represent the respiratory motion model W using the first three principal components ($\vec{\phi}_1, \vec{\phi}_2, \vec{\phi}_3$), reducing the dimensionality of input depth data.

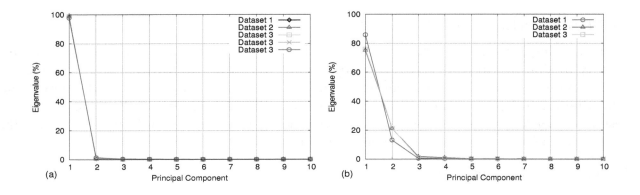

Figure 5. (**a**) Comparison of the first ten principal components using five sets of input data taken during regular breathing and (**b**) three sets of input data taken during irregular breathing. The first principal component is dominant over others and represents over 98% of data variance for regular breathing, while three principal components are needed to cover 98% of data variance for irregular breathing.

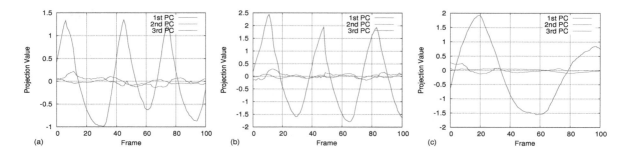

Figure 6. Projection results of 100 depth frames onto the first three PCs. Only the first PC shows a clear respiratory motion pattern for three datasets (**a,b,c**) taken during regular breathing.

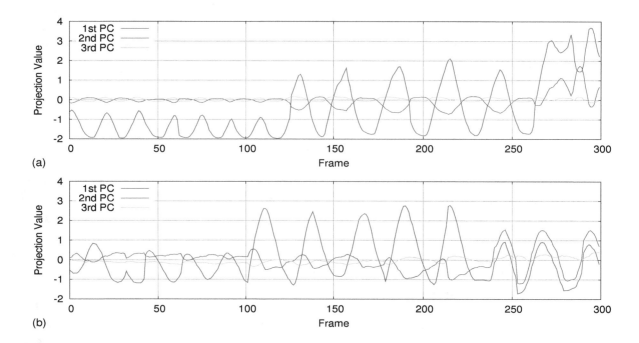

Figure 7. Projection results of 300 depth frames on the first three PCs for irregular breathing. The first two principal components show an apparent respiratory pattern, while the third one also shows a smaller respiratory signal. Graphs (**a,b**) represent two datasets.

4.4. Real-Time Respiratory Motion Measurement

After creating a respiratory motion model using the first 100 depth frames, we start the real-time respiratory motion measurement from the 101st frame. The data we use for respiratory motion modeling should cover a few complete respiratory cycles in order to generalize the input data. By following this rule, we can make sure that the motion model represents all of the statuses of the respiratory cycle. After observing all of the experiment datasets, we empirically select 100 as the number of depth frames for PCA-based motion modeling.

4.4.1. Projection and Reconstruction

We project each new depth frame d_i ($i > 100$) onto the motion model $W = \begin{bmatrix} \vec{\phi}_1 & \vec{\phi}_2 & \vec{\phi}_3 \end{bmatrix}$ in order to represent them using the first three principal components. The following equation is used as the projection operation, where $\vec{\beta}_i$ represents the projection coefficients.

$$\vec{\beta}_i = W^T(\vec{d}_i - \vec{\bar{d}})$$

(6)

Even though the calculated projection coefficients represent a clear respiratory motion, we cannot use these directly for measuring the motion as these coefficients are three separate values in the principal component domain instead of the metric domain. Therefore, the following equation is used to reconstruct the depth data $(\hat{\vec{d}}_i)$, which is in the metric domain, from the projection coefficient.

$$\hat{\vec{d}}_i \approx \vec{d} + W\vec{\beta}_i \tag{7}$$

Here, the advantage is that we do not need to apply hole-filling or denoising filters to the depth data that we use for real-time respiratory motion measurement. By reconstructing the depth images using the motion model, we can remove the spatial and temporal noise, as well as the holes in the data. Figure 8 depicts the advantage of applying bilateral filtering and hole-filling to the input depth images for PCA. Figure 8a,b shows the PCA results with and without using filtering on PCA input data, respectively. As shown in Figure 8c,d, if we use the erroneous PC for projection and reconstruction, many holes and much noise will appear on the reconstructed depth data even if there are no holes in the input data. In contrast to that, if we use an accurate PC for projection and reconstruction, we can remove the holes and noise appearing in the input depth data by reconstructing it as shown in Figure 8e,f.

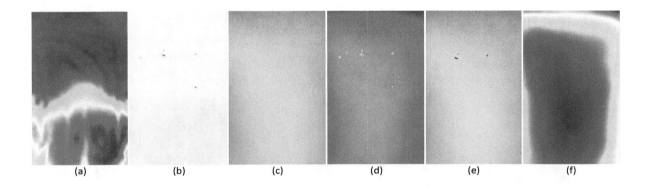

| (a) | (b) | (c) | (d) | (e) | (f) |

Figure 8. (**a**) PCA result (first eigenvector) using bilateral filtering and hole-filling; (**b**) PCA result (erroneous) without using bilateral filtering and hole-filling; (**c**) example input depth image without any holes; (**d**) reconstruction results of (**c**) using the incorrect PCA results shown in (**b**); (**e**) example input depth image with few holes; (**f**) reconstruction results of (**e**) using the PCA results shown in (**a**).

4.4.2. Motion Measurement

We use these reconstructed depth data for respiratory motion measurements. The rectangular ROI of the reconstructed depth data is further divided into smaller regions as in Figure 9a to separately measure the motion in smaller regions. Average depth values of these smaller regions along with 2D image coordinates and intrinsic camera parameters are used to calculate the 3D (X, Y and Z) coordinates of the mid-points. Then, we use these 3D coordinates to construct a surface mesh model composed of small triangles as in Figure 9b,c, which can be used to represent the chest wall surface and its motion clearly. We define the initial frame (101st frame) as the reference frame and calculate the motion of the remaining frames using the depth difference between the current frame and the reference frame.

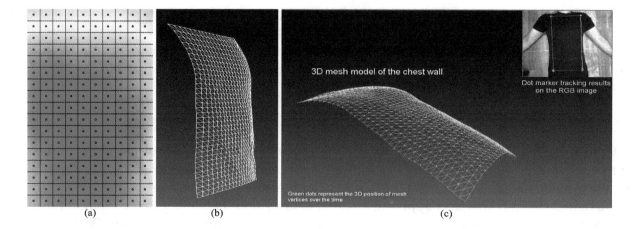

Figure 9. The surface mesh generation process. (**a**) The rectangular ROI of the reconstructed depth is further divided into smaller square ROIs; (**b**) a surface mesh is generated by finding the 3D coordinate of the midpoints of smaller ROIs using the average depth value of the region; (**c**) a selected frame of a video sequence, which shows the motion of the chest wall in a 3D viewer using a mesh model. Green dots represent the 3D position of mesh vertices over time.

4.5. Evaluation of the Accuracy

We propose an experimental setup as shown in Figure 10 for evaluating the accuracy of the proposed method. First, our proposed method is compared with a spirometer, which measures the air flow volume using a mouthpiece device, and then with a laser line scanner, which provides very accurate 3D reconstruction results.

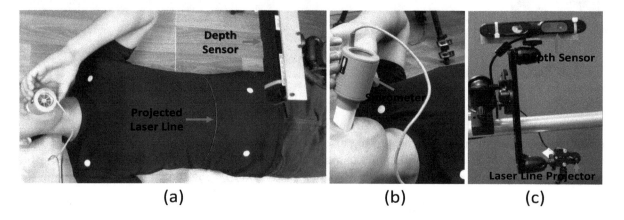

Figure 10. Experimental setup for evaluating the accuracy of the proposed method using a spirometer and a laser line scanner. (**a**) Volunteers are advised to lay down in the supine position and breath only through the spirometer. The RGB-D camera and laser line projector are placed above the volunteer, and the laser line is projected onto the abdomen area. (**b**) CareFusion SpiroUSB^{TM}spirometer. (**c**) The configuration of the RGB-D camera and laser line projector.

4.5.1. Comparison with Spirometer

We compared the respiratory motion pattern generated using the proposed method with a spirometer, which has been used for evaluating the accuracy of RGB-D camera-based respiratory function evaluation methods [41,63,64]. During this experiment, the patient breathed through a calibrated spirometer (SpiroUSB^{TM}, CareFusion) to record the airflow volume while the depth camera captured the chest wall motion simultaneously (see Figure 10a,b). The spirometer provides the air flow volume in liters, not the respiratory motion in millimeters. Therefore, with the help of surface mesh data, we developed a method to measure the volume difference of the current frame compared to a reference frame. We found the volume difference by calculating the sum of the volume of small prisms created by the triangles in the surface mesh of the current frame and their projection on the reference plane as the top and bottom surfaces.

First, these prisms were further divided into three irregular tetrahedrons. Then, the volume of a tetrahedron was calculated using Equation (8), where $a(a_x, a_y, a_z)$, $b(b_x, b_y, b_z)$, $c(c_x, c_y, c_z)$ and $d(d_x, d_y, d_z)$ represent the 3D coordinates of the four vertices.

$$V = \frac{det(A)}{6}, \quad A = \begin{bmatrix} a_x & b_x & c_x & d_x \\ a_y & b_y & c_y & d_y \\ a_z & b_z & c_z & d_z \\ 1 & 1 & 1 & 1 \end{bmatrix} \tag{8}$$

4.5.2. Comparison with Laser Line Scanning

Laser line scanning, which is well known for providing high accuracy (<0.1 mm) [65], is a 3D reconstruction method consisting of a laser line projector and a camera. We used this method to reconstruct a specific position of the chest wall accurately and to compare it with the PCA reconstruction results. The setup for this experiment consists of a laser line projector and the RGB-D camera as shown in Figure 10c. We projected the laser line onto the abdominal area of the target chest wall and captured the illuminated scene using the visual (RGB) camera of the RGB-D sensor. We prepared 15 datasets (D01, D02, ..., D15) from ten healthy volunteers ranging in age from 24 to 32 who participated in the data capturing process. Volunteer information is given in Table 1.

Table 1. Clinical and demographic information of the volunteers who participated in the experiments.

Volunteer	Gender	Age (years)	BMI (kg/m^2)	Datasets
1	M	29	26.4	D01, D02
2	M	32	28.7	D03
3	M	26	27.4	D04, D05
4	M	27	21.5	D06, D07
5	M	25	26.9	D08
6	M	28	26.5	D09
7	M	27	19.3	D10, D11
8	M	24	24.3	D12, D13
9	M	30	20.9	D14
10	M	25	24.0	D15

First, we calibrated the laser line projector and the RGB camera to find the 3D plane equation of the laser line with respect to the camera coordinate system using a checkerboard pattern [65,66]. Then, we separated the measuring area from the rest of the image by defining a rectangular ROI on the RGB images the same as on the depth images. We took the red channel of the RGB image, applied Gaussian smoothing and fit a parabola to each column of the ROI image according to the pixel intensities. Then, by finding the maximum of the parabola, which corresponds to the laser line location, we can identify the 2D image coordinates of it with sub-pixel level accuracy. We projected these image coordinates to the 3D laser plane using the intrinsic camera parameters and calculated the 3D coordinates by finding the ray-plane intersection points. These 3D coordinates are referred to as *laser reconstruction* in the remainder of this paper. Next, we projected the 2D coordinates of the laser line onto the reconstructed depth image $\hat{d}_i$ to identify the 3D coordinates of the laser line according to the proposed PCA-based method and referred to this as *PCA reconstruction*.

The purpose of the proposed method is not to reconstruct the chest wall surface, but to measure the chest wall motion accurately. Therefore, instead of comparing the direct 3D reconstruction results, we compared the respiratory motion; defined as the depth difference between the current frame and reference frame. We chose the 101st frame as the reference frame, as it is the starting frame of real-time respiratory motion measurement. To have a quantitative comparison, we selected five points $(P1, P2, ..., P5)$ across the laser line and found the motion error of each point separately for 100 frames. By taking the laser line reconstruction as the ground truth, we calculated the motion error E_{ij} of the j-th point on the laser line of i-th frame ($1 \leq j \leq 5$ and $1 \leq i \leq 100$) using:

$$E_{ij} = \left| (D_{ij}^L - D_{rj}^L) - (D_{ij}^P - D_{rj}^P) \right|, \qquad (9)$$

where D_{ij} is the depth value of the j-th point on the laser line of the i-th frame. L and P represent the laser reconstruction and PCA reconstruction, respectively, while r represents the reference frame.

5. Results

First, we present the accuracy evaluation results of the proposed respiratory motion measurement method compared to the spirometer and laser line scanner. With the use of the spirometer, we examined the respiratory pattern using volume changes. The laser line scanner was used to analyze the motion measurement accuracy of the proposed method. Later, we compared our method with bilateral filtering and then conducted isovolume maneuver to show the advantages of the proposed method over existing ones. Finally, we analyzed how the proposed method works in a condition of longer and irregular breathing. All of these experiments were performed in a general laboratory environment, and the software components were implemented using C++ language with the help of OpenCV and OpenNI libraries.

5.1. Comparison of Respiratory Pattern with Spirometer

Figure 11 depicts the volume comparison graphs of the spirometer and the proposed PCA-based method. The sample rate of the spirometer is lower than the RGB-D camera. Therefore, we applied b-spline interpolation on available spirometer data to generate a smooth motion curve to achieve a similar frame interval as the RGB-D camera.

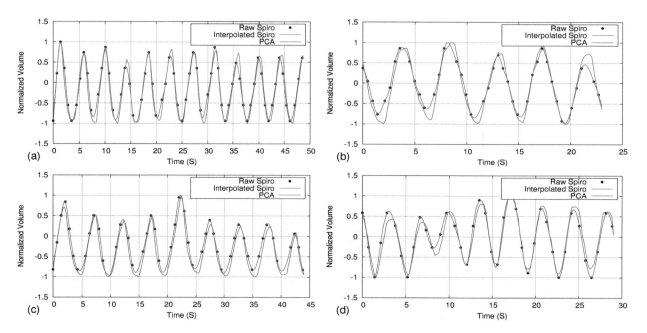

Figure 11. Comparison of respiratory volume measurement (normalized into −1:1 range) using the proposed method (PCA) and a spirometer. Graphs (**a–d**) represent the selected four different datasets. Black dots represent the original data points of the spirometer, while the blue line represents the interpolated data.

The magnitude of the respiratory volume is different between the spirometer and the proposed method, as the measuring area and methodology are different. Therefore, we compared the data by normalizing it to a $-1{:}1$ range. As shown in Figure 11, the proposed method could generate respiratory motion patterns very similar to the spirometer with a 0.97 average correlation.

5.2. Accuracy Analysis Using Laser Line Scanning

Table 2 gives the motion error results of the five points on the laser line, calculated from 15 datasets. We summarized the data on the table as the average, maximum and standard deviation of the motion error (E_{ij}) over 100 frames. The average motion error of all datasets on all five points is 0.53 ± 0.05 mm. As a qualitative comparison, motion graphs of four datasets calculated on four different points of the laser line are depicted in Figure 12. As a further analysis, we calculated the normalized cross-correlation (NCC) between the PCA motion ($D_{ix}^P - D_{rx}^P$) and laser line motion ($D_{ix}^L - D_{rx}^L$) for each x coordinate of the laser line over 100 frames. The graph in Figure 13 shows the NCC results, which was separately calculated for each X-coordinate of the laser line for all 15 datasets. The results indicate a very high correlation between the two motion estimation methods as the average NCC for all of the datasets is 0.98 ± 0.0009.

Table 2. Motion error of the proposed PCA-based method compared to laser line scanning calculated on five locations of the laser line for 15 datasets. All data are given in mm.

Position	Parameters	D01	D02	D03	D04	D05	D06	D07	D08	D09	D10	D11	D12	D13	D14	D15	Average
P1	Average	0.23	0.66	0.18	0.27	0.39	0.36	0.36	0.21	0.83	0.45	0.32	0.36	0.94	0.43	0.55	0.44
	Max.	0.92	2.69	0.66	1.14	0.96	1.41	1.41	0.77	1.91	1.45	1.05	1.47	1.89	1.24	1.51	1.37
	Standard deviation	0.19	0.66	0.13	0.24	0.22	0.32	0.32	0.16	0.47	0.31	0.23	0.29	0.50	0.27	0.38	0.31
P2	Average	0.39	0.34	0.33	0.52	0.22	1.09	0.47	0.47	0.85	0.46	0.30	0.50	0.52	0.97	0.38	0.52
	Max.	1.10	1.34	0.84	1.62	0.66	1.87	1.37	1.31	1.72	1.34	0.79	1.55	1.56	2.51	1.38	1.40
	Standard deviation	0.25	0.31	0.21	0.38	0.16	0.40	0.30	0.33	0.46	0.32	0.19	0.34	0.40	0.66	0.29	0.33
P3	Average	0.31	0.85	0.42	0.50	0.59	0.41	0.44	0.74	0.70	0.40	0.63		1.04	0.57	0.64	0.60
	Max.	1.09	1.90	1.18	1.29	1.39	1.28	1.59	1.81	1.97	1.83	1.03	1.89	2.55	1.56	1.82	1.61
	Standard deviation	0.25	0.44	0.26	0.32	0.34	0.31	0.34	0.44	0.50	0.46	0.26	0.47	0.65	0.36	0.40	0.39
P4	Average	0.42	0.27	0.28	0.51	0.34	0.40	0.36	0.38	1.18	1.55	0.69	0.50	0.74	0.49	0.41	0.57
	Max.	0.95	1.38	0.77	1.72	0.91	0.90	1.03	1.24	2.45	3.18	1.52	1.52	1.86	1.11	1.02	1.44
	Standard deviation	0.21	0.27	0.19	0.46	0.23	0.24	0.26	0.27	0.71	0.67	0.32	0.43	0.43	0.32	0.24	0.35
P5	Average	0.32	0.43	0.33	0.29	0.51	0.89	0.53	0.70	0.37	0.43	0.38	0.70	0.87	0.63	0.73	0.54
	Max.	0.89	2.23	0.96	1.61	0.97	1.68	1.46	1.59	1.27	1.35	1.02	2.04	2.16	1.63	1.79	1.51
	Standard deviation	0.22	0.49	0.21	0.27	0.23	0.37	0.40	0.40	0.29	0.33	0.25	0.59	0.56	0.37	0.42	0.36

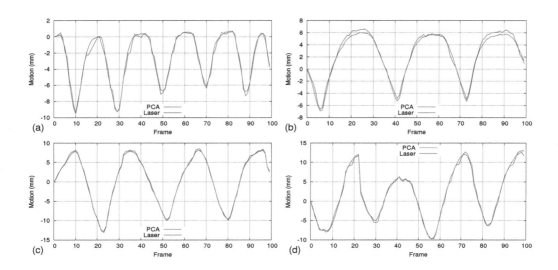

Figure 12. Comparison of respiratory motion measurement using the proposed method (PCA) and laser line scanning. Measurements are taken from different places on the projected laser line. The 101st frame of the dataset is selected as the reference frame, and we measure the motion of remaining frames with respect to it until the 200th frame. Graphs (**a–d**) show the motion measurement results of four different datasets.

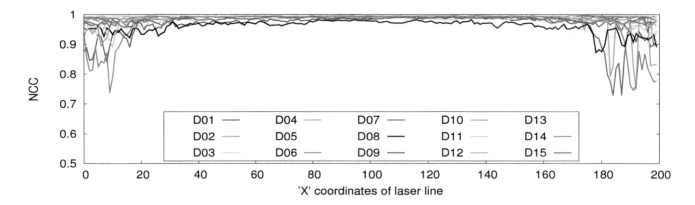

Figure 13. Normalized cross-correlation (NCC) between PCA and laser scanning across 100 frames. NCC is calculated for each point on the laser line along the X-axis separately.

5.3. Comparison with Bilateral Filtering

To show the advantages, we compared our proposed method with bilateral filtering. In our method, hole-filling and bilateral filtering are applied only to the first 100 frames that we used as the input for PCA, and we do not use this during real-time respiratory motion measurements. During this experiment, we measured the respiratory motion by applying bilateral filtering and hole-filling to all frames and without using PCA, and the results are compared with the proposed PCA-based method. Figure 14a shows a part of the motion comparison graph, where the bilateral filtering gives a rough curve with more temporal noise, while the proposed method gives a smoother curve with less temporal noise. The reason is that PCA provides both spatial and temporal filtering, not like bilateral filtering, which provides only spatial filtering.

Furthermore, Figure 14b compares the proposed method and bilateral filtering with a very accurate 3D reconstruction method of laser line scanning (details are given in Section 4.5.2). Considering the laser reconstruction as the ground truth, we calculated the motion error (Equation (9)) of the proposed method and bilateral filtering on a selected location of the chest wall. In the case of the motion comparison provided in Figure 14b, the average error is 0.35 ± 0.06 mm for the proposed method and 0.85 ± 0.08 mm for the bilateral filtering.

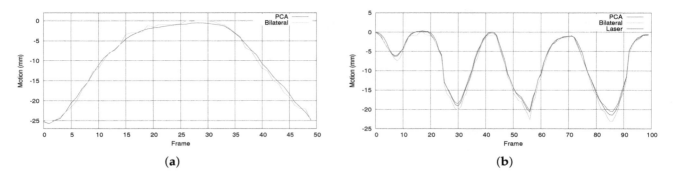

(a)   (b)

Figure 14. Comparison of the proposed PCA-based method and bilateral filtering. (a) A part of the motion comparison graph. The proposed PCA-based method provides a smooth curve, while bilateral filtering gives a rough curve with more temporal noise. (b) Comparison of the proposed PCA-based method and bilateral filtering with laser line scanning.

5.4. Isovolume Maneuver

We conducted an isovolume maneuver to emphasize the capability of the regional respiratory motion measurement of the proposed method. During the test, the subjects are advised to hold their breath without air flow, but exchanging the internal volume between thorax and abdomen. Then, we measured the motion of whole chest wall (which is covered by the four dot markers) and the regional motion of thorax and abdomen separately, presented in Figure 15. We used a few additional markers to separate the thorax and abdomen area on the chest wall. Theoretically, there should be no volume changes for the whole chest wall, but as we measure the depth difference in an ROI defined by the markers, which does not cover the entire chest wall area exactly, a motion pattern appears on the whole chest wall. However, opposite phases of the whole thorax and the whole abdomen motion with −0.99 cross-correlation reflecting the volume exchange between them, which we cannot determine using a respiratory volume-measuring devices such as the spirometer.

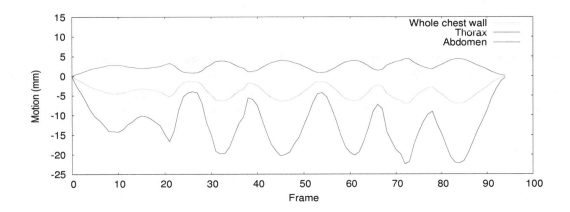

Figure 15. Respiratory motion graph of a volunteer performing the isovolume maneuver. The opposite phase of the whole thorax and the whole abdomen motion reflect the volume exchange between them.

5.5. Handling Irregular Breathing

We analyze how the motion model generated using the first 100 frames affects the accuracy during longer and irregular breathing. For regular respiration that does not have much variation in respiratory rate and volume, only the first principal component is enough to accurately measure the motion. Figure 16 shows two graphs of regular respiratory motion that were calculated over 350 frames compared with the laser line scanning (details are given in Section 4.5.2). Even though we use only the first principal component calculated over 100 depth frames, the average error is about 0.3 mm and 0.8 mm for the two graphs, respectively.

However, during irregular breathing (respiratory rate and amplitude change time to time), accuracy gets lower when we are using only the first principal component as the motion model. As shown in Figure 17, the large difference compared to the laser line scanning proves that only the first principal component is not enough for handling irregular respiratory motions. Therefore, we redo the accuracy analysis including the first three principal components of the motion model and draw the results on the same graph. Using the first three principal components, we could achieve sub-millimeter accuracy (∼0.5 mm) even if the respiratory pattern of the first 100 frames is entirely different from rest of the data.

As a further refinement step for a very long treatment duration, we can update the motion model by recalculating the principal components with a new set of depth data at regular intervals.

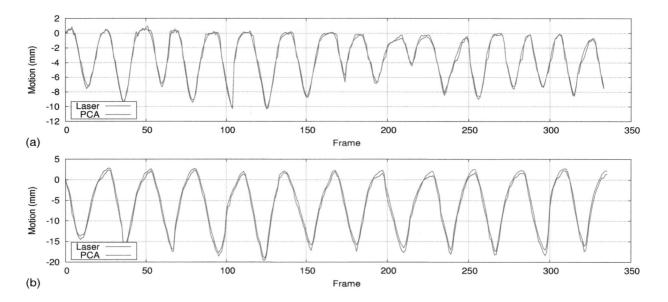

(a)

(b)

Figure 16. Motion comparison graphs generated for a regular respiratory patterns over a longer duration (350 frames). The first 100 frames are used for PCA, and only the first principal component is used as the motion model. All frames are then used for accuracy analysis. Higher accuracy could be achieved even though only the first PC is used for reconstruction. Graphs (**a,b**) show the motion comparison results of two different datasets.

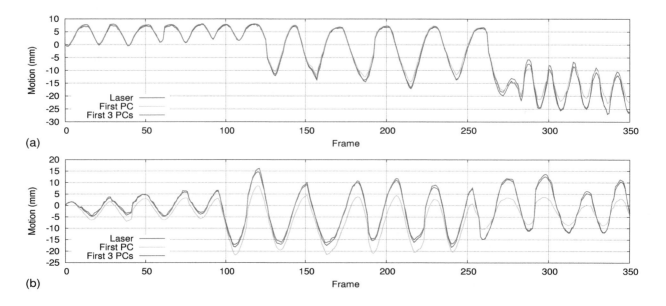

(a)

(b)

Figure 17. Motion comparison graphs generated for irregular respiratory patterns over a longer duration (350 frames). The first 100 frames are used for PCA, and the first principal component and first three principal components are used as the motion models, respectively. All frames are then used for accuracy analysis. A large difference appears between the laser scanner and PCA method when we are using only the first principal component. Higher accuracy could be achieved when we are using the first three principal components as the motion model. Graphs (**a,b**) show the motion comparison results of two different datasets.

6. Discussion and Conclusions

We have proposed a patient-specific external respiratory motion analyzing technique based on PCA. A commercial RGB-D camera was used to acquire the depth data of the target respiratory motion, and PCA was applied to find a motion model corresponding to the respiration. Four dot markers attached to the chest wall were used to define an anatomically-consistent measuring region throughout the measuring period. Using an experimental analysis, we found out that only the first three principal components are sufficient to represent the respiratory motion while the rest of the principal components represent patterns of small perturbations. Therefore, all of the depth data were projected onto the first three principal component and reconstructed removing the spatial and temporal noise existing in the input data.

For the convenience of the volunteers who participated in the laboratory-level experiments, we allowed them to wear a black-colored t-shirt and attached white color dot markers on it. Even though we use a tight-fitting t-shirt, a few wrinkles can appear within the chest wall area and affect the accuracy of the results. Therefore, we recommend not using any clothing that covers the measuring region during the clinical treatment process. We can select dot markers with an apparent color difference with the patient's skin color and directly attach them to the patient's body. Furthermore, it is advisable to attach the dot markers on four locations of the chest wall where there is no compelling motion due to the respiration, such as the end of the collar bones and hip bones.

During respiratory motion modeling using PCA, we used the first 100 depth frames as the input data. The criterion for selecting this number is that input depth data should cover a few complete respiratory cycles. All of our experiment datasets satisfy this criterion within 100 frames. The frame rate during the experiments was about 6.7 fps on average because it takes time for writing/reading data to hard disk frame by frame. However, during real respiratory motion measurement sessions, reading and/or writing data to a hard disk is not necessary; thus, we can achieve a frame rate of around 20 fps. The frame rate was very stable during the experiments with only a 0.4 fps standard deviation.

The accuracy of the proposed method was first evaluated using a spirometer, which has an accuracy level of 3%. Even though the magnitude of the measured volume was different, the spirometer and the proposed method were highly correlated in motion pattern (0.97 average correlation). Second, a laser line scanning technique, which is well known for high accuracy, was used to analyze the motion measurement accuracy of the proposed method. A laser line that was projected onto the abdominal area of the subject was reconstructed using a laser line scanning technique and compared with the proposed PCA reconstruction method. The motion of the projected laser line is measured using the both reconstruction results with respect to a reference frame. We could achieve high correlation (0.98 NCC) between the laser line scanner and the proposed method. Considering the laser scanning results as the ground truth, the measured average motion error of the proposed method is 0.53 mm, which is very comparable to commercial respiratory tracking systems according to Table 3.

Table 3. Accuracy comparison of the proposed method with related respiratory motion tracking methods.

System	Accuracy
Synchrony [17]	<1.5 mm
ExacTrac [19,67]	<1.0 mm
Calypso [18]	<1.5 mm
Yang et al. [23]	1.1 ± 0.8 mm
Chen et al. [41]	$4.25 \pm 3.49\%$
Alnowami et al. [55]	3.1 ± 0.6 mm
Proposed Method	0.53 ± 0.25 mm

The proposed method provides not only a high accuracy, but also a very simple system setup, which is very flexible and portable. With the advantage of non-contact measurement, the proposed method has no interference with the patient's respiration and, hence, provides more accurate measurements. Furthermore, the proposed method has the advantage of measuring the motion in a particular location of the chest wall, instead of measuring the motion of the whole chest wall at once.

Finding a motion model that can be used to correlate the external respiratory motion with internal tumor motion has been discussed in the literature [14–16]. Linear, polynomial, b-spline and PCA-based models are a few techniques that have been investigated so far. As future work, we are also planning to work on finding a correlation model, that can be employed to measure internal tumor motion, by using external surface motion as the surrogate input data. Furthermore, we are planning to test the proposed system in a real clinical environment using patients with different demographic and clinical properties.

Acknowledgments: This work was supported partly by 'The Cross-Ministry Giga KOREA Project' grant funded by the Korea Government (MSIT) (No.GK17P0300, Real-time 4D reconstruction of dynamic objects for ultra-realistic service), and partly by the Convergence R&D Development Project of the Small and Medium Administration, Republic of Korea (S2392741).

Author Contributions: U.W. developed the software components, conducted the experiments, analyzed the results and drafted the manuscript. S.P. supervised the study and critically revised and finalized the intellectual content of the manuscript.

References

1. Keall, P.J.; Mageras, G.S.; Balter, J.M.; Emery, R.S.; Forster, K.M.; Jiang, S.B.; Kapatoes, J.M.; Low, D.A.; Murphy, M.J.; Murray, B.R.; et al. The management of respiratory motion in radiation oncology report of AAPM Task Group 76. *Med. Phys.* **2006**, *33*, 3874–3900.
2. Ozhasoglu, C.; Murphy, M.J. Issues in respiratory motion compensation during external-beam radiotherapy. *Int. J. Radiat. Oncol. Biol. Phys.* **2002**, *52*, 1389–1399.
3. Hanley, J.; Debois, M.M.; Mah, D.; Mageras, G.S.; Raben, A.; Rosenzweig, K.; Mychalczak, B.; Schwartz, L.H.; Gloeggler, P.J.; Lutz, W.; et al. Deep inspiration breath-hold technique for lung tumors: The potential value of target immobilization and reduced lung density in dose escalation. *Int. J. Radiat. Oncol.* **1999**, *45*, 603–611.
4. Barnes, E.A.; Murray, B.R.; Robinson, D.M.; Underwood, L.J.; Hanson, J.; Roa, W.H.Y. Dosimetric evaluation of lung tumor immobilization using breath hold at deep inspiration. *Int. J. Radiat. Oncol. Biol. Phys.* **2001**, *50*, 1091–1098.
5. Davies, S.C.; Hill, A.L.; Holmes, R.B.; Halliwell, M.; Jackson, P.C. Ultrasound quantitation of respiratory organ motion in the upper abdomen. *Br. J. Radiol.* **1994**, *67*, 1096–1102.
6. Ross, C.S.; Hussey, D.H.; Pennington, E.C.; Stanford, W.; Fred Doornbos, J. Analysis of movement of intrathoracic neoplasms using ultrafast computerized tomography. *Int. J. Radiat. Oncol. Biol. Phys.* **1990**, *18*, 671–677.
7. Langen, K.M.; Jones, D.T.L. Organ motion and its management. *Int. J. Radiat. Oncol. Biol. Phys.* **2001**, *50*, 265–278.
8. Engelsman, M.; Damen, E.M.F.; De Jaeger, K.; Van Ingen, K.M.; Mijnheer, B.J. The effect of breathing and set-up errors on the cumulative dose to a lung tumor. *Radiother. Oncol.* **2001**, *60*, 95–105.
9. Malone, S.; Crook, J.M.; Kendal, W.S.; Zanto, J.S. Respiratory-induced prostate motion: Quantification and characterization. *Int. J. Radiat. Oncol. Biol. Phys.* **2000**, *48*, 105–109.
10. Lujan, A.E.; Larsen, E.W.; Balter, J.M.; Ten Haken, R.K. A method for incorporating organ motion due to breathing into 3D dose calculations. *Med. Phys.* **1999**, *26*, 715–720.
11. Jacobs, I.; Vanregemorter, J.; Scalliet, P. Influence of respiration on calculation and delivery of the prescribed dose in external radiotherapy. *Radiother. Oncol.* **1996**, *39*, 123–128.
12. Wijenayake, U.; Park, S.Y. PCA based analysis of external respiratory motion using an RGB-D camera. In Proceedings of the IEEE International Symposium on Medical Measurements and Applications (MeMeA), Benevento, Italy, 15–18 May 2016; pp. 1–6.
13. Bukovsky, I.; Homma, N.; Ichiji, K.; Cejnek, M.; Slama, M.; Benes, P.M.; Bila, J. A fast neural network approach to predict lung tumor motion during respiration for radiation therapy applications. *BioMed Res. Int.* **2015**, *2015*, 489679. doi:10.1155/2015/489679.
14. McClelland, J.; Hawkes, D.; Schaeffter, T.; King, A. Respiratory motion models: A review. *Med. Image Anal.* **2013**, *17*, 19–42.

15. McClelland, J. Estimating Internal Respiratory Motion from Respiratory Surrogate Signals Using Correspondence Models. In *4D Modeling and Estimation of Respiratory Motion for Radiation Therapy*; Ehrhardt, J., Lorenz, C., Eds.; Springer; Berlin/Heidelberg, Germany, 2013; pp. 187–213.

16. Fayad, H.; Pan, T.; Clément, J.F.; Visvikis, D. Technical note: Correlation of respiratory motion between external patient surface and internal anatomical landmarks. *Med. Phys.* **2011**, *38*, 3157–3164.

17. Seppenwoolde, Y.; Berbeco, R.I.; Nishioka, S.; Shirato, H.; Heijmen, B. Accuracy of tumor motion compensation algorithm from a robotic respiratory tracking system: A simulation study. *Med. Phys.* **2007**, *34*, 2774–2784.

18. Willoughby, T.R.; Kupelian, P.A.; Pouliot, J.; Shinohara, K.; Aubin, M.; Roach, M.; Skrumeda, L.L.; Balter, J.M.; Litzenberg, D.W.; Hadley, S.W.; et al. Target localization and real-time tracking using the Calypso 4D localization system in patients with localized prostate cancer. *Int. J. Radiat. Oncol. Biol. Phys.* **2006**, *65*, 528–534.

19. Jin, J.Y.; Yin, F.F.; Tenn, S.E.; Medin, P.M.; Solberg, T.D. Use of the BrainLAB ExacTrac X-Ray 6D System in Image-Guided Radiotherapy. *Med. Dosim.* **2008**, *33*, 124–134.

20. Fu, D.; Kahn, R.; Wang, B.; Wang, H.; Mu, Z.; Park, J.; Kuduvalli, G.; Maurer, C.R., Jr. Xsight lung tracking system: A fiducial-less method for respiratory motion tracking. In *Treating Tumors that Move with Respiration*; Springer: Berlin/Heidelberg, Germany, 2007; pp. 265–282.

21. Zhang, Y.; Yang, J.; Zhang, L.; Court, L.E.; Balter, P.A.; Dong, L. Modeling respiratory motion for reducing motion artifacts in 4D CT images. *Med. Phys.* **2013**, *40*, 041716.

22. Mori, S.; Hara, R.; Yanagi, T.; Sharp, G.C.; Kumagai, M.; Asakura, H.; Kishimoto, R.; Yamada, S.; Kandatsu, S.; Kamada, T. Four-dimensional measurement of intrafractional respiratory motion of pancreatic tumors using a 256 multi-slice CT scanner. *Radiother. Oncol.* **2009**, *92*, 231–237.

23. Yang, D.; Lu, W.; Low, D.A.; Deasy, J.O.; Hope, A.J.; El Naqa, I. 4D-CT motion estimation using deformable image registration and 5D respiratory motion modeling. *Med. Phys.* **2008**, *35*, 4577–4590.

24. Yun, J.; Yip, E.; Wachowicz, K.; Rathee, S.; Mackenzie, M.; Robinson, D.; Fallone, B.G. Evaluation of a lung tumor autocontouring algorithm for intrafractional tumor tracking using low-field MRI: A phantom study. *Med. Phys.* **2012**, *39*, 1481–1494.

25. Crijns, S.P.M.; Raaymakers, B.W.; Lagendijk, J.J.W. Proof of concept of MRI-guided tracked radiation delivery: Tracking one-dimensional motion. *Phys. Med. Biol.* **2012**, *57*, 7863.

26. Cerviño, L.I.; Du, J.; Jiang, S.B. MRI-guided tumor tracking in lung cancer radiotherapy. *Phys. Med. Biol.* **2011**, *56*, 3773.

27. Cai, J.; Chang, Z.; Wang, Z.; Paul Segars, W.; Yin, F.F. Four-dimensional magnetic resonance imaging (4D-MRI) using image-based respiratory surrogate: A feasibility study. *Med. Phys.* **2011**, *38*, 6384–6394.

28. Siebenthal, M.V.; Székely, G.; Gamper, U.; Boesiger, P.; Lomax, A.; Cattin, P. 4D MR imaging of respiratory organ motion and its variability. *Phys. Med. Biol.* **2007**, *52*, 1547.

29. Hwang, Y.; Kim, J.B.; Kim, Y.S.; Bang, W.C.; Kim, J.D.K.; Kim, C. Ultrasound image-based respiratory motion tracking. *SPIE Med. Imaging* **2012**, 83200N, doi:10.1117/12.911766.

30. Nadeau, C.; Krupa, A.; Gangloff, J. Automatic Tracking of an Organ Section with an Ultrasound Probe: Compensation of Respiratory Motion. In *Medical Image Computing and Computer-Assisted Intervention—MICCAI 2011*; Springer: Berlin/Heidelberg, Germany, 2011; pp. 57–64.

31. Nutti, B.; Kronander, A.; Nilsing, M.; Maad, K.; Svensson, C.; Li, H. *Depth Sensor-Based Realtime Tumor Tracking for Accurate Radiation Therapy*; Eurographics 2014—Short Papers; Galin, E., Wand, M., Eds.; The Eurographics Association: Strasbourg, France, 2014; pp. 10–13.

32. Tahavori, F.; Alnowami, M.;Wells, K. Marker-less respiratory motion modeling using the Microsoft Kinect forWindows. In Proceedings of Medical Imaging 2014: Image—Guided Procedures, Robotic Interventions, and Modeling, San Diego, CA, USA, 15–20 February 2014.

33. Ferrigno, G.; Carnevali, P.; Aliverti, A.; Molteni, F.; Beulcke, G.; Pedotti, A. Three-dimensional optical analysis of chest wall motion. *J. Appl. Physiol.* **1994**, *77*, 1224–1231.

34. Wijenayake, U.; Park, S.Y. Respiratory motion estimation using visual coded markers for radiotherapy. In Proceedings of the 29th Annual ACM Symposium on Applied Computing Association for Computing Machinery (ACM), Gyeongju, Korea, 24–28 March 2014; pp. 1751–1752.

35. Yan, H.; Zhu, G.; Yang, J.; Lu, M.; Ajlouni, M.; Kim, J.H.; Yin, F.F. The Investigation on the Location Effect of External Markers in Respiratory Gated Radiotherapy. *J. Appl. Clin. Med. Phys.* **2008**, *9*, 2758.

36. Alnowami, M.R.; Lewis, E.; Wells, K.; Guy, M. Respiratory motion modelling and prediction using probability density estimation. In Proceedings of the IEEE Nuclear Science Symposuim and Medical Imaging Conference, Knoxville, TN, USA, 30 October–6 November 2010; pp. 2465–2469.

37. Alnowami, M.; Lewis, E.; Wells, K.; Guy, M. Inter- and intra-subject variation of abdominal vs. thoracic respiratory motion using kernel density estimation. In Proceedings of the IEEE Nuclear Science Symposuim and Medical Imaging Conference, Knoxville, TN, USA, 30 October–6 November 2010; pp. 2921–2924.

38. Babchenko, A.; Khanokh, B.; Shomer, Y.; Nitzan, M. Fiber Optic Sensor for the Measurement of Respiratory Chest Circumference Changes. *J. Biomed. Opt.* **1999**, *4*, 224–229.

39. Allsop, T.; Bhamber, R.; Lloyd, G.; Miller, M.R.; Dixon, A.; Webb, D.; Castañón, J.D.A.; Bennion, I. Respiratory function monitoring using a real-time three-dimensional fiber-optic shaping sensing scheme based upon fiber Bragg gratings. *J. Biomed. Opt.* **2012**, *17*, 117001.

40. Aoki, H.; Koshiji, K.; Nakamura, H.; Takemura, Y.; Nakajima, M. Study on respiration monitoring method using near-infrared multiple slit-lights projection. In Proceedings of the IEEE International Symposium on Micro-NanoMechatronics and Human Science, Nagoya, Japan, 7–9 November 2005; pp. 273–278.

41. Chen, H.; Cheng, Y.; Liu, D.; Zhang, X.; Zhang, J.; Que, C.; Wang, G.; Fang, J. Color structured light system of chest wall motion measurement for respiratory volume evaluation. *J. Biomed. Opt.* **2010**, *15*, 026013.

42. Müller, K.; Schaller, C.; Penne, J.; Hornegger, J. Surface-Based Respiratory Motion Classification and Verification. In *Bildverarbeitung für die Medizin 2009*; Meinzer, H.P., Deserno, T.M., Handels, H., Tolxdorff, T., Eds.; Springer: Berlin/Heidelberg, Germany, 2009; pp. 257–261.

43. Schaller, C.; Penne, J.; Hornegger, J. Time-of-flight sensor for respiratory motion gating. *Med. Phys.* **2008**, *35*, 3090–3093.

44. Placht, S.; Stancanello, J.; Schaller, C.; Balda, M.; Angelopoulou, E. Fast time-of-flight camera based surface registration for radiotherapy patient positioning. *Med. Phys.* **2012**, *39*, 4–17.

45. Burba, N.; Bolas, M.; Krum, D.M.; Suma, E.A. Unobtrusive measurement of subtle nonverbal behaviors with the Microsoft Kinect. In Proceedings of the 2012 IEEE Virtual Reality Workshops (VRW), Costa Mesa, CA, USA, 4–8 March 2012; pp. 1–4.

46. Martinez, M.; Stiefelhagen, R. Breath rate monitoring during sleep using near-IR imagery and PCA. In Proceedings of the 21st International Conference on Pattern Recognition (ICPR2012), Tsukuba, Japan, 11–15 November 2012; pp. 3472–3475.

47. Yu, M.C.; Liou, J.L.; Kuo, S.W.; Lee, M.S.; Hung, Y.P. Noncontact respiratory measurement of volume change using depth camera. In Proceedings of the Annual International Conference of the IEEE Engineering in Medicine and Biology Society, San Diego, CA, USA, 28 August–1 September 2012; pp. 2371–2374.

48. Benetazzo, F.; Longhi, S.; Monteriù, A.; Freddi, A. Respiratory rate detection algorithm based on RGB-D camera: Theoretical background and experimental results. *Healthc. Technol. Lett.* **2014**, *1*, 81–86.

49. Bernal, E.A.; Mestha, L.K.; Shilla, E. Non contact monitoring of respiratory function via depth sensing. In Proceedings of the IEEE-EMBS International Conference on Biomedical and Health Informatics (BHI), Valencia, Spain, 1–4 June 2014; pp. 101–104.

50. Al-Naji, A.; Gibson, K.; Lee, S.H.; Chahl, J. Real Time Apnoea Monitoring of Children Using the Microsoft Kinect Sensor: A Pilot Study. *Sensors* **2017**, *17*, 286.

51. Procházka, A.; Schätz, M.; Vyšata, O.; Vališ, M. Microsoft Kinect Visual and Depth Sensors for Breathing and Heart Rate Analysis. *Sensors* **2016**, *16*, 996.

52. Seppenwoolde, Y.; Shirato, H.; Kitamura, K.; Shimizu, S.; van Herk, M.; Lebesque, J.V.; Miyasaka, K. Precise and real-time measurement of 3D tumor motion in lung due to breathing and heartbeat, measured during radiotherapy. *Int. J. Radiat. Oncol. Biol. Phys.* **2002**, *53*, 822–834.

53. Xia, J.; Siochi, R.A. A real-time respiratory motion monitoring system using KINECT: Proof of concept. *Med. Phys.* **2012**, *39*, 2682–2685.

54. Wasza, J.; Bauer, S.; Haase, S.; Hornegger, J. Sparse Principal Axes Statistical Surface Deformation Models for Respiration Analysis and Classification. In *Bildverarbeitung für die Medizin 2012*; Tolxdorff, T., Deserno, M.T., Handels, H., Meinzer, H.P., Eds.; Springer: Berlin/Heidelberg, Germany, 2012; pp. 316–321.

55. Alnowami, M.; Alnwaimi, B.; Tahavori, F.; Copland, M.; Wells, K. A quantitative assessment of using the Kinect for Xbox360 for respiratory surface motion tracking. In Proceedings of the SPIE Medical Imaging. International Society for Optics and Photonics, San Diego, CA, USA, 4 February 2012; p. 83161T-83161T-10.

56. Tahavori, F.; Adams, E.; Dabbs, M.; Aldridge, L.; Liversidge, N.; Donovan, E.; Jordan, T.; Evans, P.; Wells, K. Combining marker-less patient setup and respiratory motion monitoring using low cost 3D camera technology. In Proceedings of the SPIE Medical Imaging. International Society for Optics and Photonics, Orlando, Florida, USA, 21 February 2015; p. 94152I-94152I-7. doi:10.1117/12.2082726.

57. Gonzalez, R.C.; Woods, R.E. *Digital Image Processing*, 3rd ed.; Pearson: New York, NY, USA, 2007.

58. Gui, P.; Ye, Q.; Chen, H.; Zhang, T.; Yang, C. Accurately calibrate kinect sensor using indoor control field. In Proceedings of the 2014 Third International Workshop on Earth Observation and Remote Sensing Applications (EORSA), Changsha, China, 11–14 June 2014; pp. 9–13.

59. Daniel, H.C.; Kannala, J.; Heikkilä, J. Joint Depth and Color Camera Calibration with Distortion Correction. *IEEE Trans. Pattern Anal. Mach. Intell.* **2012**, *34*, 2058–2064.

60. Hartley, R.; Zisserman, A. *Multiple View Geometry in Computer Vision*, 2nd ed.; Cambridge University Press: Cambridge, UK, 2004.

61. Tomasi, C.; Manduchi, R. Bilateral filtering for gray and color images. In Proceedings of the Sixth International Conference on Computer Vision (IEEE Cat. No.98CH36271), Bombay, India, 4–7 January 1998; pp. 839–846.

62. Jolliffe, I. *Principal Component Analysis*; Springer: Berlin/Heidelberg, Germany, 2002.

63. Hartc, J.M.; Golby, C.K.; Acosta, J.; Nash, E.F.; Kiraci, E.; Williams, M.A.; Arvanitis, T.N.; Naidu, B. Chest wall motion analysis in healthy volunteers and adults with cystic fibrosis using a novel Kinect-based motion tracking system. *Med. Biol. Eng. Comput.* **2016**, *54*, 1631–1640.

64. Sharp, C.; Soleimani, V.; Hannuna, S.; Camplani, M.; Damen, D.; Viner, J.; Mirmehdi, M.; Dodd, J.W. Toward Respiratory Assessment Using Depth Measurements from a Time-of-Flight Sensor. *Front. Physiol.* **2017**, *8*. doi:10.3389/fphys.2017.00065.

65. Zhou, F.; Zhang, G. Complete calibration of a structured light stripe vision sensor through planar target of unknown orientations. *Imag. Vis. Comput.* **2005**, *23*, 59–67.

66. Dang, Q.; Chee, Y.; Pham, D.; Suh, Y. A Virtual Blind Cane Using a Line Laser-Based Vision System and an Inertial Measurement Unit. *Sensors* **2016**, *16*, 95.

67. Matney, J.E.; Parker, B.C.; Neck, D.W.; Henkelmann, G.; Rosen, I.I. Target localization accuracy in a respiratory phantom using BrainLAB ExacTrac and 4DCT imaging. *J. Appl. Clin. Med. Phys.* **2011**, *12*, 3296.

12

Vibration and Noise in Magnetic Resonance Imaging of the Vocal Tract: Differences between Whole-Body and Open-Air Devices

Jiří Přibil [1,*], Anna Přibilová [2] and Ivan Frollo [1]

[1]   Institute of Measurement Science, Slovak Academy of Sciences, 841 04 Bratislava, Slovak Republic; ivan.frollo@savba.sk

[2]   Faculty of Electrical Engineering and Information Technology, Slovak University of Technology in Bratislava, 812 19 Bratislava, Slovak Republic; anna.pribilova@stuba.sk

*   Correspondence: umerprib@savba.sk

Abstract: This article compares open-air and whole-body magnetic resonance imaging (MRI) equipment working with a weak magnetic field as regards the methods of its generation, spectral properties of mechanical vibration and acoustic noise produced by gradient coils during the scanning process, and the measured noise intensity. These devices are used for non-invasive MRI reconstruction of the human vocal tract during phonation with simultaneous speech recording. In this case, the vibration and noise have negative influence on quality of speech signal. Two basic measurement experiments were performed within the paper: mapping sound pressure levels in the MRI device vicinity and picking up vibration and noise signals in the MRI scanning area. Spectral characteristics of these signals are then analyzed statistically and compared visually and numerically.

Keywords: magnetic resonance imaging; acoustic noise; mechanical vibration

1. Introduction

The magnetic resonance imaging (MRI) tomograph is basically a huge intelligent sensor used for biomedical purposes. Two different types of MRI equipment were analyzed and compared in the framework of this paper. They both work with a weak stationary magnetic field B_0 up to 0.2 T but with totally different mechanical construction and different physical principle of this magnetic field creation. A pair of permanent magnets is usually incorporated in the open-air MRI device being normally used in clinical diagnostic practice for scanning smaller parts of human body such as a hand, a neck, a coxa, a knee, etc., or various biological tissues [1]. On the other hand, a resistive magnet containing a water-cooled multi-section coil is used for generation of a basic magnetic field in larger whole-body device enabling MR scans of more complex parts of the human body. Every MRI device consists of a gradient system to select x, y, and z slices of a tested subject. In the open-air MRI system, planar gradient coils [2] are mostly used to minimize space requirements. For the whole-body devices, there is typical use of cylindrical gradient coils distributed around the tube in which an examined person/object lies. There are also many differences in construction and practical realization of open-air and whole-body types of these devices. In spite of all the differences, both devices have in common undesirable production of significant mechanical pulses during execution of a scan sequence. Although magnetic translational forces and torques on diamagnetic and paramagnetic tissues are not of safety concern, this does not apply to acoustic noise as a result of rapid switching of large currents accompanied with rapid direction reversal of Lorenz forces [3]. The radiated acoustic noise can be measured by a microphone and its sound pressure level (SPL) can be mapped in the MRI neighborhood. The component frequencies of this acoustic noise fall into the standard audio frequency range, so it can be processed in the spectral domain and analyzed using methods similar to those of audio and speech signal analysis.

These MRI devices can also be successfully used for analysis of the human vocal tract structure and its dynamic shaping during speech production [4]. For this purpose, the speech signal must be recorded simultaneously in real time while the MR scan sequence is being executed [5]. The speech signal should be recorded with high signal-to-noise ratio (SNR), but an acoustic noise produced by the MRI gradient system degrades its quality [6]. Thus, noise reduction techniques must be applied to improve the SNR of the speech signal [7,8]. One group of enhancement methods is based on spectral subtraction of the estimated background noise [9]. However, noise estimation techniques based on statistical approaches are not able to track real noise variations; thereby they result in an artificial residual musical noise and a distorted speech [10]. Therefore, spectral properties of both vibration and noise generated by the gradient system of the MRI device must be analyzed with high precision so that the noise could be efficiently suppressed while preserving maximum quality of the processed speech signal [11].

The main motivation of this study was to measure and compare intensity, distribution, and spectral properties of mechanical vibration and acoustic noise produced by the low magnetic field MR imagers. As both types of investigated tomographs use the same physical principles for modulation of the basic magnetic field, we suppose comparable results of measured vibration and noise signals. These results can be generalized for next use, e.g., when direct measurement is difficult or practically impossible or undistorted values cannot be obtained. Hence, it is helpful that we can use results from the alternative type of MRI with the final aim to suppress negative influence of noise in the recorded speech signal while using a similar device. The original contribution of our paper lies in investigation and comparison of two low-field MRI devices with similar magnetic flux density differing in construction.

The study also describes measurement experiments performed in the scanning area and in the neighborhood of the MRI equipment. First, for both types of investigated MRI devices, mapping of the SPL was performed in their vicinity. The main experiment consisted of real-time recording of the vibration and noise signals which were subsequently off-line processed—the determined spectral features were statistically analyzed, and the obtained results were visually and numerically compared. Attenuation and reflection of the acoustic wave caused by the enclosing metal shielding cage, and influence of the mass of a tested person/object in the scanning area during execution of an MR scan sequence on the properties of vibration and noise signals were also discussed. Finally, the time delay between the vibration signal and the excitation impulse in the gradient coil from simultaneously recorded electrical excitation, vibration, and noise signals was analyzed and evaluated.

2. Subject and Methods

2.1. Differences in Construction of the Gradient System in the Open-Air and the Whole-Body MRI Equipment

Basic vibration and noise analysis was performed on the open-air MRI device [12] normally used in clinical diagnostic practice. This type of equipment has a stationary magnetic field with magnetic induction of 0.178 T produced by a pair of permanent magnets. The gradient system consists of 2×3 planar coils situated between the magnets and an RF receiving/transmitting coil with a tested object/subject. Different RF coils with cylindrical diameter not exceeding 18 cm are used for MR scans of a human knee, an arm, a leg, thin layers of botanical and zoological samples, or testing phantoms. Due to electromagnetic compatibility and reduction of possible RF signal interference, the whole MRI scanning equipment is located inside a metal cage. It is made of 2-mm thick steel plate with symmetrically placed holes of 2.5-mm diameter in 5-mm grid to eliminate electromagnetic field propagation to the surrounding space (control room with operator console, etc.). Such a perforated surface successfully attenuates low-frequency sound if its wavelength is much larger than perforation thickness and diameter [13,14]. The orifice together with the backing air cavity forms a Helmholtz resonator whose frequency of sound absorption depends on size of these acoustic elements [15]. Since volume of air behind the apertures (surrounding air in a room with a cage inside) is rather great, the Helmholtz resonance frequency is rather low, and this effect can be neglected. However, each flat part of the metal surface (between perforations) may reflect sound energy towards inside if the wavelength of the sound is much lower than the size of this flat part.

The situation is totally different when the whole-body MRI device is investigated. In this case, the gradient system is made up of six cylindrical coils. Size of the gradient coils is also greater, since the tube diameter must enable insertion of the patient's bed with an examined person. In the case of an experimental whole-body MR imager TMR96 used in measurements for this study, the device works with a magnetic field $B_0 = 0.1$ T created by a resistive water-cooled magnet with a diameter of 1414 mm and a length of 2240 mm. The active part of the equipment is enclosed in a shielding metal cage with the size of a small room ($550 \times 340 \times 230$ cm) made of 2-mm thin copper sheet with a smooth surface that is fully sealed except for four ventilation holes. For this reason, it is supposed to be a good acoustic reflector. On the other hand, although the pick-up sensors are arranged outside the scanning area to eliminate interaction with the working magnetic field, they are very close to the examined person lying inside the scan tube, so the effect of reflected acoustic wave superposition can be neglected in the recorded sound signal. More robust construction and greater mass of this device would inhibit its vibration. However, higher energy of the impulse current must be applied to select 3D coordinates of a tested subject, so stronger Lorentz forces [16] act in the gradient coil system. In the final effect, vibration and noise levels inside the scanning area are usually higher than those in the open-air MRI with planar gradient coils.

Preliminary performed experiments have shown that the produced vibration and acoustic noise are principally influenced by a mechanical load of a person lying in the scanning area of the open-air MRI machine [17] where the examined person lies directly on the plastic cover of the bottom gradient coil. The whole-body MRI contains a movable bed which is not directly connected with the gradient coils, but for larger volume of the sample inserted in larger gradient coils, higher electric current must flow through the gradient coils to perform equivalent change in the magnetic field to choose each of the x, y, z coordinates in the selected field of view (FOV) [18]. Higher energy used for generation of the vibration signal also has an effect on its spectral properties. From the acoustic point of view, the test person/sample/phantom placed on the patient's bed changes the overall mass and stiffness of the whole scanning system including the gradient coil structure. These changed mechanical properties result in different vibration than in the case of the plate weighted by the mass of a tested person. It means that, first of all, the spectral properties of the picked-up vibration signal are changed depending on the applied mechanical weight.

2.2. Sensors for Measurement in a Weak Magnetic Field Environment

In general, the interaction with a stationary magnetic field B_0 in the scanning area must be eliminated during measurement experiments to obtain MR images of sufficient quality without any artifacts. The same applies for measurement of noise SPL, excitation signal of the gradient coil system, and vibration and noise signals. In the case of MRI equipment working with a weak magnetic field (up to 0.2 T), the interaction problem can be solved by a proper choice of the arrangement where the measuring device (SPL meter and/or pick-up microphone) is located in an adequate distance from the noise signal source outside the magnetic field area. The choice of a suitable recording microphone was led by its good sensitivity and proper directional pickup pattern. Since the noise depends on the position of the measuring microphone, the directional pattern of the noise distribution in the MRI equipment neighborhood had to be mapped using optimal selection of the recording microphone position and parameters (distance from the central point of the MRI scanning area, direction angle, working height, type of the microphone pickup pattern). The sensors measuring vibration and electrical excitation signals must be placed inside the MRI scanning area where they are affected by a stationary magnetic field—see the documentary photo of measurement in and around the TMR96 device in Figure 1. In the scanning area, there is a high voltage generated by the excitation RF coil of the MRI device during execution of the MR sequence. This would result in large disturbance of a signal from the sensor or in damage of electronics integrated with the sensor. The vibration sensor with a piezoelectric transducer can be successfully used in these circumstances [11,12,17]. It is important that the sensor has good sensitivity and maximally flat frequency response. Its frequency range should cover harmonic frequencies of vibration and noise signals. These are concentrated in the low band due to frequency-limited gradient pulses [19], which is similar to the frequency range used for basic processing of speech signals. The above-mentioned requirements can be fulfilled by the sensor constructed for acoustic musical instrument pick up [20]. Finally, the sensing coil measuring the excitation signal must be designed with appropriate physical parameters (impedance, number of turns, mechanical construction, etc.) together with the input circuits for signal processing.

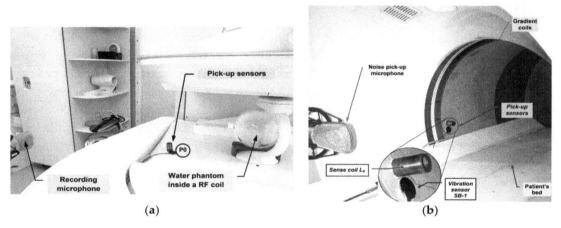

Figure 1. Photo of sensors placement for recording of vibration, noise, and electrical excitation signals in open-air and whole-body devices; (**a**) E-scan Esaote Opera with the spherical water phantom inside the knee RF coil; (**b**) MR imager TMR-96.

2.3. Features for Description of Vibration and Noise Signal Properties

For basic visual comparison of spectral properties of the recorded vibration or noise signals, a periodogram representing an estimate of a power spectral density (PSD) can be successfully used. Another useful graphical rendering is a spectrogram showing all PSD values in a time window moving through the whole analyzed signal.

Basic spectral properties of the vibration/noise are determined from the spectral envelope and subsequently histograms of spectral values are calculated and compared. MRI parameters of repetition time (TR) and echo time (TE) affect the dominant resonance F_{V0} (reciprocal of TR) and the secondary resonances $F_{V1,2}$ (first two local maxima of the spectral envelope where its gradient changes from positive to negative or poles of the linear predictive coding transfer function). Spectral decrease ($S_{decrease}$) is a parameter representing a degree of fall of the power spectrum. It can be calculated by a linear regression using the mean square method. A similar parameter is spectral tilt (S_{tilt}) as an angle between a line connecting spectral envelope values at low and high frequencies and a horizontal line. Supplementary spectral features describe a shape of the power spectrum of the analyzed signal. Spectral centroid (S_{centr}) determines a centre of gravity of the spectrum—the average frequency weighted by the values of the normalized energy of each frequency component in the spectrum. Spectral flatness (S_{flat}) determining a degree of periodicity in the signal is calculated as a ratio of geometric and arithmetic means of the power spectrum. Shannon spectral entropy (S_{entrop}) is a measure of randomness of the spectral probability density represented by normalized spectral components. Spectral spread (S_{spread}) represents the dispersion of the power spectrum around its mean value.

In the last step, relationship between the primary electrical excitation of the gradient coils and the secondary generated acoustic noise is described. For this purpose, the time delay between these two signals must be analyzed. Indirect determination is based on statistical analysis of mutual positions of signal peaks of excitation and noise signals recorded in parallel. From the obtained distances, the histograms of percentage occurrence are calculated in dependence on the signal polarity and the maximum values of time delays Td_{pos}, Td_{neg} are determined [12]. These two maxima are not equal for a non-planar surface of the lower cover of the gradient coil system. This means that vibration travels in two different paths between the point of its generation and the target position of the pick-up microphone. Then the final result is given by a median value of both maxima. The second method of time delay determination is based on direct calculation using formulae

$$c = \sqrt{\frac{\gamma \cdot R \cdot T}{M}}, \qquad \Delta t = \frac{D_{X0}}{c} = \frac{\Delta n}{f_s}, \tag{1}$$

where c is velocity of sound propagation in the air at a given temperature, $\gamma = 1.4$ is air adiabatic constant, $R = 8.31446$ J K^{-1} mol^{-1} is universal gas constant, T [K] $= t$ [°C] $+ 273.15$ is thermodynamic temperature, $M = 28.9647 \times 10^{-3}$ kg mol^{-1} is air molar mass, D_{X0} is real distance between the noise microphone location and the excitation signal measuring point Δn is corresponding number of samples, and f_s is sampling frequency. These two approaches (direct and indirect) of time delay determination can be used to compare theoretical and real distances between the vibrating gradient coils and the noise sensor. However, this time delay involves superposition of a delay between the electrical excitation signal and the consequent vibration signal. Being a small delay, it is difficult to be determined in practice, but it causes an increase of the resulting theoretical distance D_X.

3. Experiments and Results

This study encompasses three basic parts dealing with different comparisons in the area of MRI. The first part describes experiments for analysis of vibration and noise conditions in the scanning area and in the neighborhood of the open-air MRI equipment E-scan Opera by Esaote company Esaote S.p.A., Genoa, Italy [21], and the experimental whole-body experimental MR imager TMR96 device built at the Institute of Measurement Science (IMS) in Bratislava, using the Apollo (Tecmag Inc., Houston, TX, USA) console for control by the NTNMR ver. 1.4 software package [22]. Both investigated MRI devices are located at the IMS, in the laboratories of the department of imaging methods.

At first, different recording microphone positions and parameters (distance between the central point of the MRI scanning area and the microphone membrane, direction angle, working height, and microphone pickup pattern) are tested, and their effect on spectral properties of the recorded noise signal is analyzed. Next, the recorded electrical excitation, vibration, and noise signals are processed for visual comparison of spectrograms and periodograms. Then, basic and supplementary spectral features are statistically analyzed. Time delays between the electrical excitation impulses in the gradient coils and the subsequently generated mechanical vibration/acoustic noise are determined from the simultaneously picked-up signals. These delay times are visualized by histograms and occurrence density plots.

Two basic types of MR scan sequences called Spin Echo (SE) and Gradient Echo (GE) arising from physical principles of MRI [18] are used in the performed experiments. For real-time recording of the vibration signal, the piezoelectric SB-1 bass pickup was used. The acoustic noise was recorded by the 1″ dual diaphragm condenser microphone B-2 PRO (by Behringer GmbH, Kirchardt, Germany) with final choice of a cardioid pickup pattern. For sensing the excitation signal, a special coil with an inductance L_0 was designed and used—see documentary photos of measurement arrangement for both investigated MRI devices in Figure 1. The whole recording was performed by the Behringer Podcast Studio equipment used for connection to an external computer by the USB interface. A typical duration of the recorded signal was 30 s and for further signal processing the stationary parts lasting 15 s were selected using the sound editor program Sound Forge 8.0 by Sony Media Software, WI, USA.

Subsequently, spectral properties of the recorded noise signals were analyzed. The temperature was always kept by air conditioning at 23 °C, giving the sound velocity of 345 m/s.

3.1. Mapping of Vibration and Noise Conditions in the Scanning Area of the Open-Air MRI Device

Basic mapping of vibration and noise conditions in the scanning area and in the neighborhood of the open-air MRI E-Scan Opera was performed within our previous research [12]. In the framework of the present study, two additional experiments were performed:

1. Measurement of the acoustic noise SPL in the MRI neighborhood in directions of 30°, 90°, and 150°—see the overview photo together with the principal angle diagram of the MRI scanning area in Figure 2a. Discrete MRI noise SPL values measured at distances of 45, 60, and 75 cm from the central point of the scanning area are shown in Figure 3a. The detailed measurement of the directional pattern of the acoustic noise SPL distribution was practically executed in the range of <0°~165°> in 15° steps (excluding the last one because of a patient bed at the position of 180°), at the distance of $D_L = 60$ cm from the MRI device central point—see the resulting diagram in Figure 3b. In both cases, the measurement was realized with the help of the sound level meter of the multi-function environment meter Lafayette DT 8820.

2. Parallel real-time recording of the signals from the electrical excitation, the vibration sensor, the microphone and/or the sound level meter. Comparison of both MRI devices in the form of histograms and occurrence density plots of basic and supplementary spectral properties together with the calculated time delays between the electrical excitation of the gradient coils and the subsequently generated noise can be found in Section 3.3.

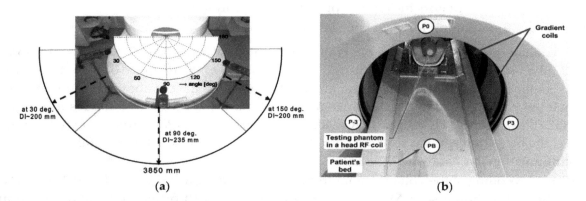

Figure 2. Arrangement of the noise and vibration measurements: in the open-air magnetic resonance imaging (MRI) device Opera together with principal angle diagram of the MRI scanning area; (**a**) sound pressure level (SPL) meter situated at 30°, 90°, and 150°; (**b**) in the whole-body imager TMR-96.

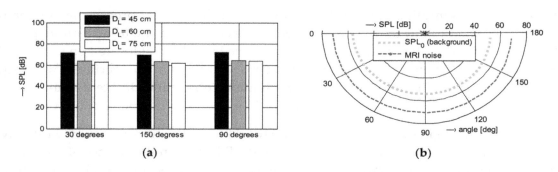

Figure 3. Visual comparison of obtained noise SPL values; (**a**) measured in the directions of 30°, 90°, and 150° at the distances of $D_L = \{45, 60, 75\}$ cm; (**b**) measured directional patterns of the noise source and the background noise SPL_0, $D_L = 60$ cm.

The baseline measurement in the open-air device Opera was carried out during the execution of 3-D and Hi-Resolution (Hi-Res) sequences that are used for scanning of a human vocal tract [11,12,17]. In order to obtain results comparable with those for the whole-body MRI device, the parameters of used Hi-Res SE HF scan sequence were set to TE = 26 ms and TR = 500 ms. The auxiliary parameters were adjusted to 10 slices of 4-mm thickness and sagittal orientation, the spherical test phantom filled with doped water was inserted in the scanning RF knee coil. The sensors of electrical excitation and vibration signals were mounted directly on the lower plastic holder of the gradient coils in the direction of 45° at the point P0—see the arrangement photo in Figure 1a.

3.2. Analysis of Vibration and Noise Conditions of the Whole-Body MRI Equipment

The second collection of experiments was aimed at mapping noise conditions in the scanning area and in the vicinity of the experimental whole-body MR imager TMR-96 [23]. These experiments consist of

1. Measurement of the acoustic noise SPL in MRI neighborhood in the direction of 0° at three heights (2, 25, and 55 cm) above the patient's bed level. Then, the SPL meter was located in ±120° (points P3 and P-3) at the height of 85 cm above the floor—see the arrangement photo in Figure 2b. The SPL meter was always placed at the distance of D_L = 60 cm from the front plastic panel to minimize interaction with the magnetic field. The measurement itself was carried out during the SE scan sequence with TE = 18 ms, TR = 400 ms under three noise conditions (obtained discrete noise SPL values are presented in Table 1).

    * SPL_{00}—the background noise when all devices are stopped,
    * SPL_{01}—the ventilators inside the copper cage are running,
    * SPL_X—the scanning MR sequence is being executed with ventilation fans running.

2. The detailed measurement of the directional pattern of the acoustic noise SPL distribution in the MRI tube vicinity in the range of 0°~180° with 15° steps, at the distance of D_L = 45 cm from the MRI center (point PC) of the scanning area, in the high h = 120 cm above the floor level (25 cm above the patient's bed)—see the arrangement photo in Figure 4a and the resulting diagram for GE/SE sequence (TE = 18 ms, TR = 400 ms) together with SPL_{01} curve in Figure 4b. In both cases, the measurement was realized with the help of the sound level meter of the multi-function environment meter Lafayette DT 8820.

3. Real-time recoding of the voltage signal from a piezoelectric transducer of the SB-1 sensor during execution of a chosen scan MR sequence (SE/GE type with different TE and TR parameter settings) and parallel recording of the electrical excitation signal (impulses from the MRI device gradient coil system) and/or the signals from the vibration sensor/pick-up microphone for time delay calculation and spectral properties comparison.

The succession of sampling, resampling to 16 kHz, off-line signal processing, and analysis of spectral properties was similar to that in the open-air device. Here, the test phantom consists of a 1-liter plastic bottle filled with doped water [24] inside the head RF coil located on the patient's bed in the middle of the MRI device scanning area. The second comparison experiment was focused on testing the influence of different locations of the vibration sensor and different scan sequences on spectral properties of the vibration signal. The succeeding analysis and comparison were aimed at:

*   Mapping of vibration in different parts of the MRI device—the sensor mounted directly on the surface of the front plastic cover at the points P0, P3, P-3, and on the surface of the patient's bed (PB). The numerical results of the basic spectral features can be seen in Table 2 and the box-plot statistics of the supplementary spectral properties in Figure 6.
*   Determination of differences between two mostly used MR scan sequences of SE and GE types; the pick-up sensor at the P3 point—see the visualization of differences of the selected signal features in Figure 5.

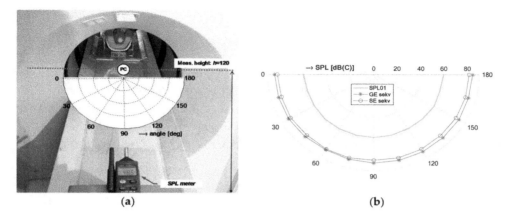

Figure 4. Arrangement of measurement of the acoustic noise SPL distribution in the vicinity of the TMR96 scanning tube; (**a**) SPL meter situated at the distance D_L = 45 cm from the scanning area center (point PC), in the height h = 120 cm above the floor level; (**b**) directional pattern for SE/GE sequences together with SPL_{01} values.

Table 1. Measured SPL [dB(C)] at different positions.

Noise Condition/Measuring Position	at 0°		at 120°	at 120°	
	$h_0{}^1$ = 55 cm	$h_0{}^1$ = 25 cm	$h_0{}^1$ = 2 cm	$h_1{}^2$ = 85 cm	$h_1{}^2$ = 85 cm
SPL_{00} silent	47.9	47.7	47.5	47.4	47.5
SPL_{01} + ventilators	54.1	56.8	56.9	61.8	59.6
SPL_X scan sequence	77	79.1	80.1	79.5	78.7

[1] Height above the patient's bed level. [2] Height above the floor.

Table 2. Mean values of basic spectral features of the recorded vibration signals [1].

Sensor Position/Feature	Signal$_{RMS}$ (-)	En$_{c0}$ (-)	S_{tilt} (°)	F_{V1} (Hz)	F_{V2} (Hz)
0° (TR = 400)	4.3	0.47	−22	429	1380
120° (TR = 400/500)	2.7/2.4	0.38/0.31	−1/−14	352/260	1105/1048
−120° (TR = 400)	2.5	0.27	−13	368	930
Patient's bed (TR = 400)	7.9	0.95	3	398	1662

[1] Used SpinEcho sequence with TE = 18 ms in all cases.

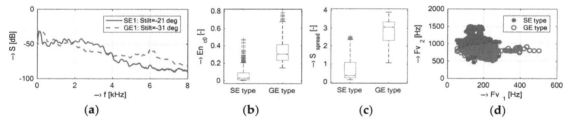

Figure 5. Visualization of differences of selected features of the recorded vibration signals; (**a**) spectral envelopes and calculated spectral tilts; (**b**) boxplot of basic statistical properties for En_{c0}; (**c**) S_{spread}; (**d**) mutual positions of F_{v1} and F_{v2} for SE/GE scan sequences with TE = 18 ms and TR = 500 ms.

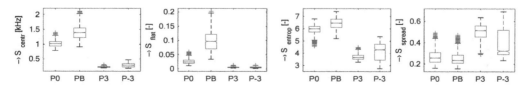

Figure 6. Box-plot of basic statistical parameters of supplementary spectral properties (centroid, flatness, entropy, spread) determined from the vibration signal picked up at different measuring positions {P0, PB, P3, P-3} during the SE sequence (TE = 18 ms, TR = 400 ms).

3.3. Comparison of Spectral Properties of Vibration and Noise Signals Recorded in Open and Closed MRI Devices

The vibration and/or noise signals recorded in the open-air Opera and the whole-body TMR96 MRI devices using the test phantom placed in the RF coil were compared graphically and grouped for both types of devices. If not stated otherwise, the signals were taken at the position P0 during execution of the MR sequence Hi-Res SE 26 HF (TR = 400 ms) for the Opera MRI device and the position P3 using the SE1-18 (TR = 400 ms) for the TMR96 device. The processed signals were used to compare

- Basic spectral properties of vibration signals including spectral density, its envelope, spectral tilt, and spectrograms presented in the set of graphs in Figure 7;
- Histograms of supplementary spectral properties of vibration signals shown in Figure 8;
- Time delays between an electrical excitation signal and a generated acoustic noise (calculated from positive and negative pulses using the statistical method described in [12])—see the set of graphs in Figure 9.

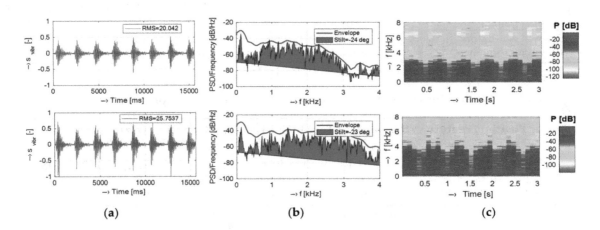

(a)   (b)   (c)

Figure 7. Visualization of basic spectral properties of recorded vibration signals; (**a**) stationary part of a normalized signal with its RMS value; (**b**) spectral density together with its envelope and calculated spectral tilt; (**c**) corresponding spectrograms for MRI Opera (upper set) and TMR96 (lower set).

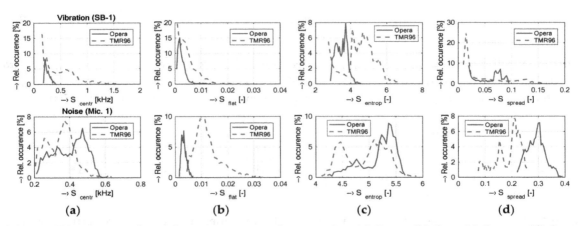

(a)   (b)   (c)   (d)

Figure 8. Histograms of supplementary spectral properties; (**a**) S_{centr}; (**b**) S_{flat}; (**c**) S_{entrop}; (**d**) S_{spread}, determined from picked-up vibration signals inside the Opera and TMR96 MRI devices.

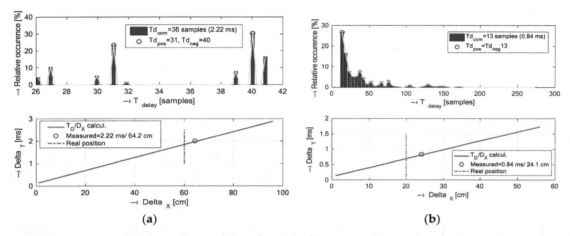

Figure 9. Histograms of evaluated time delays [samples] between electrical excitation and acoustic noise signals recorded in the MRI device (upper set), comparison of calculated and estimated mean values of time delays [ms] together with theoretical and real microphone distances (lower set); (**a**) for MRI Opera microphone Mic. 1 at a distance 60 cm and a direction 30°, sensing coil L_0 at 45°; (**b**) for TMR96 Mic. 1 at a distance 16 cm from the patient's bed position, L_0 at P3, sequence SE1-18 (TR = 400 ms); t = 23 °C, c = 346 m/s.

4. Discussion and Conclusions

The measurements in the vicinity of the open-air MRI equipment E-scan Esaote Opera have shown that the maximum sound pressure level of about 72 dB(C) was achieved for the SPL meter located in the direction of 30°, the height of 85 cm (in the middle between the upper and the lower gradient coils), and at the distance of 45 cm, while the background noise SPL_0 originating from the temperature stabilizer reached approximately 52 dB(C) measured in the time instant when no scan sequence was executed. Next, for three directions of 30°, 90°, and 150°, the noise SPL values measured with the examined person lying in the MRI scanning area were about 10 dB lower when compared with using the water phantom. The obtained noise SPL values were roughly inversely proportional to the effective weights of the male and female testing persons lying on the bottom plastic holder of the permanent magnet and gradient coils. On the other hand, the noise in the neighbourhood of the whole-body MRI device TMR96 achieved its maximum SPL of about 80 dB(C) using the SE scanning sequence and its minimum mean value of 62 dB(C) with no sequence running (the background noise generated mainly by the ventilators inside the cage) as documented by the numerical results in Table 1 and the detailed directional pattern in Figure 4b. In summary, it holds that the maximum SPL was observed for the sound level meter located at the point PB on the patient's bed level and the minimum at the point P0. Evaluations of other authors are usually aimed at high-field MRI systems. Sound noise of various pulse sequences was compared for two whole-body MRI scanners by Cho et al. [25] with the rest value 79.5 dB(C) for the 1.5-T scanner and 68.6 dB(C) for the 2-T scanner. The highest sound pressure level of about 103 dB(C) was observed during the gradient echo sequence with TE = 4 ms, TR = 250 ms in the 1.5-T scanner and TE = 35 ms, TR = 100 ms in the 2-T scanner. Prince et al. [26] investigated acoustic noise in 15 MRI scanners giving a minimum of 82.5 dB(A) for a 0.23-T device using GE sequence, TE = 5 ms, TR= 525 ms and a maximum of 118.4 dB(A) for a 3-T device using the same sequence and TE, but TR = 3000 ms.

The vibration recording experiment was arranged to map basic points on the plastic cover as well as on the surface of the patient's bed. In the case of the TMR96 device, the maximum vibration energy (expressed by RMS and/or from the first cepstral coefficient) was attained for the sensor placement on the patient's bed almost at the top of the plastic cover (point PB)—see the mean values in Table 2. As regards the spectral features, the mean values of the vibration frequencies $F_{V1,2}$ are the highest at P3 position (120°) and the lowest at the point P-3 (left bottom part of the plastic cover with the minimal vibration energy). The obtained results of the supplementary spectral properties are in good correlation with the basic ones—as documented by the visualization in Figure 6. Investigation of spectral differences between two mostly used MR scan sequences (SE/GE types) confirms our assumption that the GE sequence has more structured noise and the SE sequence generates more compact vibration with higher energy in the final effect, larger spread, and lower dispersion of $F_{V1,2}$ frequencies as shown by the graphical results in Figure 5. Due to different construction of the open-air and the whole-body MRI devices, different software tools of their control systems, different types of used phantoms, etc., it was practically impossible to use the identical MR sequences. Only similar types of sequences with similar choice of basic parameters (TE, TR, orientation, etc.) could be applied. Consequently, the analyzed vibration signals had slightly different spectral features—see histograms in Figure 8. This general assumption was confirmed by the results presented in the form of spectrograms and periodograms. On the other hand, as documented by visualization of waveforms of the picked-up vibration signals in Figure 7a, the TMR96 device produces higher vibration levels with higher energy (signal$_{RMS}$). This is in accordance with the basic physical law—greater scan volume in this device results in higher intensity of applied current in the gradient coils in spite of lower basic magnetic field (0.1 T vs. 0.178 T applied in the MRI Opera). As mentioned in the Section 2.1, the influence of different masses (volumes) in the scanning area on the intensity as well as on the spectral properties of the produced acoustic noise was analyzed in our previous research [17] using the MRI Opera device. In near future we would like to carry out similar experiments and measurements also with the TMR96 device.

In the last comparison experiment, we analyzed how the vibrations induced by the pulse current in the gradient coil travel through the holder of the MRI device, and how the actual position of the pick-up microphone corresponds with the one calculated from the determined time delay between the electrical excitation and the subsequently generated acoustic noise signals. As documented by the histogram in Figure 9a, the MRI device Opera has different time delay values determined from the positive and negative peaks of the compared signals. It means that there exist two maxima from which the final time delay was calculated as the median value. It is in agreement with the fact that the positive peaks have higher magnitude than the negative ones. This effect can be caused by the construction of the plastic cover of the gradient coils. The documentary photo in Figure 1a shows that the surface is not planar but slightly convexly curved. Hence, the mechanical force is different for positive and negative impulses originated from the gradient coils—in the case of negative ones the vibration acts against the force of the mechanical stiffness of the curved plate. In the measurement inside the TMR96 device, the sensors were mounted not on the plastic cover surface representing the front part of the whole MRI, but directly on the back part of the gradient coil surface. Though the measured surface was also curved, only one maximum of the time delay was observed in this case, see the histogram in Figure 9b. The obtained results of the backward comparison of the determined distance between the microphone picking up the noise and the origin of the vibration (sensor positions P0 for the MRI Opera and P3 for the TMR96) confirm our assumption that the distance calculated from the determined time delay values was always higher—see the bottom set of graphs in Figure 9. The detected increase of about 4–6 cm in the actual distance corresponds to the increase of the time interval by the delay during which the vibration is generated as a consequence of the excitation impulse in the gradient coil.

The results of the experiments will help to describe the process of the gradient coil electric excitation, the subsequent mechanical vibration, and the resulting acoustic noise generation in the MRI device scanning area and its vicinity. Additional measurement and analysis are necessary for better knowledge of these acoustic noise conditions. In the case of the MRI Opera, there is need for more information about the contribution of the upper gradient coil (and its plastic holder) to the resulting acoustic noise. Therefore, in near future we plan to perform parallel measurement of the vibration signal on the surface of both plastic holders. As regards the TMR96 device, the process of noise and vibration generation inside the scanning tube of the whole-body tomograph must be known. Thus, the measurement with the vibration sensor mounted in the place of the second and third gradient coils must be also performed for detailed mapping of the vibration in the whole 360° angle around the gradient coils. Critical parts (possible loose mounting to the main mass of the resistive magnet) can be found by this method, subsequently repaired, and/or some damping material might be inserted for mechanical suppression of the generated vibration and noise.

Acknowledgments: This work was supported by the Slovak Scientific Grant Agency project VEGA 2/0001/17, the Ministry of Education, Science, Research, and Sports of the Slovak Republic VEGA 1/0905/17, and within the project of the Slovak Research and Development Agency Nr. APVV-15-0029.

Author Contributions: J.P. conceived and designed the measurement and recording experiments, carried out analysis and statistical processing of the data, and evaluated all the results. A.P. cooperated in the vibration measurement with both types of MRI devices, and participated in collection of the noise, vibration, and voice signal database. I.F. reviewed the paper and provided some advice. A.P. read and corrected the English of the manuscript.

References

1. Wellard, R.M.; Ravasio, J.P.; Guesne, S.; Bell, C.; Oloyede, A.; Tevelen, G.; Pope, J.M.; Momot, K.I. Simultaneous magnetic resonance imaging and consolidation measurement of articular cartilage. *Sensors* **2014**, *14*, 7940–7958. [CrossRef] [PubMed]

2. He, Z.; He, W.; Wu, J.; Xu, Z. The novel design of a single-sided MRI probe for assessing burn depth. *Sensors* **2017**, *17*, 526. [CrossRef] [PubMed]

3. Panych, L.P.; Madore, B. The physics of MRI safety. *J. Magn. Reson. Imaging* **2018**, *47*, 28–43. [CrossRef] [PubMed]

4. Mainka, A.; Platzek, I.; Mattheus, W.; Fleischer, M.; Müller, A.S. Three-dimensional vocal tract morphology based on multiple magnetic resonance images is highly reproducible during sustained phonation. *J. Voice* **2017**, *31*, 504.e11–504.e20. [CrossRef] [PubMed]

5. Kuortti, J.; Malinen, J.; Ojalammi, A. Post-processing speech recordings during MRI. *Biomed. Signal Process. Control* **2018**, *39*, 11–22. [CrossRef]

6. Freitas, A.C.; Ruthven, M.; Boubertakh, R.; Miquel, M.E. Real-time speech MRI: Commercial Cartesian and non-Cartesian sequences at 3T and feasibility of offline TGV reconstruction to visualise velopharyngeal motion. *Phys. Med.* **2018**, *46*, 96–103. [CrossRef] [PubMed]

7. Sun, G.; Li, M.; Rudd, B.W.; Lim, T.C.; Osterhage, J.; Fugate, E.M.; Lee, J.H. Adaptive speech enhancement using directional microphone in a 4-T MRI scanner. *Magn. Reson. Mater. Phys. Biol. Med.* **2015**, *28*, 473–484. [CrossRef] [PubMed]

8. Vahanesa, C.; Reddy, C.K.; Panahi, I.M. Improving quality and intelligibility of speech using single microphone for the broadband fMRI noise at low SNR. In Proceedings of the IEEE International Conference of the Engineering in Medicine and Biology Society (EMBC), Orlando, FL, USA, 16–20 August 2016; pp. 3674–3678.

9. Han, L.; Shen, Z.; Fu, C.; Liu, C. Design and implementation of sound searching robots in wireless sensor networks. *Sensors* **2016**, *16*, 1550. [CrossRef] [PubMed]

10. Ding, H.; Soon, I.Y.; Yeo, C.K. Over-attenuated components regeneration for speech enhancement. *IEEE Trans. Audio Speech Lang. Process.* **2010**, *18*, 2004–2014. [CrossRef]

11. Přibil, J.; Přibilová, A.; Frollo, I. Analysis of acoustic noise and its suppression in speech recorded during scanning in the open-air MRI. In *Advances in Noise Analysis, Mitigation and Control*; Ahmed, N., Ed.; InTech: Rijeka, Croatia, 2016; pp. 205–228, ISBN 978-953-51-2674-4.

12. Přibil, J.; Přibilová, A.; Frollo, I. Mapping and spectral analysis of acoustic vibration in the scanning area of the weak field magnetic resonance imager. *J. Vib. Acoust. Trans. ASME* **2014**, *136*, 051005. [CrossRef]

13. Tayong, R.; Dupont, T.; Leclaire, P. Experimental investigation of holes interaction effect on the sound absorption coefficient of micro-perforated panels under high and medium sound levels. *Appl. Acoust.* **2011**, *72*, 777–784. [CrossRef]

14. Zhao, X.; Wang, X.; Yu, Y. Enhancing low-frequency sound absorption of micro-perforated panel absorbers by combining parallel mechanical impedance. *Appl. Acoust.* **2018**, *130*, 300–304. [CrossRef]

15. Gai, X.L.; Xing, T.; Li, X.H.; Zhang, B.; Wang, F.; Cai, Z.N.; Han, Y. Sound absorption of microperforated panel with L shape division cavity. *Appl. Acoust.* **2017**, *122*, 41–50. [CrossRef]

16. Moelker, A.; Wielopolski, P.A.; Pattynama, M.T. Relationship between magnetic field strength and magnetic-resonance-related acoustic noise levels. *Magn. Reson. Mater. Phys. Biol. Med.* **2003**, *16*, 52–55. [CrossRef] [PubMed]

17. Přibil, J.; Přibilová, A.; Frollo, I. Influence of the human body mass in the open-air MRI on acoustic noise spectrum. *Acta IMEKO* **2016**, *5*, 81–86. [CrossRef]

18. Liang, Z.P.; Lauterbur, P.C. *Principles of Magnetic Resonance Imaging: A Signal Processing Perspective*; Wiley-IEEE Press: New York, NY, USA, 1999; ISBN 978-0-780-34723-6.

19. Winkler, S.A.; Alejski, A.; Wade, T.; McKenzie, C.A.; Rutt, B.K. On the accurate analysis of vibroacoustics in head insert gradient coils. *Magn. Reson. Med.* **2017**, *78*, 1635–1645. [CrossRef] [PubMed]

20. Fraden, J. *Handbook of Modern Sensors. Physics, Designs, and Applications*, 4th ed.; Springer: New York, NY, USA, 2010; ISBN 978-1-4419-6466-3.

21. E-Scan Opera. *Image Quality and Sequences Manual. 830023522 Rev*; A, Esaote S.p.A.: Genoa, Italy, 2008.

22. TNMR Reference Manual, Hardware Reference Manual, DSPect User Guide. Available online: http://www.tecmag.com/support_contact/pulse_sequences/ (accessed on 10 October 2010).

23. Andris, P.; Dermek, T.; Frollo, I. Simplified matching and tuning experimental receive coils for low-field NMR measurements. *Measurement* **2015**, *64*, 29–33. [CrossRef]

24. Andris, P.; Frollo, I. Asymmetric spin echo sequence and requirements on static magnetic field of NMR scanner. *Measurement* **2013**, *46*, 1530–1534. [CrossRef]

25. Cho, Z.H.; Park, S.H.; Kim, J.H.; Chung, S.C.; Chung, S.T.; Chung, J.Y.; Moon, C.W.; Yi, J.H.; Sin, C.H.; Wong, E.K. Analysis of acoustic noise in MRI. *Magn. Reson. Imaging* **1997**, *15*, 815–822. [CrossRef]

26. Prince, D.L.; De Wilde, J.P.; Papadaki, A.M.; Curran, J.S.; Kitney, R.I. Investigation of acoustic noise on 15 MRI scanners from 0.2 T to 3 T. *J. Magn. Reson. Imaging* **2001**, *13*, 288–293. [CrossRef]

13

Monte Carlo Modeling of Shortwave-Infrared Fluorescence Photon Migration in Voxelized Media for the Detection of Breast Cancer

Tatsuto Iida [1], Shunsuke Kiya [1], Kosuke Kubota [1], Takashi Jin [2], Akitoshi Seiyama [3] and Yasutomo Nomura [1,2,*]

[1] Department of Systems Life Engineering, Maebashi Institute of Technology, Maebashi 371-0816, Japan; m1956001@maebashi-it.ac.jp (T.I.); m1771013@maebashi-it.ac.jp (S.K.); m1771014@maebashi-it.ac.jp (K.K.)

[2] Laboratory for Nano-Bio Probes, RIKEN Center for Biosystems Dynamics Research, Suita 565-0874, Japan; tjin@riken.jp

[3] Human Health Sciences, Graduate School of Medicine, Kyoto University, Kyoto 606-8507, Japan; seiyama.akitoshi.7x@kyoto-u.ac.jp

[*] Correspondence: ynomura@maebashi-it.ac.jp

Abstract: Recent progress regarding shortwave-infrared (SWIR) molecular imaging technology has inspired another modality of noninvasive diagnosis for early breast cancer detection in which previous mammography or sonography would be compensated. Although a SWIR fluorescence image of a small breast cancer of several millimeters was obtained from experiments with small animals, detailed numerical analyses before clinical application were required, since various parameters such as size as well as body hair differed between humans and small experimental animals. In this study, the feasibility of SWIR was compared against visible (VIS) and near-infrared (NIR) region, using the Monte Carlo simulation in voxelized media. In this model, due to the implementation of the excitation gradient, fluorescence is based on rational mechanisms, whereas fluorescence within breast cancer is spatially proportional to excitation intensity. The fluence map of SWIR simulation with excitation gradient indicated signals near the upper surface of the cancer, and stronger than those of the NIR. Furthermore, there was a dependency on the fluence signal distribution on the contour of the breast tissue, as well as the internal structure, due to the implementation of digital anatomical data for the Visible Human Project. The fluorescence signal was observed to become weaker in all regions including the VIS, the NIR, and the SWIR region, when fluorescence-labeled cancer either became smaller or was embedded in a deeper area. However, fluorescence in SWIR alone from a cancer of 4 mm diameter was judged to be detectable at a depth of 1.4 cm.

Keywords: shortwave-infrared light; near-infrared light; visible light; fluorescence; breast cancer; duct; visible human project; Monte Carlo simulation; voxelized media

---

1. Introduction

Ductal carcinoma is the most common type of breast cancer and tends to progress to invasive cancer. Breast conservation therapy should be considered when the cancer is less than 2.0 cm [1,2]. However, it was shown by the accuracy of the same MRI(magnetic resonance imaging)-sonography co-registration system that the mean lesion size correlated well on MRI (11.4 mm; range 6–28 mm) compared with that of sonography (10.3 mm; range 6–28 mm) [3]. Therefore, early breast cancers of only several millimeters have occasionally failed to be detected by the use of such noninvasive methods alone. However, shortwave-infrared (SWIR) fluorescence imaging for the detection of small cancers offers a higher contrast and sensitivity with deeper penetration depths in comparison with the conventional visible (VIS) and the near-infrared (NIR) fluorescence imaging, thus it has attracted much attention recently [4,5]. As radiation exposure due to SWIR is much less than that from X-rays in mammography and gamma-rays in PET, SWIR fluorescence imaging can be used repetitively, which suggests its suitability in the case of young subjects. Furthermore, it would have a higher spatial resolution than the sentinel lymph-node biopsy with VIS (Patent blue) or NIR fluorescence (Indocyanine green, ICG) because of the lower scattering property [6–9]. Indeed, a fluorescent image of a small breast cancer of several millimeters was obtained from small animal experiments [10].

Before clinical application, detailed numerical analyses of the behavior of excitation and emission photons are required, since optical parameters such as scattering and absorption coefficients differ between humans and small experimental animals. In our previous study, as the first step for the detection of early breast cancer, Monte Carlo modeling in a multi-layered media (MCML) for fluorescence photon migration of the ICG in the NIR was proposed [11]. In contrast to the VIS fluorescence of fluorescein, the NIR fluorescence of the ICG showed effectiveness in detecting a cancer of 1.0 cm in diameter at a depth of 1.0 cm. This suggests that smaller cancers are probably detected when SWIR fluorescence is utilized. However, the analytical model was composed of a spherical cancer with fluorescence in the fat layer below the flat skin surface. The results of the analysis in the approximate model of the layered structure are not always correct, because actual breast tissue has a complex three-dimensional structure, e.g., the mammary gland. Therefore, taking the high spatial resolution of the SWIR fluorescence imaging into account, an analytical model which reflected the contour of the breast surface and its internal structure was pursued. Recently, Monte Carlo modeling in voxelized media (MCVM), by which the authors could track photon migration in realistic brain tissue structure, was reported by Li et al. [12,13], where a digital anatomical dataset of the voxelized media of the Monte Carlo model was implemented in which optical parameters were set specific to regions of the human tissue. Here we developed their method to apply to a breast cancer model, as follows.

The authors predicted distribution within the tissue of light absorption in the VIS and the NIR. In this study, we developed MCVM for the analysis of excitation and emission. The intensity of fluorescence is proportional to the concentration of the fluorescent molecules as well as the excitation efficiency. The accumulation of fluorescent probes in the cancer is dependent on the expression level of the marker protein. The concentration of fluorescent molecules located in the cancer was assumed to be spatially constant. On the other hand, it was quite difficult to set the excitation efficiency to be spatially constant. When incident photons reached the cancerous cell, the fluorescent molecules within it partially absorbed the energy. Therefore, the excitation efficiency was influenced by the optical properties surrounding the cancer and its depth. When optical parameters were set, specific to the regions of the duct with a complex morphology and the fat tissue, photon migration in association with excitation and emission would reflect the internal structure faithfully. Thus, the feasibility of detecting early breast cancer was examined by analyzing the SWIR fluorescence, which was emitted by several mechanisms, using MCVM with exact distribution of the optical parameters.

2. Materials and Methods

2.1. Breast Model

Digital anatomical data in which the internal structure of the breast was reflected were pursued for the improvement of our previous Monte Carlo model [11,14–16]. In the previous studies, Li et al. used a dataset of cross-sectional cryosection images which was provided by the Visible Chinese Human (VCH) [12,13]. However, due to limited access, there was a difficulty in obtaining the dataset from VCH. Therefore we used a public-domain library of cross-sectional cryosection, CT, as well as MRI images provided by the Visible Human Project (VHP) of the US National Library of Medicine [17]. Because 3D tomography of the breast was obtained from the dataset, it permitted us to analyze photon behaviors in the Monte Carlo model set to a complex internal structure identical to the human breast. In this study, the thoracic part of an anatomical dataset built from a cadaver of an American woman who had died of heart disease at the age of 59 was used. With the permission of her husband, the body was frozen, thinly sliced more than 5000 times, and photographed. The thickness of each slice was 0.33 mm. The three-dimensional reconstruction of the thoracic part, built from thin slices as in Figure 1A, is shown in (B). When images of the slice were processed based on the anatomy of the breast as described in the next section, the mammary gland (green structure with complex morphology) was included within the thoracic part (C). As shown in (D), fluorescence-labeled cancer (red sphere) was set in the duct of the structure. To indicate the structure observed from a different angle, rotating (D) $\pi/2$ clockwise on the x-axis was performed to obtain (E). Furthermore, (F) was obtained by rotating (D) $\pi/2$ once more.

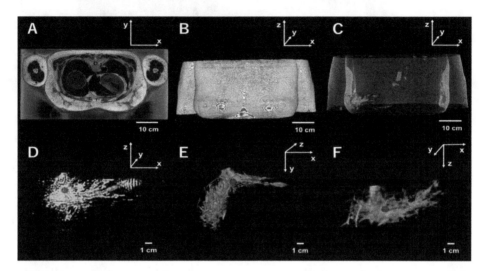

Figure 1. Visualization of the internal structure of the female breasts from the Visible Human Project (VHP). (**A**) Slice of the upper body. (**B**) Three-dimensional reconstruction of the upper body. (**C**) Internal structure in the reconstruction. (**D**) Enlarged internal structure with fluorescence-labeled cancer with 1 cm diameter. (**E**) The 3-D vision of the enlarged structure is observed from a different angle. (**F**) 3-D vision from another different angle. See text.

2.2. Image Processing and Implementation of the Model

250 slices were used from the thoracic part, with 2048×1216 pixels for each slice provided by the VHP, where the breast area of 500×220 pixels was cropped using an image processing software (ImageJ). A cropped breast image (24-bit RGB color) from the original VHP image is shown in Figure 2A. Regarding the pixel values, the cropped image in Figure 2B was allocated to areas of fat of more than 180, as well as to areas of the breast duct between 80 and 120, respectively, after conversion to an 8-bit grayscale image. The boundary between the outside and inside tissue area was extracted and the border of two pixels width was assumed to be the skin layer. Previous studies were used to set the optical parameters specific to the three areas in Table 1 [18–22]. In this study, taking medical applications into account, the excitation and emission wavelengths of the fluorescein (excitation max (Ex) 488 nm, emission max (Em) 520 nm, quantum yield (QY): 0.95, concentration (C): 0.75 mM, absorption coefficient (εC): 12 cm^{-1}) were selected, which were used for the examination of the fundus in the VIS region, as well as those of the ICG (Ex 780 nm/Em 820 nm, QY: 0.09, C: 0.2 mM, εC: 20 cm^{-1}) for the sentinel lymph-node biopsy in the NIR region [6–9,23,24]. Fluorescence imaging in the VIS region is an effective diagnostic method for transparent media such as the eyeball, but it is difficult to use in turbid media which is characteristic of the optical properties of breast tissue. For SWIR imaging, we employed lead sulfide (PbS) quantum dots (QDs) (Ex 970 nm/Em 1100 nm, QY: 0.40, C: 1.0 μM, εC: 0.63 cm^{-1}) as fluorescent probes which have been used in prior animal experiments despite the lack of medical applications of QDs [5]. As shown in Figures 2C and 3A, the optical parameters were implemented in the voxel of the 3-dimensional matrix (500, 250, 220). Each voxel was of $0.033 \times 0.033 \times 0.033$ cm^3. The fluorescence-labeled cancers with a diameter of 1, 4, 7, and 10 mm were embedded at a depth of 1 to 3 cm (Figure 2D).

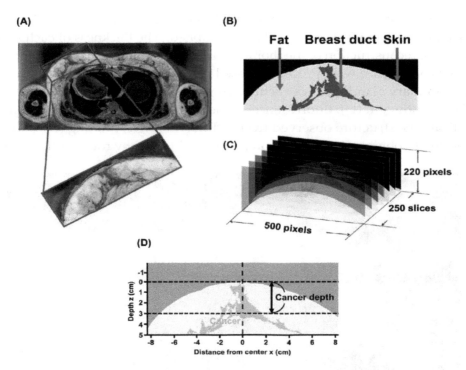

Figure 2. Implementation of the contour and the internal structures derived from breast anatomical data of the Visible Human Project (VHP). (**A**) Cropped image from a slice. (**B**) Allocation of the fat, the duct and the skin based on pixel value. (**C**) Reconstruction of a 3-D voxel model. (**D**) Setting of coordinate system in the slice containing the center and top of nipple ($x = 0$, $z = 0$). The depth denotes the distance from $z = 0$ to the upper surface of the cancer.

Table 1. Optical parameters specific to tissues in the visible (VIS), the near-infrared (NIR), and the shortwave-infrared (SWIR).

	Wavelength (nm)	Tissue	μ_a (cm^{-1})	μ_s (cm^{-1})	n
VIS	Ex 488	Skin	6.0	625	1.37
		Fat	6.0	310	1.45
		Duct	0.2	317	1.42
		Cancer	1.0	300	1.45
	Em 520	Skin	5.8	450	1.37
		Fat	4.0	300	1.45
		Duct	0.2	268	1.42
		Cancer	1.0	230	1.45
NIR	Ex 780	Skin	2.0	241	1.37
		Fat	1.4	136	1.45
		Duct	0.2	169	1.42
		Cancer	1.0	150	1.45
	Em 820	Skin	1.2	228	1.37
		Fat	1.2	132	1.45
		Duct	0.2	198	1.42
		Cancer	0.7	140	1.45
SWIR	Ex 970	Skin	1.0	210	1.37
		Fat	0.9	76.6	1.45
		Duct	0.3	122	1.42
		Cancer	0.9	75.5	1.45
SWIR	Em 1100	Skin	0.7	176	1.37
		Fat	0.6	72.3	1.45
		Duct	0.3	122	1.42
		Cancer	1.0	80.0	1.45

2.3. The Monte Carlo Simulation

The software for Monte Carlo modeling of fluorescence was developed with the use of the C programing language within the Microsoft Visual Studio program. As shown in Figure 3B, this simulation was executed by the input of an excited photon in the voxelized media, where each voxel had optical parameters specific to the three areas of the skin, duct, and fat. In Figure 3C, the computation routines described by Wang et al. were used [25]. In brief, each pathlength was considered to be the distance traveled by a photon from the original position to the next interaction site between the photon and the tissue, due to scattering and absorption. The pathlength and the direction were calculated using a random number, anisotropy g, as well as the total attenuation coefficient μ_t, which is the sum of the scattering coefficient μ_s and the absorption coefficient μ_a. Although each excitation photon had an initial weight of unity, the original weight of the photon was reduced by μ_a/μ_t during movement of the photon to the next site. Pseudo-random numbers generated using the Mersenne twister method were used [26]. Photons were reflected or transmitted based on Fresnel reflectance, calculated using refractive indices n of each layer when they crossed the boundary between two layers [25]. Random paths for photons were computed until the weight of each photon was absorbed to less than a threshold, or the photon left the medium.

The photon weight absorbed within each voxel was scored after completion in order to calculate the behavior of a million excitation photons. This was divided by μ_a of the voxel to obtain the fluence. The fluence can be considered as the weight of photons passed and the amount of energy passed per unit area (W/cm^2). Furthermore, since the fluence yielded a response to a light source 1 W/cm^2, it was converted into the response to 50 mW/cm^2 of light source, generally used in tissue spectroscopy [13,27]. The fluence was inherited by the emission photon in two ways as shown in Figure 3D. In the previous study, without the excitation gradient [14], the weight of the emission photon was set as spatially constant by the use of excitation fluency in the center of the cancer. In the present study with an excitation gradient, the emission photon had an initial weight dependent on excitation fluency in each voxel. A million emission photons were generated isotopically in a random position within the cancer.

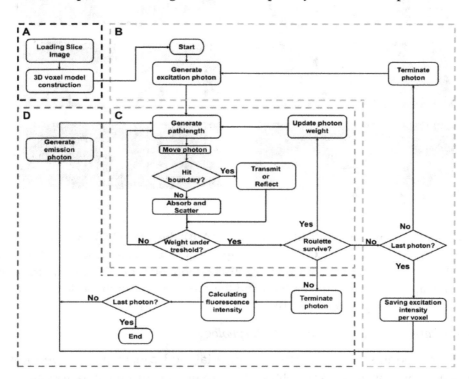

Figure 3. Flowchart of the Monte Carlo simulation in voxelized media for breast tissue. (**A**) Implementation of the breast anatomical data of the VHP. (**B**) Excitation part of the simulation. (**C**) Computation routines were based on Wang et al. [25]. (**D**) Emission part.

3. Results and Discussion

3.1. Excitation Gradient

In the previous study [11], we used the fluorescence Monte Carlo model in which spherical cancer was embedded in the fat layer below the flat skin surface for detecting of early breast cancer. Fluorescence was based on two assumptions. (1) The fluorescent probes were distributed within cancer homogeneously. (2) All probes were excited by the same intensity as the light which reached the center of the cancer. Compared with cancer near the body surface, weaker excitation light reached cancer embedded deeply. There may have been a difference in excitation light intensity between cancer in shallow and deep regions.

In this study, the Monte Carlo model was developed with or without the excitation gradient (Figure 3). The effect of the excitation gradient on VIS, NIR, and SWIR was examined. Fluence maps without and with excitation gradient are shown in Figure 4 when fluorescence-labeled cancer of 1 cm diameter in the duct was embedded $x = 0$ at a depth of 2 cm. Because high μ_s and μ_a were obstructive against reaching fluorescence-labeled cancer for VIS excitation, there was little fluorescence, with and without excitation gradient. In contrast, since the excitation of NIR and SWIR reached the fluorescence-labeled cancer, there was fluorescence with and without excitation gradient. Furthermore, taking the excitation gradient into account, the upper area of cancer shows strong signals in both NIR and SWIR. Without excitation gradient, homogeneous signals in NIR and SWIR were distributed within the entire cancer. The fluence map of SWIR simulation with excitation gradient indicated near-surface signals stronger than those of the NIR. Therefore, the previous model was improved by the use of rational mechanisms for fluorescence, further confirmed in three regions, the VIS, the NIR, and the SWIR, in this study.

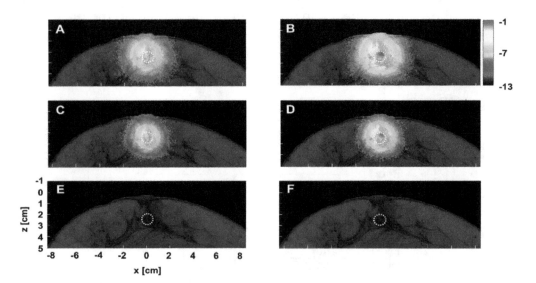

Figure 4. Effect of the excitation gradient in the SWIR (**A,B**), the NIR (**C,D**) and the VIS (**E,F**). Fluence maps without excitation gradient (**A,C,E**) and with gradient (**B,D,F**). Fluorescence-labeled cancer with a diameter of 1 cm in the duct were embedded $x = 0$ at a depth of 2 cm, denoted by circles of the white broken line. All maps share the values on the x and the z-axis of (**E**) and the scale bar, which shows the logarithmic scale of intensity (W/cm^2) in (**B**).

3.2. Setting Optical Parameters Faithful to Duct Morphology

In the previous model, spherically fluorescence-labeled cancer was embedded in the fat layer which had homogeneous optical parameters. However, the model was too simple as the actual breast tissue structure was complex. Breast cancer is frequently developed in the duct and progresses invasively. Thus, it is quite important to set optical parameters for ducts with complex morphology (Figure 1) when photon migration in the breast tissue is examined. Furthermore, the excitation and emission would be influenced by the various locations of fluorescence-labeled cancer within the duct, outside of the duct, or between the duct and the fat, due to the different optical properties that can be characteristic of each location (see Table 1).

In this study, optical parameters specific to various regions such as skin, duct, and fat were provided for the analytical model based on the breast structure data of the VHP. When the fluorescence-labeled cancer of 1 cm diameter was embedded in the duct at a depth of 2 cm, the fluorescent fluence signals from the spherical cancer had a small and vertically long shape in both the NIR and the SWIR, probably due to a higher μ_s and a lower μ_a of the duct shown in Figure 4A–D. The distortion from the perfect circle in the SWIR fluorescence signals was smaller than that in the NIR due to the low μ_s. Moreover, the signal shape on the fluence map can be attributed to the distribution of the optical parameters.

To confirm this possibility, the fluence map of excitation and emission were examined in detail when the spherical cancer of 1 mm diameter was embedded in the duct at a depth of 3 cm. Although there was no emission fluence of the VIS in Figure 4, we confirmed the effect on excitation of the faithful distribution of the optical parameters due to a higher μ_s and μ_a of the VIS than the NIR and the SWIR. As shown in Figure 5E, the VIS excitation fluence signals along the duct appeared due to the migration of photons, impeded by fat with a higher μ_a. However, no photons reached the fluorescence-labeled cancer (1 mm) embedded in the deep region of the duct at a depth of 3 cm. Then, no fluorescence probes within cancer were excited by the incident photon in Figure 5F.

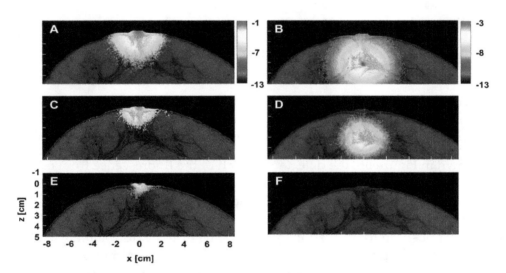

Figure 5. Fluence maps of photons associated with excitation (**A,C,E**) and emission (**B,D,F**) in the SWIR (**A,B**), the NIR (**C,D**), and the VIS (**E,F**). Fluorescence-labeled cancer with a diameter of 1 mm in the duct was embedded $x = 0$ at a depth of 3 cm. All maps share values on the x and z-axis of (**E**). (**A,C,E**) share the scale bar which shows the logarithmic scale in (**A**) and (**B,D,F**) share the scale bar in (**B**).

The excitation fluence signals of the NIR are distributed more widely than those of the VIS in Figure 5C. The signal shape of the excitation fluence of NIR was not isotropic and the signals were distributed a little downward. Although the incident photons excited the fluorescent probes within the cancer, the breast surface was not reached by any emission photon in Figure 5D. The distribution of the emission fluence signals was not isotropic either. In contrast to the excitation, the distribution was a little upward.

The excitation fluence signals of the SWIR were distributed widely than those of the NIR in Figure 5A. The distribution was downward and similar to that of the NIR. Sufficient incident photons from the SWIR reached the fluorescent probes within the cancer and emission photons reached the breast surface in Figure 5B. Therefore, the previous model was improved by a fluence signal distribution dependent on the contour of the breast tissue and the internal structure, and we confirmed this in three regions, VIS, NIR, and SWIR.

3.3. SWIR for the Detection of Small Breast Cancer in Deep Tissue

By the use of the improved Monte Carlo model improved above, photon behaviors in association with excitation and emission were examined in detail. Fluorescence-labeled cancer with a diameter of 1, 4, 7, and 10 mm was embedded at a depth of 1 to 2 cm. The fluorescence intensity detected on the tissue surface when the fluorescence-labeled cancer with a 1–10 mm diameter was embedded at a depth of 1 cm is shown in Figure 6A. In this study, a fluorescence intensity of more than 10 nW/cm^2 was detectable and the sensitivity of fluorescence image sensors reported previously was taken as the basis of the assessment [28,29]. Fluorescence from cancerous cells with a diameter of 10 mm was detectable in all regions of the VIS, the NIR, and the SWIR. The SWIR signal was the strongest; the VIS was 5.9% of the SWIR, and the NIR it was 23.5% of the SWIR. In the case of the 7 mm diameter, there was almost no VIS signal and the NIR signal was 17.2% that of the SWIR. As shown in the insert, the signal of the NIR in the 4 mm diameter was under the detection limit and was 12.6% of the SWIR. In the case of the 1 mm diameter, only the SWIR signal was detectable.

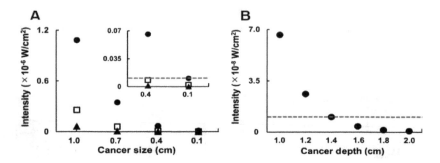

Figure 6. Effect on the detected fluorescence intensity of cancer size (**A**, 0.1–1.0 cm) and cancer depth (**B**, 1–2 cm). Insert is enlarged on the axis of the intensity. Closed circles: SWIR, Open squares: NIR, Closed triangles: VIS. The red broken line denotes the detectable intensity of 10 nW/cm^2.

Finally, as shown in Figure 6B, the detectable depth of the fluorescence from cancerous cells with a diameter of 4 mm was examined in detail. Due to the fact that no fluorescence from the VIS or the NIR from the depth of 1 cm was detectable, fluorescence-labeled cancer with SWIR alone was embedded deeper than 1 cm. At a depth of 1.2 cm, the fluorescence became weaker by 39.4% of that for 1 cm. The deepest position for cancer of a 4 mm diameter to be detectable was 1.4 cm. When the cancer was embedded deeper, the fluorescence was under the detection limit. Therefore, when the fluorescence-labeled cancer became smaller or was embedded in a deeper area, the fluorescence signal in all regions, the VIS, the NIR, and the SWIR, became weaker. However, fluorescence in the SWIR alone from cancerous cells with a diameter of 4 mm was detectable at a depth of 1.4 cm. The results show that SWIR fluorescence molecular imaging can be expected to detect breast cancer (4 mm), which is smaller than the cancer size (6 mm) detectable by MRI and sonography so far reported. Compared to the depth at which the diagnostic accuracy of sonography can be maintained (4 cm) [30], SWIR fluorescence molecular imaging may be more limited in detecting cancer, due to the depth. However, SWIR fluorescence molecular imaging has the potential advantage of distinguishing between benign and malignant tumors by the use of markers for the cancer. Furthermore, compared to MRI-sonography, the SWIR imaging system is expected to be the more practical diagnostic instrument with small size at a low running cost.

In addition to our SWIR molecular imaging for detecting early breast cancer, recently there have been remarkable advances in diagnostic methods. One of these was the early detection of circulating tumor cells in blood, an eagerly awaited noninvasive diagnosis or prognosis method [31]. In vitro assays confirmed the real time detection of cancer cells at 49 cells/mL [32]. Using a DNA biosensor based on gold nanoparticles-modified graphene oxide, breast cancer markers in the early stage were detected at a sub-nanomolar level [33]. Furthermore, when the ensemble discrete wavelet transformation as a new image processing technology was introduced to conventional mammography, the benign/malignant ROIs (regions of interest) were predicted at a precision rate of more than 97% by microcalcification cluster classification [34]. When the SWIR molecular imaging proposed in this study is applied clinically, it can be regarded as a noninvasive diagnostic method for primary breast cancer in women, without radiation exposure.

4. Conclusions and Perspectives

In the Monte Carlo model where optical parameters were set faithfully to the internal structure of the breast tissue, photon migration in association with excitation and emission was examined in detail based on the rational mechanisms for fluorescence. SWIR fluorescence molecular imaging proved the promising for the detection of small breast cancer (4 mm) at a depth of 1.4 cm, which was difficult for MRI and sonography to detect. Our results show that it is possible to predict the presence of early-stage breast cancer with high spatial resolution using SWIR and a phantom model in which the optical parameters are accurately set in the breast structure. The SWIR molecular imaging proposed in this study is suitable as a noninvasive diagnostic method for primary breast cancer in women, without radiation exposure.

Author Contributions: Conceptualization, Y.N., T.J. and A.S.; methodology, T.J.; software, T.I.; validation, T.I. and Y.N.; data curation, T.I.; writing—original draft preparation, T.I. and Y.N.; writing—review and editing, T.J. and A.S. All authors have read and agreed to the published version of the manuscript.

Acknowledgments: The authors would like to thank Enago (www.enago.jp) for the English language review.

References

1. van Dongen, J.A.; Voogd, A.C.; Fentiman, I.S.; Legrand, C.; Sylvester, R.J.; Tong, D.; van der Schueren, E.; Helle, P.A.; van Zijl, K.; Bartelink, H. Long-Term Results of a Randomized Trial Comparing Breast-Conserving Therapy with Mastectomy: European Organization for Research and Treatment of Cancer 10801 Trial. *J. Natl. Cancer Inst.* **2000**, *92*, 1143–1150. [CrossRef]

2. Silverstein, M.J.; Cohlan, B.F.; Gierson, E.D.; Furmanski, M.; Gamagami, P.; Colburn, W.J.; Lewinsky, B.S.; Waisman, J.R. Duct Carcinoma in Situ: 227 Cases without Microinvasion. *Eur. J. Cancer* **1992**, *28*, 630–634. [CrossRef]

3. Causer, P.A.; Piron, C.A.; Jong, R.A.; Plewes, D.B. Preliminary In Vivo Validation of a Dedicated Breast MRI and Sonographic Coregistration Imaging System. *Am. J. Roentgenol.* **2008**, *191*, 1203–1207. [CrossRef]

4. Wilson, R.H.; Nadeau, K.P.; Jaworski, F.B.; Tromberg, B.J.; Durkin, A.J. Review of Short-Wave Infrared Spectroscopy and Imaging Methods for Biological Tissue Characterization. *J. Biomed. Opt.* **2015**, *20*, 030901. [CrossRef] [PubMed]

5. Tsukasaki, Y.; Morimatsu, M.; Nishimura, G.; Sakata, T.; Yasuda, H.; Komatsuzaki, A.; Watanabe, T.M.; Jin, T. Synthesis and Optical Properties of Emission-Tunable PbS/CdS Core/Shell Quantum Dots for In Vivo Fluorescence Imaging in the Second Near-Infrared Window. *RSC. Adv.* **2014**, *4*, 41164–41171. [CrossRef]

6. Tong, M.; Guo, W.; Gao, W. Use of Fluorescence Imaging in Combination with Patent Blue Dye versus Patent Blue Dye Alone in Sentinel Lymph Node Biopsy in Breast Cancer. *J. Breast Cancer* **2014**, *17*, 250–255. [CrossRef] [PubMed]

7. Sugie, T.; Kassim, K.A.; Takeuchi, M.; Hashimoto, T.; Yamagami, K.; Masai, Y.; Toi, M. A Novel Method for Sentinel Lymph Node Biopsy by Indocyanine Green Fluorescence Technique in Breast Cancer. *Cancers* **2010**, *2*, 713–720. [CrossRef] [PubMed]

8. Pitsinis, V.; Wishart, G.C. Comparison of Indocyanine Green Fluorescence and Blue Dye Methods in Detection of Sentinel Lymph Nodes in Early-Stage Breast Cancer. *Ann. Surg. Oncol.* **2017**, *24*, 581–582. [CrossRef] [PubMed]

9. Kitai, T.; Inomoto, T.; Miwa, M.; Shikayama, T. Fluorescence Navigation with Indocyanine Green for Detecting Sentinel Lymph Nodes in Breast Cancer. *Breast Cancer* **2005**, *12*, 211–215. [CrossRef]

10. Tsuboi, S.; Jin, T. Shortwave-infrared (SWIR) Fluorescence Molecular Imaging Using Indocyanine Green–Antibody Conjugates for the Optical Diagnostics of Cancerous Tumours. *RSC. Adv.* **2020**, *10*, 28171–28179. [CrossRef]

11. Iida, T.; Jin, T.; Nomura, Y. Monte Carlo Modeling of Near-Infrared Fluorescence Photon Migration in Breast Tissue for Tumor Prediction. *Adv. Biomed. Eng.* **2020**, *9*, 100–105. [CrossRef]

12. Li, T.; Li, Y.; Sun, Y.; Duan, M.; Peng, L. Effect of Head Model on Monte Carlo Modeling of Spatial Sensitivity Distribution for Functional Near-Infrared Spectroscopy. *J. Innov. Opt. Health Sci.* **2015**, *8*, 1550024. [CrossRef]

13. Li, T.; Xue, C.; Wang, P.; Li, Y.; Wu, L. Photon Penetration Depth in Human Brain for Light Stimulation and Treatment: A Realistic Monte Carlo Simulation Study. *J. Innov. Opt. Health Sci.* **2017**, *10*, 1743002. [CrossRef]

14. Iida, T.; Yamato, H.; Jin, T.; Nomura, Y. Optimal Focus Evaluated Using Monte Carlo Simulation in Non-Invasive Neuroimaging in the Second near-Infrared Window. *MethodsX* **2019**, *6*, 2367–2373. [CrossRef] [PubMed]

15. Yamato, H.; Iida, T.; Jin, T.; Nomura, Y. Monte Carlo Evaluation of In Vivo Neuroimaging Using Quantum Dots with Fluorescence in the Second Window of Near Infrared Region. *Adv. Biomed. Eng.* **2019**, *8*, 105–109. [CrossRef]

16. Hasegawa, Y.; Yamada, Y.; Tamura, M.; Nomura, Y. Monte Carlo Simulation of Light Transmission through Living Tissues. *Appl. Opt.* **1991**, *30*, 4515–4520. [CrossRef]

17. Visible Human Project. Available online: https://www.nlm.nih.gov/research/visible/visible_human.html (accessed on 15 August 2020).

18. Salomatina, E.; Jiang, B.; Novak, J.; Yaroslavsky, A.N. Optical Properties of Normal and Cancerous Human Skin in the Visible and Near-Infrared Spectral Range. *J. Biomed. Opt.* **2006**, *11*, 064026. [CrossRef]

19. Jacques, S.L. Optical Properties of Biological Tissues: A Review. *Phys. Med. Biol.* **2013**, *58*, R37–R61. [CrossRef]

20. Troy, T.L.; Page, D.L.; Sevick-Muraca, E.M. Optical Properties of Normal and Diseased Breast Tissues: Prognosis for Optical Mammography. *J. Biomed. Opt.* **1996**, *1*, 342–355. [CrossRef]

21. Ding, H.; Lu, J.Q.; Wooden, W.A.; Kragel, P.J.; Hu, X.H. Refractive Indices of Human Skin Tissues at Eight Wavelengths and Estimated Dispersion Relations between 300 and 1600 nm. *Phys. Med. Biol.* **2006**, *51*, 1479–1489. [CrossRef]

22. Prince, S.; Malarvizhi, S. Monte Carlo Simulation of NIR Diffuse Reflectance in the Normal and Diseased Human Breast Tissues. *BioFactors* **2007**, *30*, 255–263. [CrossRef] [PubMed]

23. Hayreh, S.S. Recent Advances in Fluorescein Fundus Angiography. *Br. J. Ophthalmol.* **1974**, *58*, 391–412. [CrossRef]

24. Altan-Yaycioglu, R.; Akova, Y.A.; Akca, S.; Yilmaz, G. Inflammation of the Posterior Uvea: Findings on Fundus Fluorescein and Indocyanine Green Angiography. *Ocul. Immunol. Inflamm.* **2006**, *14*, 171–179. [CrossRef] [PubMed]

25. Wang, L.; Jacques, S.L.; Zheng, L. MCML—Monte Carlo Modeling of Light Transport in Multi-Layered Tissues. *Comput. Methods Programs Biomed.* **1995**, *47*, 131–146. [CrossRef]

26. Matsumoto, M.; Nishimura, T. Mersenne Twister: A 623-Dimensionally Equidistributed Uniform Pseudo-Random Number Generator. *ACM Trans. Model. Comput. Simul.* **1998**, *8*, 3–30. [CrossRef]

27. Jacques, S.L. Light Distributions from Point, Line and Plane Sources for Photochemical Reactions and Fluorescence in Turbid Biological Tissues. *Photochem. Photobiol.* **1998**, *67*, 23–32. [CrossRef]

28. Nan, L.; Zhiliang, H.; Ran, L. A CMOS Detector System for Fluorescent Bio-Sensing Application. In Proceedings of the 2008 IEEE Asian Solid-State Circuits Conference (ASSCC), Fukuoka, Japan, 3–5 November 2008.

29. Murari, K.; Ralph, E.C.; Nitish, V.T.; Cauwenberghs, G. A CMOS In-Pixel CTIA High-Sensitivity Fluorescence Imager. *IEEE. Trans. Biomed. Circuits Syst.* **2011**, *5*, 449–458. [CrossRef]

30. Guo, R.; Lu, G.; Qin, B.; Fei, B. Ultrasound Imaging Technologies for Breast Cancer Detection and Management: A Review. *Ultrasound Med. Biol.* **2018**, *44*, 37–70. [CrossRef]

31. De Mattos-Arruda, L.; Cortes, J.; Santarpia, L.; Vivancos, A.; Tabernero, J.; Jorge S Reis-Filho, J.S.R.; Seoane, J. Circulating Tumour Cells and Cell-free DNA as Tools for Managing Breast Cancer. *Nat. Rev. Clin. Oncol.* **2013**, *10*, 377–389. [CrossRef]

32. Loyez, M.; Hassan, E.M.; Lobry, M.; Liu, F.; Caucheteur, C.; Wattiez, R.; DeRosa, M.C.; Willmore, W.G.; Albert, J. Rapid Detection of Circulating Breast Cancer Cells using a Multiresonant Optical Fiber Aptasensor with Plasmonic Amplification. *ACS Sens.* **2020**, *5*, 454–463. [CrossRef]

33. Saeed, A.A.; Sánchez, J.L.A.; O'Sullivan, C.K.; Abbas, M.N. DNA biosensors based on gold nanoparticles-modified graphene oxide for the detection of breast cancer biomarkers for early diagnosis. *Bioelectrochemistry* **2017**, *118*, 91–99. [CrossRef] [PubMed]

34. Fanizzi, A.; Basile, T.M.; Losurdo, L.; Bellotti, L.; Bottigli, U.; Campobasso, F.; Didonna, V.; Fausto, A.; Massafra, R.; Tagliafico, A.; et al. Ensemble Discrete Wavelet Transform and Gray-Level Co-Occurrence Matrix for Microcalcification Cluster Classification in Digital Mammography. *Appl. Sci.* **2019**, *9*, 5388. [CrossRef]

Optical Detection of Ketoprofen by its Electropolymerization on an Indium Tin Oxide-Coated Optical Fiber Probe

Robert Bogdanowicz [1], Paweł Niedziałkowski [2], Michał Sobaszek [1], Dariusz Burnat [3], Wioleta Białobrzeska [2], Zofia Cebula [2], Petr Sezemsky [4], Marcin Koba [3,5], Vitezslav Stranak [4], Tadeusz Ossowski [2] and Mateusz Śmietana [3,*]

[1] Faculty of Electronics, Telecommunications and Informatics, Gdansk University of Technology, Narutowicza 11/12, 80-233 Gdansk, Poland; rbogdan@eti.pg.gda.pl (R.B.); micsobas@pg.edu.pl (M.S.)
[2] Department of Analytical Chemistry, Faculty of Chemistry, University of Gdansk, Wita Stwosza 63, 80-308 Gdansk, Poland; pawel.niedzialkowski@ug.edu.pl (P.N.); wioleta.bialobrzeska@phdstud.ug.edu.pl (W.B.); zofia.jelinska@phdstud.ug.edu.pl (Z.C.); tadeusz.ossowski@ug.edu.pl (T.O.)
[3] Institute of Microelectronics and Optoelectronics, Warsaw University of Technology, Koszykowa 75, 00-662 Warszawa, Poland; drkbrt@o2.pl (D.B.); marcinkoba@gmail.com (M.K.)
[4] Institute of Physics and Biophysics, Faculty of Science, University of South Bohemia, Branisovska 1760, 370 05 Ceske Budejovice, Czech Republic; petr.sezemsky@gmail.com (P.S.); stranv00@centrum.cz (V.S.)
[5] National Institute of Telecommunications, Szachowa 1, 04-894 Warszawa, Poland
* Correspondence: M.Smietana@elka.pw.edu.pl

Abstract: In this work an application of optical fiber sensors for real-time optical monitoring of electrochemical deposition of ketoprofen during its anodic oxidation is discussed. The sensors were fabricated by reactive magnetron sputtering of indium tin oxide (ITO) on a 2.5 cm-long core of polymer-clad silica fibers. ITO tuned in optical properties and thickness allows for achieving a lossy-mode resonance (LMR) phenomenon and it can be simultaneously applied as an electrode in an electrochemical setup. The ITO-LMR electrode allows for optical monitoring of changes occurring at the electrode during electrochemical processing. The studies have shown that the ITO-LMR sensor's spectral response strongly depends on electrochemical modification of its surface by ketoprofen. The effect can be applied for real-time detection of ketoprofen. The obtained sensitivities reached over 1400 nm/M (nm·mg^{-1}·L) and 16,400 a.u./M (a.u.·mg^{-1}·L) for resonance wavelength and transmission shifts, respectively. The proposed method is a valuable alternative for the analysis of ketoprofen within the concentration range of 0.25–250 μg mL^{-1}, and allows for its determination at therapeutic and toxic levels. The proposed novel sensing approach provides a promising strategy for both optical and electrochemical detection of electrochemical modifications of ITO or its surface by various compounds.

Keywords: ketoprofen; anti-inflammatory drug; drug analysis; optical fiber sensor; reactive magnetron sputtering thin film; indium tin oxide (ITO); lossy-mode resonance (LMR); electrochemistry; electropolymerization

---

1. Introduction

Demand for nonprescription drugs, such as 2-(3-benzoylphenyl)-propanoic acid (ketoprofen, KP) is expected to increase in the near future. KP is a nonsteroidal anti-inflammatory drug, widely used for the treatment of various kinds of pains, rheumatoid arthritis and osteoarthritis [1]. KP exhibits analgesic and antipyretic activity, which is mainly caused by the inhibition of prostaglandin synthesis by inhibiting cyclooxygenase [2]. The widespread and growing volume of human and veterinary prescriptions needs to be followed by the development of analytical techniques allowing for detection of KP traces in various biofluids or sludge water.

Several methods have already been reported for quantitative determination of KP, including liquid chromatography-mass spectrometry [3], UV-fluorescence [4], ion chromatography [5], flow injection with chemiluminescence [6], or electrochemical detection [7]. Both chromatographic and non-chromatographic techniques usually require rigorous sample preparation and expensive extraction methods (including solid-phase extraction) when real samples are considered. Mass spectrometry in turn requires analyte signal suppression or enhancement during electrospray ionization, especially for analysis of multi-compound samples. Application of all these methods is time-consuming and requires expensive and highly specialized setups which are only available in well-equipped research laboratories. Among other techniques, fluorescence at porous SnO_2 nanoparticles was applied for KP detection using combined ion chromatography with photodetection. The limit of detection (LOD) in human serum, urine, and canal water samples was 0.1 µg/kg, 0.5 µg/kg, and 0.39 µg/kg, respectively [5]. However, photometric UV and fluorescence-based methods commonly suffer from low sensitivity and selectivity, while the latter require specific chemicals or compounds (e.g., nanoparticles) in the detection procedure.

Electrochemical studies of KP have already been performed using the polarographic method [8,9] or simultaneously cyclic voltammetry and coulometry techniques at the mercury dropping electrode surface [8,10]. Kormosh et al. [11] developed ion-selective electrodes for potentiometric analysis of KP in piroxicam based on Rhodamine 6G in a membrane plasticizer. The measurements of KP using direct current stripping voltammetry as well as spectrophotometric methods were also reported by Emara et al. [9]. With dropping mercury electrode and using different supporting electrolytes at different pH values it was possible to reach a LOD as low as 5.08×10^{-4} ng mL^{-1}. A similar electrode was utilized by Ghoneim and Tawfik [10], and in a Britton-Robinson buffer (pH 2.0) the LOD was 0.10 ng mL^{-1}. Next, a setup containing glassy carbon (GC) electrode with multiwalled carbon nanotubes/ionic liquid/chitosan composite for covalent immobilization of the ibuprofen by specific aptamer was proposed [7].

It can be concluded that the electrochemical methods offer reliability and accuracy, enabling development of simple, rapid, and cost-effective approaches for the detection of electroactive compounds. However, electrodes for KP detection usually need complex pre-treatment in order to reach high repeatability and environmental stability. Furthermore, KP shows poor solubility in water, a tendency to adsorb and block electrodes, and a rapid metabolization to by-products [12]. Thus, conventional electrochemical assay procedures are not well-suited for this specific application.

To overcome the limitations listed above, we propose a novel approach for KP detection, where together with an electrochemical method an indium tin oxide (ITO)-coated optical fiber sensor is used. ITO is known for its high optical transparency and low electrical resistivity. Moreover, thanks to its band-gap, it is a good candidate for an electrochemical electrode, and it can be used for optical measurements as well. Contrary to other transparent electrode materials, such as boron-doped diamond, thin ITO films can be deposited at a relatively low temperature on various substrates and shapes [13]. Plasma-assisted deposition is often used for obtaining high quality ITO films. An ITO overlay was applied as a standard working electrode, where KP was electropolymerized with the cyclic voltammetry technique. Thanks to the adjustment of both ITO's electrochemical and optical properties, lossy-mode resonance (LMR) effect in optical fiber sensor can also be applied for KP detection. LMR is a thin-film-based optical effect, which takes place when a certain relation between electric permittivity of the film, substrate, and external medium is fulfilled, namely the real part of the film's electric permittivity must be positive and higher in magnitude than both the thin film's permittivity imaginary part and the permittivity of the analyte [14]. Any variation in optical properties of the analyte, especially its refractive index (RI), has an influence on resonance conditions and can thus be detected. Since in visible spectral range ITO shows relatively high RI (n_D ~2 RIU) and non-zero extinction coefficient (corresponding to optical absorption), it has already been successfully applied in LMR-based sensing devices [15]. There have been reported applications of other thin films supporting the LMR effect such as diamond-like carbon [16] , SiN_x [17], TiO_2 [18], and polymers [19], but among these materials only ITO offers low electrical resistivity and can be applied as an electrode material. Until now both the electrical conductivity of ITO and supported by its thin film LMR effect have been applied only with the purpose of inducing a high voltage change in properties of an electro-optic material deposited on ITO surface [20], and for electropolymerization of a chemical compound on the ITO surface [21]. As an alternative to the conventional assay procedures, the developed opto-electrochemical probe can offer a KP detection method free from pre-treatment of the electrode's surface, as well as prolonged analysis time and sophisticated experimental setup.

The application of opto-electrochemical probes is a novel approach. To the best of our knowledge, in this paper we discuss for the first time the application of LMR phenomenon at the ITO-coated optical fiber for electrochemically-induced KP detection. The developed opto-electrochemical probe offers capability for label-free KP detection with no need of the electrode's surface pre-treatment. Additionally, the GC electrode has been modified by KP for reference.

2. Materials and Methods

KP (2-(3-benzoylphenyl) propionic acid) of purity greater than 98% was obtained from Cayman Company (Ann Arbor, MI, USA) and used without any further purification. A KP solution with a concentration of 2 mM was prepared in a 0.1 M phosphate buffer saline (pH = 7.0). Na_2SO_4 and $K_3[Fe(CN)_6]$ were purchased from POCh (Gliwice, Poland).

2.1. ITO Optical Probe Fabrication and Testing

The LMR structures were fabricated using approx. 15 cm-long polymer-clad silica fiber samples of 400/840 μm core/cladding diameter, where 2.5 cm of polymer cladding was removed in the fiber central section [22]. Next, the electrically conductive and optically transparent ITO films were deposited by reactive magnetron sputtering of ITO target (In_2O_3-SnO_2—90/10 wt % and purity of 99.99%). The magnetron, whose axis was perpendicular to the substrate, was supplied by a Cito1310 (13.56 MHz, 300 W) RF source (Comet AG, Flamatt, Switzerland). The experiments were carried out at pressure p = 1.0 Pa in a reactive N_2/Ar atmosphere, gas flows were 15 and 0.5–1.0 sccm for Ar and N_2, respectively. The overlays were deposited on fibers rotated in the chamber during the process. Simultaneously, Si wafers and glass slides were also coated for reference. Both of the end-faces of the fiber sample were mechanically polished before the optical testing.

To determine RI sensitivity of the fabricated ITO-LMR devices, they were investigated in the air and mixtures of water/glycerin with n_D = 1.33–1.45 RIU. The RI of the mixtures was measured using an AR200 automatic digital refractometer (Reichert Inc., Buffalo, NY, USA). The optical transmission of the ITO-LMR structure was interrogated in the range of λ = 350–1050 nm using an HL-2000 white light source (Ocean Optics Inc., Largo, FL, USA) and an Ocean Optics USB4000 spectrometer. The optical transmission (T) in the specified spectral range was detected as counts in specified integration time (up to 100 ms). The temperature of the solutions was stabilized at 25 °C to avoid thermal shift of the RI.

2.2. Electrochemical Setup and Electropolymerization of KP

Cyclic voltammetry measurements were performed with a PGSTAT204 potentiostat/galvanostat (Metrohm, Herisau, Switzerland) controlled by Nova 1.1 software, and using the ITO-LMR probe as a working electrode (WE), a platinum wire as counter electrode (CE), and an Ag/AgCl/0.1 M KCl as a reference electrode (REF). The ITO-LMR working electrode was electrochemically processed in 0.1 M phosphate buffer saline containing from 1×10^{-6} to 1×10^{-3} M of KP at scan rate 50 mV·s^{-1} for 6 cycles. The process allowed for anodic electrooxidation of KP in the potential ranging from 0.3 to 2.0 V vs. Ag/AgCl/0.1 M KCl electrode. The reference GC and ITO electrodes were processed under the same conditions as the ITO-LMR electrode, but for the GC electrode the modification took

10 cycles. Next, the electrodes were washed in water and methanol, and dried under a stream of air. The electrode examinations before and after modification with cyclic voltammetry were performed in 5 mM of $K_3[Fe(CN)_6]$ in 0.5 M Na_2SO_4 solution at scan rate of 100 mV$\cdot$s^{-1}. The setup used in this experiment is schematically shown in Figure 1.

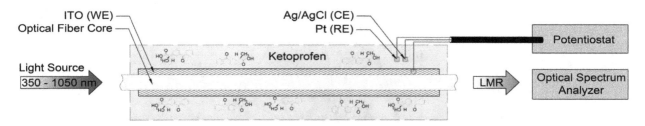

Figure 1. The schematic representation of the experimental setup with ITO-LMR probe used for combined optical and electrochemical KP detection. The electrodes were denoted as working (WE), reference (RE), and counter (CE).

2.3. X-ray Photoelectron Spectroscopy Surface Studies

X-ray Photoelectron Spectroscopy (XPS) studies were carried out using an ESCA300 XPS setup (Scienta Omicron GmbH, Taunusstein, Germany) with a high resolution spectrometer equipped with a monochromatic Kα source. Measurements were done at 10 eV pass energy and 0.05 eV energy step size. A flood gun was used for charge compensation purpose. Finally, the calibration of XPS spectra was performed for carbon peak C1s at 284.6 eV [23,24].

3. Results and Discussion

3.1. The RI Sensitivity of the ITO-LMR Probe

First, the optical probes were studied in an optical setup only. This part of the experiment was done in order to estimate the sensitivity of the device to changes of optical properties at the ITO surface. The probes were installed in a setup allowing one to record the transmission spectra, while the sensor was consecutively immersed in different RI solutions. In Figure 2 a well-defined resonance can be seen that experiences a shift towards higher wavelengths when the external RI increases. It is worth noting that the applied ITO coatings provide relatively narrow resonance. The full width at half maximum (FWHM) obtained for the resonances is approx. 110 nm. When the probe is immersed in the higher RI, the FWHM of the resonance slightly increases. Based on the obtained results, two ways of sensor interrogation can be selected, namely tracking of resonance wavelength (λ_R) or monitoring transmission at discrete wavelength, the most effectively chosen at the resonance slope. In the case of this experiment, the transmission was monitored at λ = 600 nm (T_{600}). Both the λ_R and T_{600} were plotted vs. RI in the inset of Figure 2. The shift is positive for both of the interrogation schema, but for tracking λ_R the dependence is less linear (the sensitivity increases with RI) than for the T_{600}.

The measurements of reference Si samples allowed to estimate the thickness of the coating to 260 nm. According to theoretical studies [25], a low order LMR may be observed for such thickness of ITO. It is known that low order LMRs offer the highest sensitivity to changes in external RI [14], as well as changes in properties of a layer formed on the ITO surface [26].

The standard commercial ITO electrodes undergo thermal annealing to decrease both optical absorption and electrical resistivity, most likely due to the crystallization processes [27]. The LMR-satisfying properties of non-annealed, as fabricated ITO films are attributed to unique advantages of the applied discharge during deposition process. Our previous research clearly showed that optimization of the deposition pressure 0.5 Pa < p < 1.0 Pa induces collisions of the sputtered particles [28,29]. The application of magnetron sputtering is advantageous and allows to tailor the optical and electrical properties of the deposited ITO films with no additional post-deposition annealing as it is often required in case of other deposition methods [30].

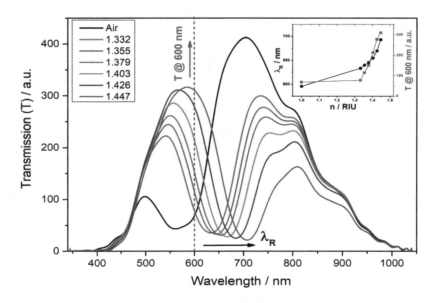

Figure 2. Spectral response of ITO-LMR probe to changes in external RI (n). The changes of resonance wavelength (λ_R) and transmission (T) at λ = 600 nm are shown in the inset.

3.2. Electrodeposition of KP on GC, ITO and ITO-LMR Electrodes

The electrochemical deposition of KP on GC, ITO and ITO-LMR electrodes was made by anodic oxidation. The redox behavior of KP molecule at the GC and ITO electrode has not been reported yet. However, the anodic oxidation of KP was observed at the boron doped diamond electrode. The current peak measured for this electrode during the electrodeposition processes is associated with the oxidation of carboxyl group in KP [31]. Moreover, the mechanism of the electrochemical reduction of KP have been until now examined only at the mercury electrode and requires transfer of two electrons. This reduction leads to formation of 2-(3-benzhydrolyl)-propionic acid [8] (Scheme 1). The mechanism of reduction of KP—benzophenone-3 has been described elsewhere [32].

(ketoprofen)
2-(3-benzoylphenyl)propanoic acid

$+ 2H^+, + 2\ e$

2-(3-benzhydrolyl)-propionic acid

Scheme 1. Chemical structure of KP and mechanism of its electrochemical reduction.

Anodic oxidation by electron transfer leads to deactivation of electrode surface and its modification by adsorption of oxidized polymeric products of the reaction. This effect has been used in this work for modification of different types of electrodes, i.e., GC, ITO, and ITO-LMR. It must be emphasized that only ITO-LMR electrode allows for simultaneous optical and electrochemical monitoring of the modification processes by KP.

The cyclic voltammetry is a very valuable and convenient tool to monitor the electrode surface properties before and after each step of modification [33]. The electrochemical responses of the bare GC, ITO and ITO-LMR electrodes were investigated in a solution of 0.5 M Na_2SO_4 containing 5 mM $[Fe(CN)_6]^{3-/4-}$. The comparison of cyclic voltammograms of modified and bare electrodes is presented in Figure 3. For the bare GC electrode, well-defined reversible redox peaks corresponding to one-electron reversible reaction and the peak to peak separation value of 95 mV were reported [34]. This redox reaction of KP completely blocked the GC electrode after 10 scans. The current peak observed in the first scan (Figure 3a) can be attributed to the oxidation of carboxyl group of the KP [35]. The absence of any current for the GC electrode cycled in presence of KP suggests that KP-based layer was formed on the GC surface (Figure 3b). Polymerized KP film the most likely prevents from the penetration of the electroactive substance towards the electrode surface [36]. This phenomenon has been commonly observed for a series of compounds and different electrode material [37,38].

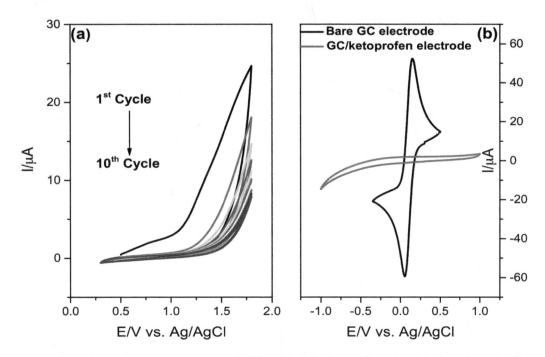

Figure 3. Cyclic voltammetry curves recorded for (**a**) GC electrode in 0.1 M phosphate buffer saline containing 2 mM of KP for 10 cycles, scan rate of 50 mV·s^{-1}; and (**b**) bare GC and GC/KP electrode in 0.5 M Na$_2$SO$_4$ containing of 5 mM [Fe(CN)$_6$]$^{3-/4-}$. The scan rate was set to 100 mV·s^{-1}.

Next, a reference ITO electrode deposited on a glass slide underwent a similar modification procedure. In Figure 4a the cyclic voltammetry curves recorded for ITO electrode in 0.1 M phosphate buffer saline containing 2 mM of KP in 10 cycles are shown. For the bare ITO electrode a redox response with peak to peak potential separation reached 245 mV. Significant differences between the electrochemical response for bare and modified electrodes recorded in 0.5 M Na$_2$SO$_4$ solution containing 5 mM [Fe(CN)$_6$]$^{3-/4-}$ were observed. The decrease in peak current and increase in peak to peak potential separation of up to 511 mV, indicate that the modification of the electrode surface by KP was effective (Figure 4b). This phenomenon also suggests that the surface of the ITO electrode was blocked by KP, which is observed in the disappearance of the anodic and cathodic peak [39].

The ITO-LMR probe was coated with KP during only six anodic oxidation cycles in the potential range from 0.3 to 2.0 V and with a scan rate of 50 mV·s^{-1} (Figure 5a). After this process, the electrode was extensively washed with water and methanol. It is worth noting that for the modification by KP of GC and ITO electrodes, 10 cycles were applied. In the case of ITO-LMR electrode, six cycles were enough to completely cover the electrode. In Figure 5b the cyclic voltammetry response to 0.5 M Na$_2$SO$_4$ containing 5 mM [Fe(CN)$_6$]$^{3-/4-}$ is shown for bare and KP-modified ITO-LMR electrode. Bare and modified ITO-LMR electrodes show redox responses with peak to peak potential separation reaching 419 mV and 628 mV, respectively. Moreover, for the KP-modified ITO-LMR electrode the redox current peaks significantly increased. This effect suggests that the electrode has a more developed active surface area than the one before modification [40]. This was only observed for anodic oxidation of

KP on the ITO-LMR electrode. In the other cases, namely reference ITO and GC electrodes, the current peaks for redox couple decreased significantly as a result of modification by KP.

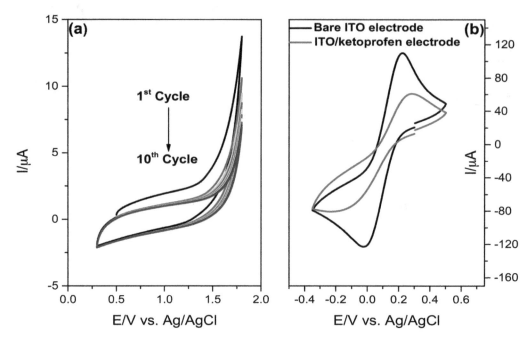

Figure 4. Cyclic voltammetry curves recorded for (**a**) ITO electrode in 0.1 M phosphate buffer saline containing 2 mM of KP (10 cycles, scan rate of 50 mV·s^{-1}) and (**b**) ITO and ITO/KP electrode in 0.5 M Na$_2$SO$_4$ containing 5 mM [Fe(CN)$_6$]$^{3-/4-}$, scan rate 100 mV·s^{-1}.

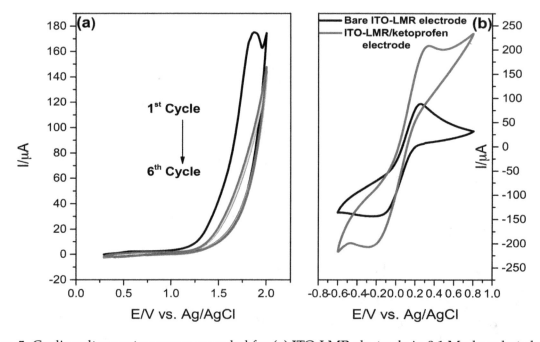

Figure 5. Cyclic voltammetry curves recorded for (**a**) ITO-LMR electrode in 0.1 M phosphate buffer saline containing 2 mM of KP for 6 cycles at scan rate of 50 mV·s^{-1}; and (**b**) bare for and KP-modified ITO-LMR in 0.5 M Na$_2$SO$_4$ containing 5 mM [Fe(CN)$_6$]$^{3-/4-}$, scan rate 100 mV·s^{-1}.

In Table 1 are summarized the electrochemical results obtained for the samples before and after KP modification. The peak splitting difference between bare ITO and ITO-LMR electrodes, i.e., ΔE reaching 245 mV and 419 mV, respectively, can originate from two effects. First, the ITO deposition on cylindrical shape, such as optical fiber, is more challenging than on a flat surface and has an impact on size, crystallinity and morphology of the electrode active surface. Second, the KP modifies the shape of the cyclic voltammetry curves and the peak to peak separations ΔE from 511 to 628 mV for ITO and ITO-LMR electrode, respectively. The diffusion of electrons through the KP is disturbed, revealing slightly reduced electrocatalytic activities, which can be attributed to its structural features and electrochemical properties.

Table 1. Electrochemical parameters of the reactions for $[Fe(CN)_6]^{3-/4-}$ on the surface of bare and KP modified ITO electrodes.

Sample	E_{red} (mV)	E_{ox} (mV)	ΔE (mV)	$E_{1/2}$ (mV)
Bare ITO electrode	−24	221	245	123
KP/ITO electrode	−230	281	511	230
Bare ITO-LMR electrode	−165	254	419	210
KP/ITO-LMR electrode	−285	343	628	314

3.3. XPS Studies of KP-Modified ITO Surface

High-resolution XPS spectra, analyzed within the energy range of C1s and O1s peaks, make it possible to verify successful KP modification of ITO surface at the level of 10^{-3} M. Survey of the XPS spectrum presented in Figure 6 reveals significant contribution from ITO background seen as tin, indium, and oxygen peaks, and smaller contribution from electropolymerized thin KP layer on ITO surface. The high-resolution XPS spectra were also acquired, in the energy range characteristic for C1s and O1s peaks. The high-resolution analysis allows for verification of successful KP modification of ITO surface at the level of 10^{-3} M. Recorded spectra with their deconvolution are shown in the inset of Figure 6 and extracted data are summarized in Table 2.

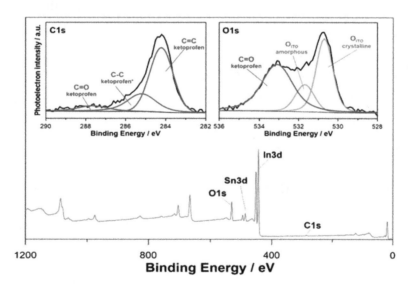

Figure 6. XPS survey spectrum and high-resolution XPS spectra registered for C1s and O1s energy range. Peaks underwent spectral deconvolution are superimposed with colors depending on their origination (blue for KP and green for ITO). The KP concentration was 1×10^{-3} M.

The C1s spectrum was deconvoluted with three peaks, each denoting a different chemical state of carbon. The primary component is located at +284.2 eV and is characteristic for aromatic C=C bonds in KP. The second and third type of interaction can be associated with aliphatic C-C and C=O bonds. Their energy shift versus the primary spectral component is +1.0 for C–C and +3.5 eV for C=O type of bonds and highly correlates with other results found in the literature [41–43]. Furthermore, the XPS analysis carried out within the O1s energy region confirmed the pronounced presence of peak located at 533.1 eV, which is characteristic for carbonyl bonds. Finally, the acquired C=C:C–C:C=O ratio of 6.5:2.8:1 corresponds to the known for KP 6:1:1. A slight excess of C–C contribution can be explained by the presence of adventitious carbon coming from sample storage in atmospheric conditions. The amount of adventitious carbon found at bare ITO electrode did not exceed 5 at.% and was excluded from further analysis.

Table 2. Comparison of chemical composition of bare ITO and ITO/KP electrode.

XPS Photopeak	Chemical State	Binding Energy (eV)	Chemical Composition (at.%)	
			Bare ITO Electrode	ITO/KP Electrode
C1s	C=C	284.2	-	27.8
	C–C *	285.2	-	9.9
	C=O	287.7	-	4.3
O1s	ITO$_{cryst}$	530.7	40.5	13.6
	ITO$_{amorph}$	531.7	12.8	5.5
	C=O	533.1	-	17.3
In	ITO$_{cryst}$	444.1	29.8	9.8
	ITO$_{amorph}$	445.1	11.8	9.2
Sn	ITO$_{cryst}$	486.1	3.7	1.4
	ITO$_{amorph}$	487.0	1.4	1.2

* Indicates the influence of adventitious carbon in total chemical composition of C–C chemical state.

We have also performed detailed XPS analysis of peaks located in In3d5 and Sn3d5 energy range. The results of the analysis were also summarized in Table 2. According to literature survey, ITO analysis are typically based on spectral deconvolution using two sub-peaks—often ascribed to be contribution from crystalline and amorphous ITO. The observed peak shift between crystalline and amorphous phases—1.0 eV for In and 0.9 eV for Sn peaks—was found to stay in agreement with literature survey [44–46].

3.4. ITO-LMR-Based KP Electropolymerization Monitoring

The electrochemically-induced polymerization of KP was monitored optically using ITO-LMR probe. As shown in Figure 7, there were changes in the spectral response during cyclic voltammetry electropolymerization of KP for its two concentrations in the solution, i.e., the lowest and the highest. Obviously, for high KP concentration (1×10^{-3} M) results in electropolymerization of denser film which is followed by more pronounced changes in the optical spectrum (Figure 7B). Nevertheless, as low KP concentration as 1×10^{-6} M can be observed in optical response (Figure 7A). For all the applied concentrations, the most noticeable changes in the spectrum can be observed for the resonance at approx. λ_R ~650 nm, where a shift towards longer wavelengths takes place with the process progress. On top of tracking the resonant wavelength shift, in the discussed case also changes in T can be monitored at specific wavelength. For these resonance conditions, as previously when response to RI has been analyzed, we picked $\lambda = 600$ nm that is in the middle of the resonance slope. Due to the limited resolution of the spectrometer, T monitoring may deliver more accurate data than λ_R.

The saturation of KP polymerization process was noticed for the ITO-LMR probe during the second CV cycle. The scan rate was set to 100 mV·s^{-1} in the range 0–2 V what resulted in 40 s per one cycle. The full range optical transmission was recorded with integration time up to 100 ms for 3500 data set. Thus, the entire optical analysis took 6 minutes. However, the wavelength range could be limited to e.g., 50 nm (approx. 250 data points) resulting in 25 seconds-long analysis. Summarizing, the result of KP determination was achieved with response time below 1 minute with no additional pretreatment, labeling, or incubation required.

Variations of the two parameters, namely λ_R and T versus progress in the electrodeposition process are shown for all the KP concentrations in Figure 8. As in the case of an increase in external RI, both of them increase with progress of the electrodeposition process. The effect can be explained as a mass transfer of KP, i.e., densification of the medium at the ITO surface, resulting in the growth of the KP polymer film. A similar shift has already been reported for aptamer immobilization or swelling of poly-acrylic acid (PAA) and polyallylamine hydrochloride (PAH) polymeric coatings on ITO deposited on a fiber [26,47]. The increase in both parameters depends on the concentration of KP and surely has an impact on the thickness of the electrodeposited film. The effect of KP deposition on the electrode was revealed earlier by XPS studies (Figure 6) and recognized by a shift of peaks characteristic for aromatic C=C and aliphatic C–C and C=O bonds existing in this compound.

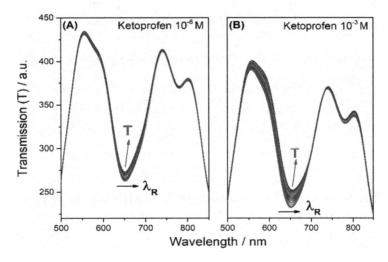

Figure 7. Changes in optical response of the ITO-LMR probe recorded during electropolymerization of KP on ITO surface for two KP concentrations, namely (**A**) 1×10^{-6} M and (**B**) 1×10^{-3} M.

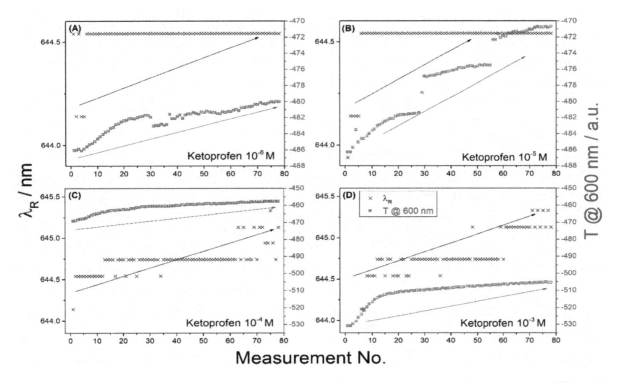

Figure 8. Change in resonance wavelengths (λ_R) {×} and transmission (T) at 600 nm {□} with progress of KP electropolymerization process on ITO-LMR probe for KP concentration (**A**) 1×10^{-6} M; (**B**) 1×10^{-5} M; (**C**) 1×10^{-4} M; and (**D**) 1×10^{-3} M.

The relative changes of λ_R and T at $\lambda = 600$ nm are summarized in Table 3 using data shown in Figure 8. The final values of the achieved parameters after 80 measurements (approx. 120 s) were plotted versus the KP concentration. It must be noted that both the parameters linearly depend on the concentration with an average correlation coefficient R^2 higher than 0.93. The sensitivities have been considered as ratios of the slopes reaching 1400.86 nm/M (nm·mg^{-1}·L) and 16,422.46 a.u./M (a.u·mg^{-1}·L) for resonance wavelengths (λ_R) and T, respectively. The calculated LOD of KP is 0.536 or 0.575 mM using λ_R and T, respectively. The application of enhanced resolution equipment and standardized solutions at lower concentration would allow us to enhance this value as well as the LOD. The KP detection experiments were performed three times using separately deposited ITO-LMR probes. They were used to determine 1 mM KP solution with an average RSD value 8.5%, which indicates the satisfactory reproducibility and repeatability of the approach.

Table 3. The relative changes of λ_R and T at 600 nm of ITO-LMR probe recorded vs. KP concentration.

KP Concentration	ΔT (a.u.)	$\Delta\lambda$ (nm)
1×10^{-3} M	255.2	1.98
1×10^{-4} M	123.2	0.99
1×10^{-5} M	113.9	0.6
1×10^{-6} M	60.4	0.4

Analytical capability for KP determination with bare ITO-LMR electrode and other previously used nanomaterials is compared in Table 4. It can be concluded that the measurements with the ITO-LMR probe offer competitive sensitivity mainly when higher KP concentrations are considered. At these conditions standard electrochemical sensors are not effective due to adsorption at the electrode surface. The sensing concept can be further developed towards detection of other polymerizing agents. Fabrication of such sensors can be easily scaled-up keeping physical homogeneity and electrochemical performance. Summarizing, the application of the ITO-LMR probe offers competitive response toward KP detection mainly when larger concentrations are considered and standard electrochemical sensors are oversaturated by adsorption. The sensing concept can be further developed for future studies of other polymerizing agents.

Table 4. Comparison of KP linear measurement range and LOD achieved with different methods.

Technique	Details	Linear Range	Limit of Detection	Reference
Adsorptive Stripping Square Wave	Mercury electrode	1×10^{-8}–3×10^{-7} M	0.1 ng mL^{-1}	[10]
LC-APCI-MS	Single Ion Monitoring mode (SIM)	100–500 ng/mL	1.0 ng/mL	[3]
IC-FLD	SnO$_2$ nanoparticles	0.1 μg/kg	0.2–1.5 mg/kg	[5]
Differential Pulse Voltammetry	Aptamer and glassy carbon electrode	70 pM–6 μM	20 pM	[7]
Potentiometry	PVC electrode	0.0001–0.05 mol/L	6.3×10^{-5} mol/L	[11]
Microdialisys	Short polymeric columns (SPE)	25–5000 ng/mL	3 ng/mL	[48]
Flow injection	Flow injection with chemiluminescence	5.0×10^{-8}–3.0×10^{-6} mol/L	2.0×10^{-8} mol/L	[6]
High-Performance Liquid Chromatography	Single-pass intestinal perfusion method	12.5–200 ng/mL	0.05 ng/mL	[49]
Rp-HPLC	PDA detector	872.5 nM	4.85–9.7×10^5	[7]
Differential Pulse Polarography	Dropping-mercury electrode	1×10^{-5}–5×10^{-4} M	9.8×10^{-6} mol/L	[8]
Polarography	Dropping-mercury electrode	10^{-8}–10^{-6}M	2.0×10^{-9} mol/L	[8]
Stripping voltammetry	Mercury electrode	1×10^{-8}–1×10^{-7} M	2.0×10^{-9} mol/L	[9]
ITO-LMR probe	ITO electrode	1×10^{-6}–1×10^{-3} M	0.5×10^{-3} mol/L	This work

4. Conclusions

In this study we have developed an optical fiber sensor based on the LMR effect supported by a thin ITO overlay and used it for real-time optical monitoring of electrochemical deposition of KP. The developed highly conductive ITO overlay was deposited on an optical fiber core and applied as a working electrode in cyclic voltammetry electrochemical setup. We have found that electrodeposition of KP on the ITO surface induces a significant change in the LMR response. The variation in optical transmission for the ITO-LMR sensor gradually follows the progress in the electrochemical deposition process. The sensor can be interrogated by tracing transmission at discrete wavelength as well as resonant wavelength shifts. Optical setup enables LMR monitoring of the KP concentration down to 1×10^{-6} M. Thus, the proposed method is a valuable alternative for the analysis of KP within the concentration range of 0.25–250 μg mL^{-1}, allowing its determination at therapeutic and toxic levels. The sensing concept can be applied for detection of various other pharmaceuticals, as well as organics or biocompounds that are capable for electropolymerization at ITO surface. It is worth noting that this effect was obtained at bare ITO electrodes fabricated by magnetron sputtering. This deposition method is known for scalability and thus is widely applied as an industrial technology for a wide range of applications. The obtained devices are cheap in large-scale production, disposable, and can be applied in low-power, portable point-of-care devices or microchips. Moreover, the probes can be interrogated with simplified and limited in wavelength range systems based on LED source and Si photodiode with a bandpass filter.

Author Contributions: R.B., P.N., M.S., V.S., T.O. and M.Ś. conceived and designed the experiments; D.B., W.B., Z.C. and P.S. performed the experiments; R.B., P.N. and M.Ś. analyzed the data; M.K. developed measurement setup elements and data acquisition and analysis tools; R.B., P.N. and M.Ś. wrote the paper.

References

1. Sakeena, M.H.F.; Yam, M.F.; Elrashid, S.M.; Munavvar, A.S.; Aznim, M.N. Anti-inflammatory and Analgesic Effects of Ketoprofen in Palm Oil Esters Nanoemulsion. *J. Oleo Sci.* **2010**, *59*, 667–671. [CrossRef] [PubMed]

2. Asanuma, M.; Asanuma, S.N.; Gómez-Vargas, M.; Yamamoto, M.; Ogawa, N. Ketoprofen, a non-steroidal anti-inflammatory drug prevents the late-onset reduction of muscarinic receptors in gerbil hippocampus after transient forebrain ischemia. *Neurosci. Lett.* **1997**, *225*, 109–112. [CrossRef]

3. Abdel-Hamid, M.E.; Novotny, L.; Hamza, H. Determination of diclofenac sodium, flufenamic acid, indomethacin and ketoprofen by LC-APCI-MS. *J. Pharm. Biomed. Anal.* **2001**, *24*, 587–594. [CrossRef]

4. Patrolecco, L.; Ademollo, N.; Grenni, P.; Tolomei, A.; Barra Caracciolo, A.; Capri, S. Simultaneous determination of human pharmaceuticals in water samples by solid phase extraction and HPLC with UV-fluorescence detection. *Microchem. J.* **2013**, *107*, 165–171. [CrossRef]

5. Muhammad, N.; Li, W.; Subhani, Q.; Wang, F.; Zhao, Y.-G.; Zhu, Y. Dual application of synthesized SnO_2 nanoparticles in ion chromatography for sensitive fluorescence determination of ketoprofen in human serum, urine, and canal water samples. *New J. Chem.* **2017**, *41*, 9321–9329. [CrossRef]

6. Zhuang, Y.; Song, H. Sensitive determination of ketoprofen using flow injection with chemiluminescence detection. *J. Pharm. Biomed. Anal.* **2007**, *44*, 824–828. [CrossRef] [PubMed]

7. Roushani, M.; Shahdost-fard, F. Covalent attachment of aptamer onto nanocomposite as a high performance electrochemical sensing platform: Fabrication of an ultra-sensitive ibuprofen electrochemical aptasensor. *Mater. Sci. Eng. C* **2016**, *68*, 128–135. [CrossRef] [PubMed]

8. Amankwa, L.; Chatten, L.G. Electrochemical reduction of ketoprofen and its determination in pharmaceutical dosage forms by differential-pulse polarography. *Analyst* **1984**, *109*, 57–60. [CrossRef] [PubMed]

9. Emara, K.M.; Ali, A.M.; Abo-El Maali, N. The polarographic behaviour of ketoprofen and assay of its capsules using spectrophotometric and voltammetric methods. *Talanta* **1994**, *41*, 639–645. [CrossRef]

10. Ghoneim, M.M.; Tawfik, A. Voltammetric studies and assay of the anti-inflammatory drug ketoprofen in pharmaceutical formulation and human plasma at a mercury electrode. *Can. J. Chem.* **2003**, *81*, 889–896. [CrossRef]

11. Kormosh, Z.; Hunka, I.; Bazel, Y.; Matviychuk, O. Potentiometric determination of ketoprofen and piroxicam at a new PVC electrode based on ion associates of Rhodamine 6G. *Mater. Sci. Eng. C* **2010**, *30*, 997–1002. [CrossRef]

12. Cheng, Y.; Xu, T.; Fu, R. Polyamidoamine dendrimers used as solubility enhancers of ketoprofen. *Eur. J. Med. Chem.* **2005**, *40*, 1390–1393. [CrossRef]

13. Paine, D.C.; Whitson, T.; Janiac, D.; Beresford, R.; Yang, C.O.; Lewis, B. A study of low temperature crystallization of amorphous thin film indium–tin–oxide. *J. Appl. Phys.* **1999**, *85*, 8445–8450. [CrossRef]

14. Villar, I.D.; Hernaez, M.; Zamarreño, C.R.; Sánchez, P.; Fernández-Valdivielso, C.; Arregui, F.J.; Matias, I.R. Design rules for lossy mode resonance based sensors. *Appl. Opt.* **2012**, *51*, 4298–4307. [CrossRef] [PubMed]

15. Zamarreño, C.R.; Hernaez, M.; Del Villar, I.; Matias, I.R.; Arregui, F.J. Tunable humidity sensor based on ITO-coated optical fiber. *Sens. Actuators B Chem.* **2010**, *146*, 414–417. [CrossRef]

16. Śmietana, M.; Dudek, M.; Koba, M.; Michalak, B. Influence of diamond-like carbon overlay properties on refractive index sensitivity of nano-coated optical fibres. *Phys. Status Solidi A* **2013**, *210*, 2100–2105. [CrossRef]

17. Michalak, B.; Koba, M.; Śmietana, M. Silicon Nitride Overlays Deposited on Optical Fibers with RF PECVD Method for Sensing Applications: Overlay Uniformity Aspects. *Acta Phys. Pol. A* **2015**, *127*, 1587–1591. [CrossRef]

18. Burnat, D.; Koba, M.; Wachnicki, Ł.; Gierałtowska, S.; Godlewski, M.; Śmietana, M. Refractive index sensitivity of optical fiber lossy-mode resonance sensors based on atomic layer deposited TiO$_x$ thin overlay. In Proceedings of the 6th European Workshop on Optical Fibre Sensors, Limerick, Ireland, 31 May–3 June 2016.

19. Zamarreño, C.R.; Hernáez, M.; Del Villar, I.; Matías, I.R.; Arregui, F.J. Optical fiber pH sensor based on lossy-mode resonances by means of thin polymeric coatings. *Sens. Actuators B Chem.* **2011**, *155*, 290–297. [CrossRef]

20. Ascorbe, J.; Corres, J.M.; Arregui, F.J.; Matías, I.R. Optical Fiber Current Transducer Using Lossy Mode Resonances for High Voltage Networks. *J. Light. Technol.* **2015**, *33*, 2504–2510. [CrossRef]

21. Sobaszek, M.; Dominik, M.; Burnat, D.; Bogdanowicz, R.; Stranak, V.; Sezemsky, P.; Śmietana, M. Optical monitoring of thin film electro-polymerization on surface of ITO-coated lossy-mode resonance sensor. In Proceedings of the 25th International Conference on Optical Fiber Sensors, Jeju, Korea, 24–28 April 2017.

22. Smietana, M.; Szmidt, J.; Dudek, M.; Niedzielski, P. Optical properties of diamond-like cladding for optical fibres. *Diam. Relat. Mater.* **2004**, *13*, 954–957. [CrossRef]

23. Miller, D.J.; Biesinger, M.C.; McIntyre, N.S. Interactions of CO2 and CO at fractional atmosphere pressures with iron and iron oxide surfaces: One possible mechanism for surface contamination? *Surf. Interface Anal.* **2002**, *33*, 299–305. [CrossRef]

24. Wysocka, J.; Krakowiak, S.; Ryl, J. Evaluation of citric acid corrosion inhibition efficiency and passivation kinetics for aluminium alloys in alkaline media by means of dynamic impedance monitoring. *Electrochim. Acta* **2017**, *258*, 1463–1475. [CrossRef]

25. Villar, I.D.; Zamarreño, C.R.; Sanchez, P.; Hernaez, M.; Valdivielso, C.F.; Arregui, F.J.; Matias, I.R. Generation of lossy mode resonances by deposition of high-refractive-index coatings on uncladded multimode optical fibers. *J. Opt.* **2010**, *12*, 095503. [CrossRef]

26. Zubiate, P.; Zamarreño, C.R.; Sánchez, P.; Matias, I.R.; Arregui, F.J. High sensitive and selective C-reactive protein detection by means of lossy mode resonance based optical fiber devices. *Biosens. Bioelectron.* **2017**, *93*, 176–181. [CrossRef] [PubMed]

27. Dominik, M.; Siuzdak, K.; Niedziałkowski, P.; Stranak, V.; Sezemsky, P.; Sobaszek, M.; Bogdanowicz, R.; Ossowski, T.; Śmietana, M. Annealing of indium tin oxide (ITO) coated optical fibers for optical and electrochemical sensing purposes. In Proceedings of the 2016 Electron Technology Conference, Wisla, Poland, 11–14 September 2016.

28. Śmietana, M.; Sobaszek, M.; Michalak, B.; Niedziałkowski, P.; Białobrzeska, W.; Koba, M.; Sezemsky, P.; Stranak, V.; Karczewski, J.; Ossowski, T.; et al. Optical Monitoring of Electrochemical Processes with ITO-Based Lossy-Mode Resonance Optical Fiber Sensor Applied as an Electrode. *J. Light. Technol.* **2018**, *36*, 954–960. [CrossRef]

29. Stranak, V.; Bogdanowicz, R.; Sezemsky, P.; Wulff, H.; Kruth, A.; Smietana, M.; Kratochvil, J.; Cada, M.; Hubicka, Z. Towards high quality ITO coatings: The impact of nitrogen admixture in HiPIMS discharges. *Surf. Coat. Technol.* **2018**, *335*, 126–133. [CrossRef]

30. Del Villar, I.; Zamarreño, C.R.; Hernaez, M.; Sanchez, P.; Arregui, F.J.; Matias, I.R. Generation of Surface Plasmon Resonance and Lossy Mode Resonance by thermal treatment of ITO thin-films. *Opt. Laser Technol.* **2015**, *69*, 1–7. [CrossRef]

31. Feng, L.; Oturan, N.; Hullebusch, E.D.; van Esposito, G.; Oturan, M.A. Degradation of anti-inflammatory drug ketoprofen by electro-oxidation: Comparison of electro-Fenton and anodic oxidation processes. *Environ. Sci. Pollut. Res.* **2014**, *21*, 8406–8416. [CrossRef] [PubMed]

32. Vidal, L.; Chisvert, A.; Canals, A.; Psillakis, E.; Lapkin, A.; Acosta, F.; Edler, K.J.; Holdaway, J.A.; Marken, F. Chemically surface-modified carbon nanoparticle carrier for phenolic pollutants: Extraction and electrochemical determination of benzophenone-3 and triclosan. *Anal. Chim. Acta* **2008**, *616*, 28–35. [CrossRef] [PubMed]

33. Wu, B.; Zhao, N.; Hou, S.; Zhang, C. Electrochemical Synthesis of Polypyrrole, Reduced Graphene Oxide, and Gold Nanoparticles Composite and Its Application to Hydrogen Peroxide Biosensor. *Nanomaterials* **2016**, *6*. [CrossRef] [PubMed]

34. Sun, Y.; Ren, Q.; Liu, X.; Zhao, S.; Qin, Y. A simple route to fabricate controllable and stable multilayered all-MWNTs films and their applications for the detection of NADH at low potentials. *Biosens. Bioelectron.* **2013**, *39*, 289–295. [CrossRef] [PubMed]

35. Murugananthan, M.; Latha, S.S.; Bhaskar Raju, G.; Yoshihara, S. Anodic oxidation of ketoprofen—An anti-inflammatory drug using boron doped diamond and platinum electrodes. *J. Hazard. Mater.* **2010**, *180*, 753–758. [CrossRef] [PubMed]

36. Yang, H.; Zhu, Y.; Chen, D.; Li, C.; Chen, S.; Ge, Z. Electrochemical biosensing platforms using poly-cyclodextrin and carbon nanotube composite. *Biosens. Bioelectron.* **2010**, *26*, 295–298. [CrossRef] [PubMed]

37. Kannan, P.; Chen, H.; Lee, V.T.-W.; Kim, D.-H. Highly sensitive amperometric detection of bilirubin using enzyme and gold nanoparticles on sol–gel film modified electrode. *Talanta* **2011**, *86*, 400–407. [CrossRef] [PubMed]

38. Oztekin, Y.; Tok, M.; Bilici, E.; Mikoliunaite, L.; Yazicigil, Z.; Ramanaviciene, A.; Ramanavicius, A. Copper nanoparticle modified carbon electrode for determination of dopamine. *Electrochim. Acta* **2012**, *76*, 201–207. [CrossRef]

39. Radi, A.-E.; Muñoz-Berbel, X.; Lates, V.; Marty, J.-L. Label-free impedimetric immunosensor for sensitive detection of ochratoxin A. *Biosens. Bioelectron.* **2009**, *24*, 1888–1892. [CrossRef] [PubMed]

40. Rahman, M.M.; Jeon, I.C. Studies of electrochemical behavior of SWNT-film electrodes. *J. Braz. Chem. Soc.* **2007**, *18*, 1150–1157. [CrossRef]

41. Nikitin, L.N.; Vasil'kov, A.Y.; Banchero, M.; Manna, L.; Naumkin, A.V.; Podshibikhin, V.L.; Abramchuk, S.S.; Buzin, M.I.; Korlyukov, A.A.; Khokhlov, A.R. Composite materials for medical purposes based on polyvinylpyrrolidone modified with ketoprofen and silver nanoparticles. *Russ. J. Phys. Chem. A* **2011**, *85*, 1190–1195. [CrossRef]

42. Bosselmann, S.; Owens, D.E.; Kennedy, R.L.; Herpin, M.J.; Williams, R.O. Plasma deposited stability enhancement coating for amorphous ketoprofen. *Eur. J. Pharm. Biopharm.* **2011**, *78*, 67–74. [CrossRef] [PubMed]

43. Zhuo, N.; Lan, Y.; Yang, W.; Yang, Z.; Li, X.; Zhou, X.; Liu, Y.; Shen, J.; Zhang, X. Adsorption of three selected pharmaceuticals and personal care products (PPCPs) onto MIL-101(Cr)/natural polymer composite beads. *Sep. Purif. Technol.* **2017**, *177*, 272–280. [CrossRef]

44. Thøgersen, A.; Rein, M.; Monakhov, E.; Mayandi, J.; Diplas, S. Elemental distribution and oxygen deficiency of magnetron sputtered indium tin oxide films. *J. Appl. Phys.* **2011**, *109*, 113532. [CrossRef]

45. Brumbach, M.; Veneman, P.A.; Marrikar, F.S.; Schulmeyer, T.; Simmonds, A.; Xia, W.; Lee, P.; Armstrong, N.R. Surface Composition and Electrical and Electrochemical Properties of Freshly Deposited and Acid-Etched Indium Tin Oxide Electrodes. *Langmuir* **2007**, *23*, 11089–11099. [CrossRef] [PubMed]

46. Li, Y.; Zhao, G.; Zhi, X.; Zhu, T. Microfabrication and imaging XPS analysis of ITO thin films. *Surf. Interface Anal.* **2007**, *39*, 756–760. [CrossRef]

47. Sanchez, P.; Zamarreño, C.R.; Hernaez, M.; Villar, I.D.; Fernandez-Valdivielso, C.; Matias, I.R.; Arregui, F.J. Lossy mode resonances toward the fabrication of optical fiber humidity sensors. *Meas. Sci. Technol.* **2012**, *23*, 014002. [CrossRef]

48. Pickl, K.E.; Magnes, C.; Bodenlenz, M.; Pieber, T.R.; Sinner, F.M. Rapid online-SPE-MS/MS method for ketoprofen determination in dermal interstitial fluid samples from rats obtained by microdialysis or open-flow microperfusion. *J. Chromatogr. B* **2007**, *850*, 432–439. [CrossRef] [PubMed]

49. Zakeri-Milani, P.; Barzegar-Jalali, M.; Tajerzadeh, H.; Azarmi, Y.; Valizadeh, H. Simultaneous determination of naproxen, ketoprofen and phenol red in samples from rat intestinal permeability studies: HPLC method development and validation. *J. Pharm. Biomed. Anal.* **2005**, *39*, 624–630. [CrossRef] [PubMed]

15

An Objective Balance Error Scoring System for Sideline Concussion Evaluation Using Duplex Kinect Sensors

Mengqi Zhu, Zhonghua Huang, Chao Ma and Yinlin Li *

School of Mechatronical Engineering, Beijing Institute of Technology, Beijing 100081, China;
vivian_zmq@yahoo.com (M.Z.); huangzh@bit.edu.cn (Z.H.); 20081124@bit.edu.cn (C.M.)
* Correspondence: liyinlin@bit.edu.cn

Abstract: Sports-related concussion is a common sports injury that might induce potential long-term consequences without early diagnosis and intervention in the field. However, there are few options of such sensor systems available. The aim of the study is to propose and validate an automated concussion administration and scoring approach, which is objective, affordable and capable of detecting all balance errors required by the balance error scoring system (BESS) protocol in the field condition. Our approach is first to capture human body skeleton positions using two Microsoft Kinect sensors in the proposed configuration and merge the data by a custom-made algorithm to remove the self-occlusion of limbs. The standing balance errors according to BESS protocol were further measured and accessed automatically by the proposed algorithm. Simultaneously, the BESS test was filmed for scoring by an experienced rater. Two results were compared using Pearson coefficient r, obtaining an excellent consistency ($r = 0.93$, $p < 0.05$). In addition, BESS test–retest was performed after seven days and compared using intraclass correlation coefficients (ICC), showing a good test–retest reliability (ICC = 0.81, $p < 0.01$). The proposed approach could be an alternative of objective tools to assess postural stability for sideline sports concussion diagnosis.

Keywords: concussion evaluation; postural stability; balance error scoring system; Kinect sensor

1. Introduction

Sports-related concussion is common in most sports with a higher incidence in American football, hockey, rugby, soccer, and basketball, of which 78% occur during games as opposed to training [1,2]. The Centers for Disease Control estimates that 1.6 to 3.8 million concussions occur in the US per year in competitive sports and recreational activities [3]. Failure of early recognition and removal of the concussed athlete from play may put the individual at risk for potential complications and long-term consequences [4]. This often requires a rapid and accurate sideline assessment in the midst of competition by certified athletic trainers and team physicians [5].

Since 1997, a multidimensional approach consisting of the systematic assessment of cognition, balance and symptoms has been recommended for the diagnosis and management of sports concussion (SC) [2,6,7]. The multidimensional approach emphasizes multiple diagnostic elements including a physical examination, a survey of post-concussion symptoms, performance-based measures of acute mental status and postural stability, and careful consideration of clinical history [5,8]. Unfortunately, this approach is neither time- nor cost-effective, making them difficult to employ at varying levels of sport. A recent survey of certified athletic trainers indicated that only 21% of respondents used the recommended multidimensional approach to assess SC [9]. When used in isolation, each of the aforementioned clinical measures of cognition, balance, and/or symptoms has been demonstrated to have suboptimal reliability and validity [10–12].

As an alternative to the multidimensional approach, the Balance Error Scoring System (BESS) provides an objective measure of balance with the nature of being time- and cost-effective [13]. The BESS relies on the observational skills of trained sports administrator to count the total number of predefined balance errors that a subject makes during three standing stances on firm and foam surfaces. The BESS has been adopted as the current clinical standard of care for balance assessment in concussed athletes on the sideline [14]. However, several studies have addressed the measurement properties of the BESS showing variable inter-rater and test–retest reliability [4,15,16], which are partially based on the raters' subjective interpretations of errors committed throughout the test and different strictness of the scoring criteria.

To overcome the subjective nature of the BESS, technologies have been used to automate the assessment of postural stability. Such efforts can be divided into two main approaches: postural sway and error scoring [14,17]. The first has been evaluated by using force plate [17–19] or wearable devices [14,20,21]. Different from the scores of BESS, the metrics of postural sway are quantified by measured changes in body sway amplitude, velocity, frequency and direction of anterior-posterior, medial-lateral or trunk-rotation movements [20]. The primary clinical balance test for concussion assessment and most often used clinically and described in the literature is the BESS [14]. Therefore, the automated approach of error scoring with increased objectivity and subsequent reliability and validity could have great utility. Brown et al. provided insight into the relationship between inertial sensor-based kinematic outcomes and BESS errors' scores [22]. Potentially being able to track the six balance errors [23] as they are defined in the BESS standard, the Microsoft Kinect®sensor V1 [24] and V2 [23] have been investigated for the purpose. The use of a single Kinect sensor in the previous studies, however, has been called into the problem of self-occlusion happening when some parts of a human body are hidden. In addition, none of the previous studies have accounted for the error of eye-opening. As such, a large level of variability of the counted errors can result, leading to inaccurate BESS scores. Self-occlusion may be addressed by using multiple Kinect sensors instead of one [25–27]. The configuration of two Kinect sensors has been demonstrated to enhance the recognition rate, therefore limiting the issue of self-occlusion [28,29]. Nevertheless, the use of multiple Kinect sensors has not been explored or validated specifically as a way to count the BESS errors.

The aim of the current study is to present and validate a portable, untethered, and affordable solution for sideline sports concussion BESS test using two Kinect sensors. A custom algorithm is developed to automatically score errors committed during each BESS trial from duplex-views. The system is verified by concurrent validity and test–retest reliability in healthy participants. We hypothesized that the use of two Kinect sensors will effectively address the issue of self-occlusion, leading to strong concurrent validity and test–retest reliability when compared to a human rater.

2. Methods

2.1. Balance Error Scoring System (BESS) and Test Protocol

The BESS is a clinical accepted measure of postural stability prior to and following a sport concussion. To complete the BESS test, participants are required to maintain balance in three different stances, as shown in Figure 1. Each stance is performed on firm ground and pad form, respectively. The foam pad is medium density and measured 40 cm × 40 cm × 8 cm in size [30]. All trials are 20 s in length. During the completion of each trial, participants are asked to maintain a double leg, single leg or tandem stance with their hands on their iliac crests and with their eyes closed. The BESS errors consist of removal of hands from hips (balance error a), opening of the eyes (balance error b), stepping, stumbling, or falling (balance error c), abduction or flexion of the hip beyond 30° (balance error d), lifting the forefoot or heel off of the firm or foam surface (balance error e), and/or remaining out of the testing position or more than 5 s (balance error f). A maximum of 10 errors could be committed during each trial. If a subject committed multiple errors simultaneously, only one error was recorded. For example, if a subject stumbled, removed his or her hands from their hips and opened their eyes simultaneously, only one error is counted [13]. The balance error is identified by human skeleton data from two Kinect sensors and the final test score is counted. Testing consists of two parts separated by 7 days.

To complete the BESS, subjects are asked to stand at 2.5 m away from the sensors. Each participant is then instructed on how to complete the BESS. Following instruction and assurance of participant understanding, each participant completes the BESS test as previously described. After each trial, a 30 s rest period is employed. An experienced rater (over 60 h of grading experience) simultaneously counts the number of BESS errors for each trial. All trials are video recorded for a follow-up proof counting in order to ensure the accuracy of error numbers. The same testing protocol is administered seven days after the first session.

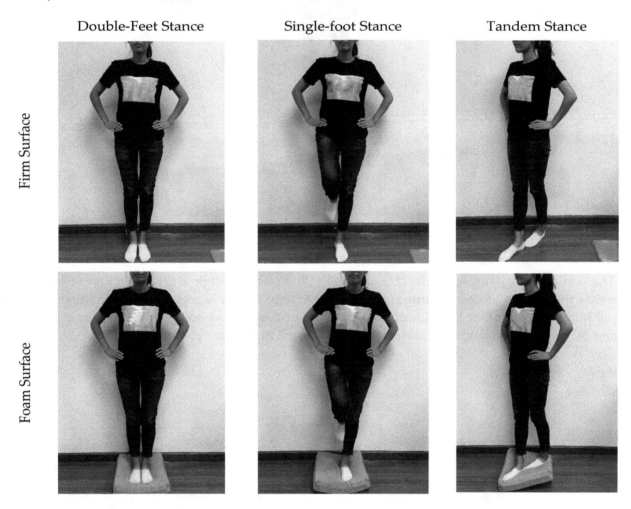

Figure 1. Trials of BESS test in three different stances (double feet, single foot and tandem) on two different surfaces (firm and foam).

2.2. Instrumentation and Configurations

The Kinect V2 sensors (Microsoft Corporation, Redmond, WA, USA) were deployed to measure the 3D coordinates of the skeletons and joints of the human body, which were then being used to judge the aforementioned balance errors a–f using custom-made algorithms. Though the camera is capable of obtaining 25 human skeletal joints through the depth image, only wrists, hips, ankles, spine, shoulder and hip center are used in the method, as denoted by the nine white circles in Figure 2. Experimental equipment includes two Kinect V2 cameras and two laptop computers with Windows 8.1 operating system (Microsoft Corporation, Redmond, WA, USA), Intel Core i5 processor and 4 GB memory. The algorithms were implemented in Visual Studio 2013 (Microsoft Corporation, Redmond, WA, USA) and Kinect SDK 2.0 (Microsoft Corporation, Redmond, WA, USA).

The basic configuration consideration for a Kinect sensor is to put the subject conducting the trial stances in the field of view (FOV), even when the movement of the hip is up to 30° of abduction. Moreover, the nine skeletal joints, as denoted in Figure 2, should not be occluded by body parts in the camera vision, or there should be no self-occlusion, for all three of the stances.

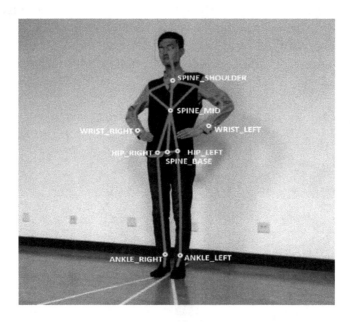

Figure 2. The selected joints used for the BESS test.

The vertical FOV of a single Kinect is up to 60°, illustrated as angle $\angle C'K1B'$ in Figure 3a; Point K1 represents the Kinect sensor mounted at height of 65 cm, which is regarded as the ideal operating value of Microsoft Xbox One floor mounting stand; Point B is the test position where the subject stands, and line BC denotes the height of subject, herein taking 2 m as the representative value.

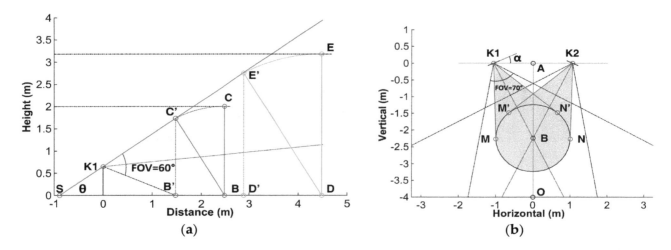

Figure 3. Illustration of duplex Kinect sensor placements. (a) the vertical field of view (FOV) of single Kinect sensor and setup for a 2 m high subject; (b) the positions, horizontal FOVs and required space (gray color) of the two sensors.

When the subject leans the hip maximally to 30°, the projection height in the vertical axis is under the curve CC' in math. The point C' corresponds to the subject's head position at the abduction angle 30°, which determines the upward tilt angle of the Kinect sensor and the minimal camera to subject distance (MCSD) that is able to watch the whole body skeletons. Under the prescribed condition, the distance is computed to be 2.48 m and the radius BB′ of the test area is 1 m mathematically. The duplex sensor setup in horizontal view is shown in Figure 3b, in which *K1* and *K2* denote the two Kinect sensors. The distance between the two sensors is 2.12 m and the required test space as illustrated by a gray color in Figure 3b is 5.21 square meters. Since the horizontal FOV of the camera is 70°, the horizontal rotation angle of the camera, *α*, is allowed to be between 15° and 36°.

Although the above configurations are determined supposing 2 m as the height of participant, the sensor can track the whole body skeletons of shorter subjects as well, without any alteration of the setup parameters. When the subject is taller than 2 m, the mathematical expression between the MCSD value *d* and the subject height h can be described as

$$\begin{cases} d = \left(\frac{\sqrt{3}}{2} \cot \theta + 0.5 \right) \times h - H_s \cot \theta \\ \frac{\cot(60° - \theta)}{\cot \theta} = \frac{\frac{\sqrt{3}}{2} H_r - H_s}{H_s} \end{cases}, \tag{1}$$

where θ is the angle $\angle C'SB'$ as denoted in the Figure 3a, H_s and H_r are the sensor mounting height of 0.65 m and the reference subject height of 2 m, respectively. Equation (1) is obtained according to the triangular relationships of the sensor setup, as shown in Figure 3a, in which the setup parameters including the tilt angle, horizontal rotation angle and mounting height of the sensors are all the same as the case of the 2 m high subject. Typical numerical solutions of Equation (1) are present in Table 1. In the situation, the subject would simply move a distance referring to Table 1, along line AO toward point O as denoted in Figure 3b. The fixed installation parameters will help to ease the use of the system.

Table 1. The height of the subject and the required minimal camera to subject distance.

Height h (m)	MCSD d (m)
2.1	2.65
2.2	2.82
2.3	2.99
2.4	3.12
2.5	3.32
2.6	3.49
2.7	3.67
2.8	3.83
2.9	3.99

It is noteworthy that the above setup parameters are the worst case values. For example, there is less chance that one can fall like a rigid body without flexing one's hip, and hence the test area diameter should be less than 2 m. Therefore, in a real situation when these values are smaller, the system will have better performance in terms of required installation space and MCSD distance.

2.3. Algorithm Development

Microsoft Kinect SDK 2.0 provides all the methods or functions to acquire the skeletal joints coordinates of recognized users. In the tracking loop, *NuiSkeletonTrackingEnable* method is called to enable the tracking and *NuiSkeletonGetNextFrame* method is to access the members of the *NUI_SKELETON_FRAME* structure to receive information about the users. In the members of the skeleton frame structure, the *NUI_SKELETON_DATA* structure has a *SkeletonPositionTrackingState* array, which contains the tracking state for each joint. A tracking state of a joint can be "tracked" for a clearly visible joint, "inferred" when a joint is not clearly visible and Kinect is inferring its position, or "non-tracked". In addition, the *SkeletonPositions* array in the skeleton frame structure contains the position of each joint.

Once the positions and tracking states of the participants are obtained, the data from two Kinect sensors will be fed into a custom-made algorithm to compute BESS scores. It is mainly composed of two parts: error motion recognition and scoring algorithm.

2.3.1. Error Motion Recognition Algorithm

The error motion recognition algorithm (EMRA) functions to determine whether the balance errors occur during the BESS test. Specifically, the EMRA obtains the coordinates of skeletal joints from the two Kinect sensors and then extracts the feature vectors of the predefined balance errors, which is further processed by comparing the deviation of the joints away from its original position. Subsequently, the EMRA merges the results of two cameras by weighting a fusion coefficient in order to choose the best candidate of the skeletal joints from the two Kinect sensors, especially when one is self-occluded or incurred poor accuracy. Supposing the coordinate of a joint at time t is $p_i^t = (x_i^t, y_i^t, z_i^t)$, the vector between joint i and joint j at time t can be expressed as $p_{i,j}^t = p_i^t - p_j^t$. Then, the error equation $\delta^t(i,j)$ for balance error a, c, e is described as follows:

$$\delta^t(i,j) = \begin{cases} 1, & \|p_i^t - p_j^t\| > H, \|p_i^{t-1} - p_j^{t-1}\| \leq H \\ 0, & otherwise \end{cases}, \tag{2}$$

where H is the predefined threshold. When the $\delta^t(i,j)$ is computed to be 1, a balance error is found. In the case of balance error a, the p_i and p_j are the coordinates of the joint wrist and hip, respectively; the term $\|p_i^t - p_j^t\|$ is $\|p_{wrist}^t - p_{hip}^t\|$, and the H equals to $\|p_{wrist}^0 - p_{hip}^0\|$, which means the distance between joint wrist and hip at the initial time. For the balance error c, the p_i is joint spine_mid and p_j is its initial value, and the term $\|p_i^t - p_j^t\|$ is then $\|p_{spine\_mid}^t - p_{spine\_mid}^0\|$. For the balance error e, the p_i is joint ankle and the term $\|p_i^t - p_j^t\|$ becomes $\|p_{ankle}^t - p_{ankle}^0\|$. The threshold H is set to 10 cm in the study for balance error c and e, the amount of which is determined by experiments and set to be large enough to reflect slight balance error motion meanwhile suppressing the jitter caused by the camera vision noise.

The error equation of balance error d is defined by:

$$\delta^t(i,j) = \begin{cases} 1, & \cos(p_{i,j}^{t-1}, v) > H, \cos(p_{i,j}^t, v) \leq H \\ 0, & otherwise \end{cases}, \tag{3}$$

where $p_{i,j}$ is the vector from joint spine_base to spine_shoulder, v means a vertical vector, and threshold H is 0.866 corresponding to the cosine $30°$ of the maximal allowed hip flexion angle.

The error recognition fusion equation is expressed as:

$$\varphi^t = \begin{cases} 1, & \omega_A^t(i,j) \cdot \delta_A^t(i,j) + \omega_B^t(i,j) \cdot \delta_B^t(i,j) \geq 1 \\ 0, & \omega_A^t(i,j) \cdot \delta_A^t(i,j) + \omega_B^t(i,j) \cdot \delta_B^t(i,j) < 1 \end{cases}, \tag{4}$$

where $\delta_A^t(i,j)$ and $\delta_B^t(i,j)$ represent the results of error recognition at time t from Kinect sensor A and B, and $\omega_A^t(i,j)$ and $\omega_B^t(i,j)$ are the weight coefficients of sensor A and B at time t, respectively. The values of $\omega_A^t(i,j)$ and $\omega_B^t(i,j)$ are determined according to the capture state of joint (well tracked, inferred and not tracked), which are provided by the Microsoft Kinect SDK. The values of $\omega(i,j)$ are shown in Table 2.

As for the balance error b, it can be achieved directly by calling the *GetFaceProperties* function of the Microsoft Kinect SDK to recognize the states of the eye (open, closed and unknown).

Table 2. The weight coefficient for error recognition fusion.

i	j	$\omega(i,j)$
Not tracked	Not tracked	0
Not tracked	Inferred	0
Not tracked	Well tracked	0
Inferred	Inferred	0.25
Inferred	Well tracked	0.5
Well tracked	Inferred	0.5
Well tracked	Well tracked	1

2.3.2. Scoring Algorithm

In addition to the error motion recognition, the software should also be able to score the BESS trials automatically. As one error might be accompanied by multiple simultaneous or subsequent errors, redundant errors count should be screened out. For the balance errors α and β, $t^{\alpha}_{i,begin}$ is the start time of the i-th occurrence of the balance error α, and the end time is $t^{\alpha}_{i,end}$; $t^{\beta}_{j,begin}$ is the start time of the j-th occurrence of the balance error β, and the end time is $t^{\beta}_{j,end}$. Whether the balance error α and β occur simultaneously is determined by the following equation:

$$\begin{cases} t^{\alpha}_{i,begin} - t^{\beta}_{j,begin} < 0 \\ t^{\alpha}_{i,end} - t^{\beta}_{j,begin} \geq 0 \end{cases} \quad or \quad \begin{cases} t^{\beta}_{j,begin} - t^{\alpha}_{i,begin} < 0 \\ t^{\beta}_{j,end} - t^{\alpha}_{i,begin} \geq 0 \end{cases}. \tag{5}$$

If simultaneous errors are detected, the later one will be ignored.

A total of six stances are performed in sequence (double feet, one foot, tandem) on the firm surface followed by the foam surface. For each stance, there are six types of balance errors a–f. The equation of BESS test score at j-th stance is defined as follows:

$$Score_j = \begin{cases} \sum_{i=1}^{6} \varphi_i - \gamma, & 0 \leq \sum_{i=1}^{6} \varphi_i - \gamma + \varepsilon < 10 \\ 10, & \sum_{i=1}^{6} \varphi_i - \gamma + \varepsilon \geq 10 \end{cases}, \tag{6}$$

where φ_i is the number of occurrences of balance error i, and γ represents the number of simultaneous errors that should be ignored. The constant ε is to indicate whether or not the subject fails to maintain the testing stance less than 5 s or remains out of a proper testing position for longer than 5 s. If so, ε is 0; otherwise, ε is 10. The maximum score of each stance is limited to 10, and the total BESS score is the sum of $Score_j$ counted during all six stances. The total score acquired automatically using the above algorithm is then compared with the rater score to verify the Duplex Kinects System's validity and reliability.

2.4. Subjects

The current study was approved by the institutional academic board. Thirty healthy and physically active subjects (12 female and 18 male) between the 22 and 31 years (yr) of age (25.6 ± 2.56 yr), and who were 158 to 190 cm tall (171.1 ± 6.72 cm) participated in the current study. Exclusion criteria included neurological or musculoskeletal conditions, respiratory or cardiovascular problems, and pregnancy. All subjects were informed of the purpose, methods and instructions to complete the BESS and signed informed consent.

2.5. Analysis

Concurrent validity of scores obtained by the custom-made duplex Kinect BESS software and by the rater were assessed using Pearson correlation coefficients. In addition, intraclass correlation coefficients ICC (2,1) (2-way random effect, single measure model) were used to assess the test–retest reliability of the custom-made duplex Kinect BESS software between days 1 and 8. A modified version of BESS (mBESS) using only three stance conditions on the firm surface, which is currently included in the SCAT3 protocol and the Official NFL Sideline Tool [31], has also been accessed. All analyses were conducted with $p < 0.05$ as the significance level and performed using SPSS Version 20.0 (IBM Corporation, Armonk, NY, USA). For the Pearson coefficient r, it was excellent relationship if r was greater than 0.90, good relationship if r was between 0.8 and 0.89, a fair degree if r was between 0.7 and 0.79, and poor if r was below 0.70 [32]. Regarding the ICC coefficients, it was excellent if ICC was greater than 0.90, good if ICC was between 0.75 and 0.90, moderate if ICC was between 0.50 and 0.75, and poor if ICC was below 0.50 [33].

3. Results

In order to validate the self-occlusion of the proposed sensor configuration, representative images captured by sensors are shown in Figure 4. Direct view indicates the image captured by the sensor placed at position A in Figure 3b, facing directly to the subject; left and right view shows images captured by sensors placed at position K1 and K2 in Figure 3b, respectively, facing to the subject in the same way as depicted in Figure 3b. In Figure 4a, the rear ankle is occluded by the front one during tandem stance in direct view, resulting in a self-occlusion joint denoted as E in the figure. However, the rear ankle joint occluded in direct view is tracked properly in the right view. The same result could be found in the other three stance situations. The red dots overlaid on the eyes were generated by software automatically in case the eyes were tracked by the sensor, as shown in Figure 4.

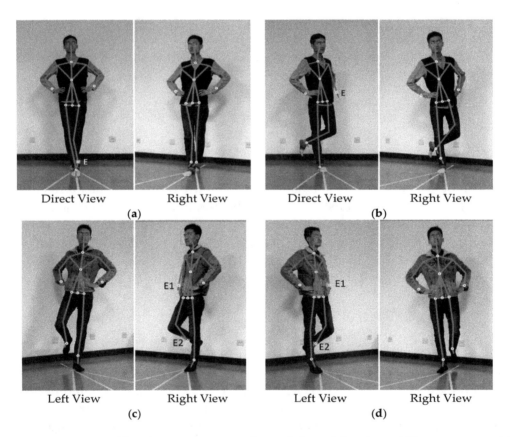

Figure 4. Representative self-occlusion images in direct, left or right view of Kinect sensors. (**a**) in the direct view, the rear ankle joint E is occluded whereas not in the right view; (**b**) in the direct view, the left wrist joint E is occluded when the body twisted, whereas not in the right view; (**c**) in the right view, the joints E1 and E2 are occluded, whereas not in the left view; (**d**) in the left view, joints E1 and E2 are occluded whereas not in the right view.

Further experiments were performed to examine the performance of the system for the purpose gof the BESS test. Table 3 shows the statistical results of the system measurements and the rater counting of the six balance conditions. In each condition, balance errors a–f committed by the subject were counted, including the error b of eye opening. Concurrent validity of the system and the rater counting shows that the system's BESS total score is 11.83 ± 7.62, and the rater's is 11.33 ± 7.89, and the Pearson coefficient r is 0.93 ($p < 0.05$). The total mBESS scores counted by system and rater are 4.67 ± 3.13 and 4.43 ± 3.40, respectively, indicating that the system score accurately fits the rater's ($r = 0.92, p < 0.05$) in the subset of balance conditions (firm surface only).

Table 3. The statistical results of the system and rater scores with Pearson coefficient value of each condition ($p < 0.05$).

Balance Condition	System Score	Rater Score	Pearson Coefficient r
Double feet firm	0.10 ± 0.40	0.10 ± 0.40	0.78
Single foot firm	3.37 ± 2.38	3.10 ± 2.34	0.89
Tandem firm	1.20 ± 2.34	1.23 ± 2.50	0.93
Double feet foam	0.33 ± 0.61	0.10 ± 0.30	0.55
Single foot foam	4.43 ± 3.13	4.30 ± 3.19	0.82
Tandem foam	2.37 ± 2.85	2.50 ± 3.08	0.87
BESS total	11.83 ± 7.62	11.33 ± 7.89	0.93
mBESS total (only firm)	4.67 ± 3.13	4.43 ± 3.40	0.92

A scatter plot is also presented in Figure 5, indicating that the system and rater score correlated positively and agreed with each other.

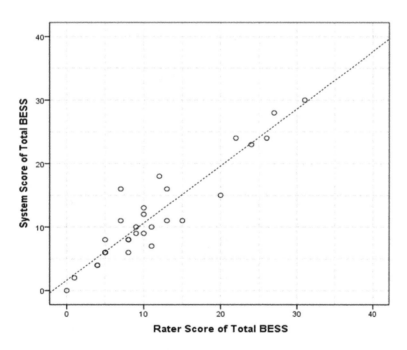

Figure 5. BESS score for rater and system.

Test–retest reliability of the system measurements on the first and eighth day as well as the ICC value in each condition shows that the first day total score of the BESS test is 12.07 ± 7.75, the eighth day total score of the BESS test is 11.47 ± 6.93, and the ICC was 0.81 ($p < 0.001$). The mBESS test score is 4.73 ± 3.17 on day 1 while 4.70 ± 3.76 on day 8, with ICC value of 0.84 ($p < 0.001$). The detail is illustrated in Table 4. The scatter plot of the BESS score for the first day and the eighth day is shown in Figure 6.

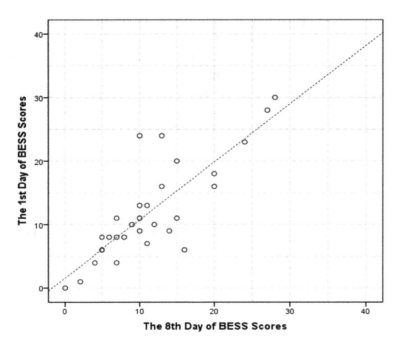

Figure 6. BESS score for day 1 and day 8.

Table 4. The statistical results of system score on the first and eighth day as well as the ICC value of each condition.

Balance Condition	Day 1	Day 8	ICC	p
Double feet firm	0.13 ± 0.30	0.10 ± 0.30	0.83	<0.001
Single foot firm	3.37 ± 2.36	3.67 ± 2.95	0.78	<0.001
Tandem firm	1.23 ± 2.36	0.93 ± 2.18	0.57	0.012
Double feet foam	0.33 ± 0.61	0.23 ± 0.50	0.58	0.010
Single foot foam	4.57 ± 3.21	4.40 ± 3.22	0.68	0.001
Tandem foam	2.40 ± 2.89	2.10 ± 2.93	0.87	<0.001
BESS total	12.07 ± 7.75	11.47 ± 6.93	0.81	<0.001
mBESS total (only firm)	4.73 ± 3.17	4.70 ± 3.76	0.84	<0.001

4. Discussion

The BESS is recognized as the current standard for the evaluation of sports related concussion. However, the intra- and inter-raters reliability of BESS scores has been questioned. In an attempt to overcome the subjective limitations of the BESS, the proposed method used two Kinect sensors along with a custom-made algorithm to track the postural balance errors committed by the participant. The primary findings derived from the results include: (1) the duplex views from two Kinect sensors can compensate for each other and track the key human body skeletal joints without blind spot or self-occlusion, even during the challenging tandem stance; and, (2) due to the constraint of the sensor's field of view, placement parameters including sensor separation distance, tilt angle and mounting height, etc., should be properly determined by taking into consideration the portability, installation space and ease of setup.

Our proposed custom-made algorithm for duplex Kinect BESS yielded excellent correlation coefficients to the human rater's BESS scores ($r = 0.93$, $p < 0.05$) and test–retest reliability (ICC = 0.81, $p < 0.05$) across an eight-day test–retest interval. Our method has greater test–retest reliability compared to that of human rater's BESS scores present by Finnoff et al. (ICC = 0.74) [16] and by Valovich et al. for high school participants (ICC = 0.70) [34]. These results indicate that the suggested duplex Kinect BESS method may be an objective and reliable measure of postural stability.

Brown et al. employed inertial sensors to evaluate the oBESS scores using a custom-made equation in an effort to overcome the subjectivity of the BESS scoring system [22]. Even though their oBESS was able to produce scores with accurate fit to raters in certain conditions, it didn't match well (ICC = 0.68) when using data from the subset of conditions (firm surface only). Contrary to the result of Brown et al., our system's mBESS scores are able to accurately fit the rater's ($r = 0.92$, $p < 0.05$) in the subset of balance conditions (firm surface only) as well. The support for the mBESS test of our method implies a time-saving test of postural stability when required. Moreover, the methodology by Brown et al didn't take into consideration the error of eye opening, which results in further discrepancy relative to the BESS standard.

Dave's study [24] using Kinect sensor V1 can only recognize three balance errors out of a total of six BESS test errors. In our study, we expanded on Dave's work by using a second Kinect sensor which tracked the six total BESS errors, resulting in system-derived scores with accurate fit to raters ($r = 0.93$, $p < 0.05$) compared to Dave's ($r = 0.38$) [24]. Furthermore, in Dave's study, the subject's balance loss may introduce unwanted error detection or may not detect errors during the BESS test, due to the joints' location outside the FOV of the Kinect sensor. In this regard, our work suggested a method to determine the advisable sensor configuration size and hence successfully removed the problem. Moreover, Dave only used a single Kinect sensor V1 and found the camera was limited to detect eye opening during the completion of each balance trial [24]. However, the use of the Kinect V2 improved upon the its predecessors' capability and was able to detect eye-opening, potentially as a result of an improvement of the Kinect V2 camera's resolution from 640×480 to 1920×1080 pixels of color image, and from 320×240 to 512×424 pixels of depth image. These results suggest that the proposed methodology is an improvement over previous attempts at automating error counting while participants complete the BESS.

In addition, Napoli et al. developed an automated assessment of postural stability (AAPS) algorithm based on a single Kinect Sensor V2 to evaluate the BESS errors [23], in which low AAPS performance levels were detected in single-leg and tandem stances on foam. In a separate paper on the same work, they reported the issues detecting the back leg that is hidden behind the other leg during the tandem stance [35]. Their works were only validated by comparing the level of agreement of system's BESS scores with that of rates and a professional camera. In our study, however, the aforementioned limitations have been addressed and verified by concurrent validity and test–retest reliability metrics.

Our study was limited to healthy normal subjects with a mean BESS score of 11.83 ± 7.62 errors. The thresholds used in the error detection algorithm, which influences the sensitivity of the BESS scoring, were determined through experiment and selection of optimal values. Therefore, the threshold values should be further considered when applied to the concussed participants. Our future research will also validate the duplex Kinect system in a clinical setting to assess errors in a large amount of concussed samples.

5. Conclusions

In the current study, we presented a novel Balance Error Scoring System by using duplex Kinect sensors and a custom-made algorithm. Our approach overcomes the self-occlusion problem of a previous solution using the Kinect sensor, realizing the recognition of balance error and the automatic administration of the BESS test, with a stronger test–retest reliability and concurrent validity compared to previous works. The current methodology provides a contactless clinic-based concussion administration and scoring approach that accurately detects all balance errors as per BESS instructions. Our method could be used as an affordable, portable and reliable tool for the concussion assessment in the field.

Acknowledgments: We would like to thank Jacob E. Resch from the Exercise and Sport Injury Laboratory at the University of Virginia for his idea of using Kinect to measure BESS errors, guidance and revision of the current manuscript.

Author Contributions: Mengqi Zhu built the system, designed the algorithm, performed the experiments, and also contributed to the data collection, analysis and writing of the corresponding paragraphs; Zhonghua Huang provided many useful comments and constructive discussions; Cao Ma helped in the experiment and manuscript formatting; Yinlin Li conceived of the technical solution of the study and contributed to the drafting of the manuscript. All authors read and approved the final manuscript.

References

1. Ravdin, L.D.; Barr, W.B.; Jordan, B.; Lathan, W.E.; Relkin, N.R. Assessment of cognitive recovery following sports related head trauma in boxers. *Clin. J. Sport Med.* **2003**, *13*, 21–27. [CrossRef] [PubMed]

2. Harmon, K.G.; Drezner, J.A.; Gammons, M.; Guskiewicz, K.M.; Halstead, M.; Herring, S.A.; Kutcher, J.S.; Pana, A.; Putukian, M.; Roberts, W.O. American Medical Society for Sports Medicine position statement: Concussion in sport. *Br. J. Sports Med.* **2013**, *47*, 15–26. [CrossRef] [PubMed]

3. Langlois, J.A.; Rutland-Brown, W.; Wald, M.M. The epidemiology and impact of traumatic brain injury: A brief overview. *J. Head Trauma Rehabil.* **2006**, *21*, 375–378. [CrossRef] [PubMed]

4. Valovich McLeod, T.C.; Barr, W.B.; McCrea, M.; Guskiewicz, K.M. Psychometric and measurement properties of concussion assessment tools in youth sports. *J. Athl. Train.* **2006**, *41*, 399–408. [PubMed]

5. Putukian, M. Clinical Evaluation of the Concussed Athlete: A View From the Sideline. *J. Athl. Train.* **2017**, *52*, 236–244. [CrossRef] [PubMed]

6. Kelly, J.P.; Rosenberg, J.H. Diagnosis and management of concussion in sports. *Neurology* **1997**, *48*, 575–580. [CrossRef] [PubMed]

7. Broglio, S.P.; Cantu, R.C.; Gioia, G.A.; Guskiewicz, K.M.; Kutcher, J.; Palm, M.; Valovich McLeod, T.C. National Athletic Trainers' Association position statement: management of sport concussion. *J. Athl. Train.* **2014**, *49*, 245–265. [CrossRef] [PubMed]

8. Lovell, M.R.; Iverson, G.L.; Collins, M.W.; Podell, K.; Johnston, K.M.; Pardini, D.; Pardini, J.; Norwig, J.; Maroon, J.C. Measurement of symptoms following sports-related concussion: Reliability and normative data for the post-concussion scale. *Appl. Neuropsychol.* **2006**, *13*, 166–174. [CrossRef] [PubMed]

9. Lynall, R.C.; Laudner, K.G.; Mihalik, J.P.; Stanek, J.M. Concussion-Assessment and -Management Techniques Used by Athletic Trainers. *J. Athl. Train.* **2013**, *48*, 844–850. [CrossRef] [PubMed]

10. Broglio, S.P.; Macciocchi, S.N.; Ferrara, M.S. Sensitivity of the concussion assessment battery. *Neurosurgery* **2007**, *60*, 1050–1057. [CrossRef] [PubMed]

11. Register-Mihalik, J.K.; Guskiewicz, K.M.; Mihalik, J.P.; Schmidt, J.D.; Kerr, Z.Y.; McCrea, M.A. Reliable change, sensitivity, and specificity of a multidimensional concussion assessment battery: Implications for caution in clinical practice. *J. Head Trauma Rehabil.* **2013**, *28*, 274–283. [CrossRef] [PubMed]

12. Resch, J.E.; Brown, C.N.; Schmidt, J.; Macciocchi, S.N.; Blueitt, D.; Cullum, C.M.; Ferrara, M.S. The sensitivity and specificity of clinical measures of sport concussion: Three tests are better than one. *BMJ Open Sport Exerc. Med.* **2016**, *2*, e000012. [CrossRef] [PubMed]

13. Riemann, B.L.; Guskiewicz, K.M. Assessment of mild head injury using measures of balance and cognition: A case study. *J. Sport Rehabil.* **1997**, *6*, 283–289. [CrossRef]

14. Alberts, J.L.; Thota, A.; Hirsch, J.; Ozinga, S.; Dey, T.; Schindler, D.D.; Koop, M.M.; Burke, D.; Linder, S.M. Quantification of the Balance Error Scoring System with Mobile Technology. *Med. Sci. Sports Exerc.* **2015**, *47*, 2233–2240. [CrossRef] [PubMed]

15. Hunt, T.N.; Ferrara, M.S. Age-Related Differences in Neuropsychological Testing Among High School Athletes. *J. Athl. Train.* **2009**, *44*, 405–409. [CrossRef] [PubMed]

16. Finnoff, J.T.; Peterson, V.J.; Hollman, J.H.; Smith, J. Intrarater and Interrater Reliability of the Balance Error Scoring System (BESS). *PM&R* **2009**, *1*, 50–54.

17. Chang, J.O.; Levy, S.S.; Seay, S.W.; Goble, D.J. An Alternative to the Balance Error Scoring System: Using a Low-Cost Balance Board to Improve the Validity/Reliability of Sports-Related Concussion Balance Testing. *Clin. J. Sport Med.* **2014**, *24*, 256–262. [CrossRef] [PubMed]

18. Merchant-Borna, K.; Jones, C.M.; Janigro, M.; Wasserman, E.B.; Clark, R.A.; Bazarian, J.J. Evaluation of Nintendo Wii Balance Board as a Tool for Measuring Postural Stability After Sport-Related Concussion. *J. Athl. Train.* **2017**, *52*, 245–255. [CrossRef] [PubMed]

19. Alsalaheen, B.A.; Haines, J.; Yorke, A.; Stockdale, K.; Broglio, S.P. Reliability and concurrent validity of instrumented balance error scoring system using a portable force plate system. *Physician Sportsmed.* **2015**, *43*, 221–226. [CrossRef] [PubMed]

20. King, L.A.; Mancini, M.; Fino, P.C.; Chesnutt, J.; Swanson, C.W.; Markwardt, S.; Chapman, J.C. Sensor-Based Balance Measures Outperform Modified Balance Error Scoring System in Identifying Acute Concussion. *Ann. Biomed. Eng.* **2017**, *45*, 2135–2145. [CrossRef] [PubMed]

21. King, L.A.; Horak, F.B.; Mancini, M.; Pierce, D.; Priest, K.C.; Chesnutt, J.; Sullivan, P.; Chapman, J.C. Instrumenting the Balance Error Scoring System for Use With Patients Reporting Persistent Balance Problems after Mild Traumatic Brain Injury. *Arch. Phys. Med. Rehabil.* **2014**, *95*, 353–359. [CrossRef] [PubMed]

22. Brown, H.J.; Siegmund, G.P.; Guskiewicz, K.M.; Van Den Doel, K.; Cretu, E.; Blouin, J.S. Development and validation of an objective balance error scoring system. *Med Sci Sports Exerc* **2014**, *46*, 1610–1616. [CrossRef] [PubMed]

23. Napoli, A.; Glass, S.M.; Tucker, C.; Obeid, I. The Automated Assessment of Postural Stability: Balance Detection Algorithm. *Ann. Biomed. Eng.* **2017**. [CrossRef] [PubMed]

24. Dave, P.T. Automated BESS Test for Diagnosis of Post-Concusive Symptoms Using Microsoft Kinect. Master's Thesis, Temple University, Philadelphia, PA, USA, 2014.

25. Asteriadis, S.; Chatzitofis, A.; Zarpalas, D.; Alexiadis, D.S.; Daras, P. Estimating human motion from multiple Kinect sensors. In Proceedings of the 6th International Conference on Computer Vision/Computer Graphics Collaboration Techniques and Applications, Berlin, Germany, 6–7 June 2013.

26. Azis, N.A.; Choi, H.J.; Iraqi, Y. Substitutive Skeleton Fusion for Human Action Recognition. In Proceedings of the International Conference on Big Data and Smart Computing (BigComp), Jeju, Korea, 9–11 February 2015; pp. 170–177.

27. Kaenchan, S.; Mongkolnam, P.; Watanapa, B.; Sathienpong, S. Automatic multiple kinect cameras setting for simple walking posture analysis. In Proceedings of the IEEE International Computer Science and Engineering Conference, Nakorn Pathom, Thailand, 4–6 September 2013; pp. 245–249.

28. Yeung, K.Y.; Kwok, T.H.; Wang, C.C.L. Improved Skeleton Tracking by Duplex Kinects: A Practical Approach for Real-Time Applications. *J. Comput. Inf. Sci. Eng.* **2013**, *13*, 041007. [CrossRef]

29. Gao, Z.; Yu, Y.; Zhou, Y.; Du, S. Leveraging Two Kinect Sensors for Accurate Full-Body Motion Capture. *Sensors* **2015**, *15*, 24297–24317. [CrossRef] [PubMed]

30. Bell, D.R.; Guskiewicz, K.M.; Clark, M.A.; Padua, D.A. Systematic review of the balance error scoring system. *Sports Health* **2011**, *3*, 287–295. [CrossRef] [PubMed]

31. Herring, S.A.; Cantu, R.C.; Guskiewicz, K.M.; Putukian, M.; Kibler, W.B.; Bergfeld, J.A.; Boyajian-O'Neill, L.A.; Franks, R.R.; Indelicato, P.A.; American College of Sports Medicine. Concussion (mild traumatic brain injury) and the team physician: A consensus statement—2011 update. *Med. Sci. Sports Exerc.* **2011**, *43*, 2412–2422. [PubMed]

32. Cicchetti, D.V. The precision of reliability and validity estimates re-visited: distinguishing between clinical and statistical significance of sample size requirements. *J. Clin. Exp. Neuropsychol.* **2001**, *23*, 695–700. [CrossRef] [PubMed]

33. Koo, T.K.; Li, M.Y. A Guideline of Selecting and Reporting Intraclass Correlation Coefficients for Reliability Research. *J. Chiropr. Med.* **2016**, *15*, 155–163. [CrossRef] [PubMed]

34. Valovich, T.C.; Perrin, D.H.; Gansneder, B.M. Repeat Administration Elicits a Practice Effect With the Balance Error Scoring System but Not With the Standardized Assessment of Concussion in High School Athletes. *J. Athl. Train.* **2003**, *38*, 51–56. [PubMed]

35. Napoli, A.; Ward, C.R.; Glass, S.M.; Tucker, C.; Obeid, I. Automated assessment of postural stability system. *Conf. Proc. IEEE Eng. Med. Biol. Soc.* **2016**, *2016*, 6090–6093. [PubMed]

16

Biomechanical Modeling of Pterygium Radiation Surgery

Bojan Pajic [1,2,3,4], **Daniel M. Aebersold** [5], **Andreas Eggspuehler** [6], **Frederik R. Theler** [7] and **Harald P. Studer** [1,8,*]

[1] Eye Clinic Orasis, Swiss Eye Research Foundation, CH-5734 Reinach, Switzerland; bpajic@datacomm.ch
[2] Department of Physics, Faculty of Sciences, University of Novi Sad, 21000 Novi Sad, Serbia
[3] Division of Ophthalmology, Department of Clinical Neurosciences, Geneva University Hospitals, CH-1205 Geneva, Switzerland
[4] Faculty of Medicine of the Military Medical Academy, University of Defence, 11000 Belgrade, Serbia
[5] Department of Radiation Oncology, Inselspital, Bern University Hospital, University of Bern, CH-3010 Bern, Switzerland; daniel.aebersold@insel.ch
[6] Department of Neurology, Schulthess Klinik, CH-8008 Zuerich, Switzerland; a.eggspuehler@gmx.net
[7] Optimo Medical, CH-2503 Biel, Switzerland; frederik.theler@optimo-medical.com
[8] OCTlab, Department of Ophthalmology, University of Basel, CH-4001 Basel, Switzerland
*   Correspondence: harald.studer@gmail.com

Academic Editors: Dragan Indjin and Małgorzata Jędrzejewska-Szczerska

Abstract: Pterygium is a vascularized, invasive transformation on the anterior corneal surface that can be treated by Strontium-/Yttrium90 beta irradiation. Finite element modeling was used to analyze the biomechanical effects governing the treatment, and to help understand clinically observed changes in corneal astigmatism. Results suggested that irradiation-induced pulling forces on the anterior corneal surface can cause astigmatism, as well as central corneal flattening. Finite element modeling of corneal biomechanics closely predicted the postoperative corneal surface (astigmatism error -0.01D; central curvature error -0.16D), and can help in understanding beta irradiation treatment. Numerical simulations have the potential to preoperatively predict corneal shape and function changes, and help to improve corneal treatments.

Keywords: pterygium; radiation; cornea surgery; biomechanics; finite element modeling; simulation

1. Introduction

Pterygium, also called Surfer's Eye, is a vascularized, invasive transformation growing on the anterior corneal surface, starting in the conjunctiva near the limbal region and with expanding towards the corneal center. The Bowmann's membrane, underneath the epithelium, thereby serves as a controlling structure for the pterygium. Besides UV light, the following co-factors promoting the development of a pterygium have been reported in literature: chronic exposure to ultraviolet light in combination with hot and dry climate, chronic irritation by dust, and frequent exposure to wind [1]. The in-growth almost exclusively starts nasally (92%) [2], possibly because in that area the rays from the sun pass laterally through the cornea, intensifying the tissues' exposure to UV light.

Even though co-factors are named, the main etiological reason for developing a pterygium is ultraviolet light exposure [3,4], as a recent mathematical model demonstrated that ultraviolet irradiation can lead to limbal stem cell dysfunction [5–7]. The fact that Fibroblast Growth Factor (FGF), Vascular Endothelial Growth Factor (VEGF), Transforming Growth Factor β (TGF β), and Stem Cell Factor (SCM) are increased in pterygial tissue [8–10], while IGFBP3 is decreased, further suggests that growth proliferation is not controlled in the same way as in tumor cells and, as a consequence, that pterygium is not neoplasia. Rather, it is a degenerative alteration [11], as VEGF leads to angiogenesis and SCM to the modulation of mast cells.

Various surgical treatments for pterygium have been suggested in the past and have been frequently employed in the field. However, depending on the technique, the recurrence rate of pterygium used to be relatively high, in a range from 35% to 68% [12–14]. More modern surgical procedures involving the implementation of antimetabolites, such as Mitomycin C, or the introduction of radiotherapy, decrease the recurrence rate down to a level of 1.7% to 12.5% [2,6,15–18]. Furthermore, therapy concepts such as pterygium excision with conjunctival autografts and subconjunctival amniotic membranes also reduce this rate down to a level of ~1% [19].

In their previous research [5–7,10,20], the authors of these papers showed that with the introduction of Strontium-/Yttrium-90 beta-irradiation as an exclusive, non-surgical treatment, no recurrences have occurred to date. Even though the result of beta-irradiation treatment is an inactive pterygium without vessels, the procedure may induce certain amounts of corneal astigmatism [5–7,10,20]. The authors hypothesized that the observed changes in cylinder value may stem from pulling forces placed the cornea by the retracting pterygium. Hence, it is of great importance to understand the underlying biomechanical connection between beta-irradiation and its pterygium reduction, as well as the induction of corneal astigmatism. The goal of this study is to develop a mathematical model to describe the governing biomechanical processes.

2. Materials and Methods

The right eye of a 56-year-old female subject, diagnosed with pterygium, was treated with Strontium-/Yttrium-90 irradiation treatment (see Figure 1a). Preoperative Pentacam (Oculus Optikgeräte GmbH, Wetzlar, Germany) measurements were taken to create a subject-specific finite element model. The model was numerically simulated using the Optimeyes software (Optimo Medical AG, Biel, Switzerland), employing an earlier published [21–25] constitutive material model. Optimeyes is a comprehensive technology platform for the simulation and prediction of corneal shape and function changes, caused by mechanical interferences with the tissue. The software allowed us to create patient-specific finite element models from anterior segment tomography measurement data, compute initial stress-distribution, and run numerical simulations of cornea surgical treatments. Simulation results were then compared to the 25-month postoperative follow-up Pentacam measurements. Comparison included corneal shape and corneal function analysis.

2.1. Pterygium Surgery with Beta Irradiation

A convex plate with a diameter of 12 mm, attached to a pen-like holder, was used as a Strontium-/Yttrium-90 applicator. The radioactive substance was attached to the inner surface of the plate, and softly put onto the eye, well centered over the pterygium. To reduce irradiation exposure of the surrounding tissue, a surround of 0.002 mm stainless steel and 0.01 mm aluminum, fitted to the edge of the applicator plate, filtered the original Strontium-90 irradiation down to 3%, and the Yttrium-90 down to 60%. The irradiation application scheme was as follows: A dosage of 6 gray (1 Gy = 1 J/kg) of the ionizing radiation was applied twice a week, for three consecutive weeks. Hence, a total dose of 6×6 Gy was administered to the pterygium.

2.2. Constitutive Material Model

Biomechanically, corneal tissue is known for being nearly incompressible, having non-linear elastic characteristics, being highly inhomogeneous in-plane as well as over its thickness, and for revealing a high degree of anisotropy. In this work, we used a previously published biomechanical model [21–25] which used additive terms in a non-linear, hyper elastic strain energy function to describe the tissue characteristics. Generally speaking, strain-energy functions are derived from the laws of thermodynamics, and relate deformation (right-hand side of the equation) to deformation energy (left-hand side of the equation). The formulation used in this work was already available in the Optimeyes software, and is given as:

$$\Psi = U + \overline{\Psi}_m[C_{10}] + \frac{1}{\pi} \int \Phi \cdot \left(\overline{\Psi}_{f1}[\gamma_m, \mu_m] + \overline{\Psi}_{f2}[\gamma_k, \mu_k] \right) d\theta \qquad (1)$$

where U is a penalty-term, preventing volume changes and therefore modeling the incompressibility of corneal tissue, $\overline{\Psi}_m$ is a non-linear adaptation of Hooke's law—called neo-hookean—representing the tissue matrix with its proteoglycans and glycosaminoglycans, and $\overline{\Psi}_{f1}$ and $\overline{\Psi}_{f2}$ are anisotropic polynomial material functions [26] modeling the main collagen fibers and the cross-links, respectively. The probability distribution function Φ defines a realistic fiber distribution, as has been assessed through X-ray scattering by Aghamohammadzadeh et al. [27]. The distribution is defined in the model by assigning a weighting to each possible direction ($0°$ to $180°$) for any location in the model, and as a function of corneal depth. Material constants (Table 1) were determined using three sets of experimental data: one from button inflation experiments [28] and two (one superior-inferior strip, one superonasal-inferotemporal strip) from strip extensometry [29] experiments. The inverse finite element method was used to fit the above strain energy function to the experimental data from our earlier work [21].

Table 1. Material coefficients, matching the age of the study subjects, that have been used in conjunction with the constitutive material model implementation. C_{10} is the material constant of the neo-hookean hyper elastic material model for tissue matrix (proteoglycans and glycosaminoglycans, etc.), γ_m, μ_m are material constants of the polynomial material function Ψ_{f1}, introduced by Markert et al. [26], which model the main corneal collagen fibers, and γ_k, μ_k are material constants of the polynomial material function Ψ_{f2}, which model the collagen cross-links. Material coefficients were obtained from our earlier work [21].

$C_{10}[\mathbf{MPa}]$	γ_m	$\mu_m[\mathbf{MPa}]$	γ_k	$\mu_k[\mathbf{MPa}]$
0.06	0.13	24.0	0.08	95.0

2.3. Patient-Specific Radiation Surgery Simulation

A patient-specific finite element model for the patient in the study was obtained with a three-step algorithm, available in the Optimeyes software: (i) The geometrical information obtained from spatial elevation data of the front and back surface of the patient's cornea (acquired with the Scheimpflug tomography system Pentacam HR, Oculus Optikgeräte GmbH, Germany) was used to warp a spherical template cornea model to create a patient-specific finite element mesh containing 35,000 elements and over 44,000 nodes. (ii) The initial stress distribution in the model was then computed with an iterative approach [30,31]. (iii) Finally, the effects of the surgery were simulated. The anterior and posterior surfaces, computed by the finite-element (FE) model, were then compared to the postoperative surfaces to assess the accuracy and reliability of FE modeling. The details of the algorithm steps i–iii are described below:

(i)   Mesh warping: In our earlier work [23], we showed that a model with patient-specific geometry of the human cornea can be obtained by warping a spherical finite element mesh such that its anterior and posterior surfaces match the respective surfaces of the tomography measurements. Thereby, the tomography surfaces are expressed as the coefficients obtained from Zernike expansion (up to the twelfth order, and over the central 8.0 mm optical zone of the cornea), and the inside mesh nodes proportionally follow the deformation of the respective surface nodes. This way, the template mesh was warped to match the patient's cornea, without producing distorted elements (which is crucial for finite element analysis).

(ii) Calculation of initial stress distribution: Since the Pentacam Scheimpflug camera measures corneal geometry in vivo, whereby the corneal tissue is under mechanical stress, the shape in the absence of acting forces is a priori not known. An iterative approach to calculate the initial stress distribution in the model, as was previously published [30,31], was employed in this study.

(iii) Surgery simulation: A specific, three-dimensional, finite element model was created in the finite element software package ANSYS 17.1 (ANSYS Inc., Canonsburg, PA, USA). The model represents the full cornea, plus a 4-mm wide rim of scleral tissue. The model was fixed at the edge of the scleral rim, and a pressure of 15 mmHg on the models inside represented the intraocular pressure. The anterior surface of the model cornea is prepared such that a specific part exactly corresponds to the shape and position of the subject's pterygium (see Figure 1b). Pressure was applied to that specific part, modeling the pulling forces of the retracting pterygium, tangentially to the corneal surface and towards the limbus (see Figure 2). This simulation approach reproduces the pulling effects placed onto the corneal surface when radiation-induced tissue shrinking in pterygium tissue occurs. The pterygium tissue itself was not modelled.

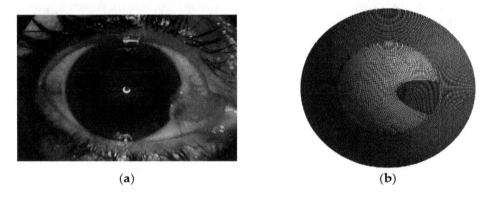

(a)   (b)

Figure 1. (a) Top-view image of the study subject with pterygium in-growth in the cornea; (b) Three-dimensional finite element model of the cornea and parts of the sclera, as seen from the top. The specific area (shown in red), representing where the pterygium pulls on the anterior corneal surface.

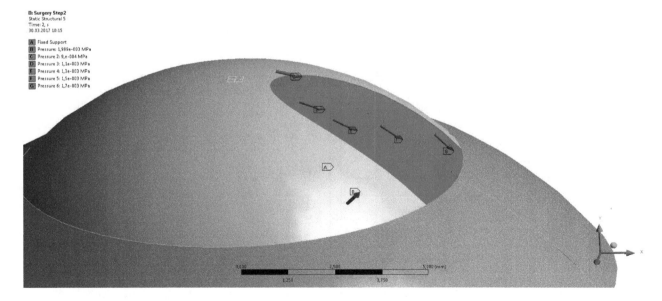

Figure 2. Three-dimensional finite element model of the cornea and the 4-mm scleral rim. The red area represents the specific part of the anterior surface of the cornea model where the tangential pulling forces were applied.

The anterior and posterior surface final geometry after finite element simulation were automatically imported, and then analyzed in the user interface of the Optimeyes software. The software uses an 8.0-mm region of interest for Zernike decomposition of the anterior and posterior corneal surface in the model, and the keratometric index $n = 1.3375$ for curvature calculation. Thereby, the sagittal curvature was calculated as $C_S = (n-1)/R$, where R is the radius of the curvature, the normal distance between a surface point and the central axis of the cornea. From the sagittal curvatures, corneal astigmatism was calculated as the difference between the steep and flat simulated keratometry values over a central annulus of a 0.5- to 2.0-mm radius. Elevation data were calculated as the normal distance between the cornea and a reference surface, a best-fit sphere fitted over a central 8.0-mm diameter zone.

Corneal shape was compared by analyzing sagittal curvature maps of the anterior corneal surface. Color-coded curvature maps, provided by the Pentacam software as well as by the Optimeyes software, were used to calculate anterior corneal astigmatism, as well as central and paracentral corneal curvatures. Astigmatism was thereby calculated on an apex-centered annulus of 0.5 mm < r < 2.5 mm. Central corneal curvature is the average curvature on an apex-centered disk with a 2.0-mm radius. Paracentral corneal curvature is the average curvature on an apex-centered annulus of 2.0 mm < r < 3.5 mm. Corneal function was compared by analyzing anterior corneal wavefront indices over a central wavefront pupil with a 6-mm diameter.

Besides postoperative geometrical shape, the deformed finite element model also provides full-field biomechanical stress information for every simulation step as part of the software package. The average stress (and standard deviation) was calculated from the simulation within the central 3.0-mm zone.

3. Results

Results from the patient-specific finite element simulations were compared to the actual clinical follow-up anterior segment tomography measurements. The simulation results showed a close match to the clinical data. While the simulation predicted an increase in astigmatism cylinder of +0.32D, in clinics, an increase of +0.31D was observed (see Figure 3a). The astigmatism axis did not change. The central corneal curvature decreased from 44.15D to 43.70D post-surgically. The simulation predicted a decrease to 43.86D. Furthermore, while the paracentral curvature decrease from 43.28D to 43.15D, the simulation predicted a decrease to 43.10D (see Figure 3b).

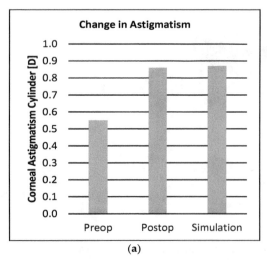 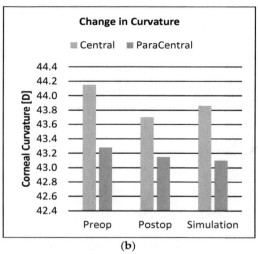

(a)   (b)

Figure 3. (a) Comparison of postoperative astigmatism cylinder and predicted cylinder. The simulation predicted the postoperative cylinder values very closely; (b) Comparison of postoperative central and paracentral curvatures and predicted curvature. Postoperative central and paracentral curvatures were well predicted by the simulation model.

While Figure 4 compares the postoperative corneal sagittal curvature map to the predicted curvature map, Figure 5 shows the postoperative corneal pachymetry next to the predicted pachymetry map. Pachymetry slightly increased in clinics, as central corneal thickness went up from 512 to 528 micron, but remained stable in the simulation.

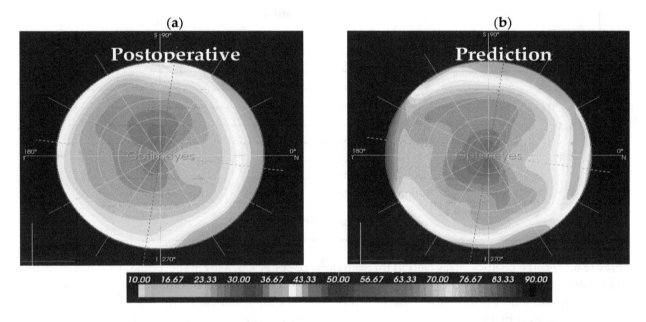

Figure 4. Sagittal anterior corneal curvature maps in Diopters [D] for the central 10.0-mm optical zone. (a) The left map is the post-surgical follow-up map, assessed by the Pentacam HR; (b) The right map shows the simulated prediction after the numerical simulation of pulling forces.

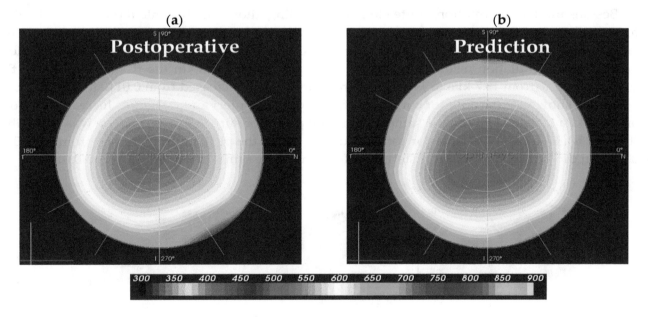

Figure 5. Corneal pachymetry maps, with a scale from 300 to 900 micrometers for the central 10.0-mm optical zone. (a) The left-hand side represents the postoperative pachymetry map; (b) The right-hand side depicts the simulated prediction of corneal thickness.

3.1. Corneal Function

Corneal function was analyzed by comparison of anterior corneal wavefront coefficients between the postsurgical and the simulated cornea. Figure 6 depicts spherical, astigmatic, coma, trefoil, and tetrafoil aberrations, as well as the root means square of higher order aberrations (Zernike order 4 and higher). Predicted spherical, astigmatic, and coma aberrations were close to the clinical follow-up measurements. The more irregular terms of trefoil and tetrafoil did not show a good match.

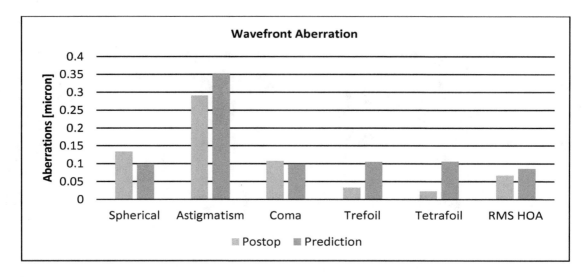

Figure 6. Zernike coefficients, given in micrometers, of spherical, astigmatic, coma, trefoil, tetrafoil, and root means square of higher order (RMS-HOA) wavefront aberrations. While the predicted values were comparable to postoperative wavefront coefficients for spherical (-26%), astigmatic ($+21\%$), coma (-8%), and higher order aberrations ($+28\%$), trefoil ($+217\%$) and tetrafoil ($+360\%$) were not well predicted.

3.2. Corneal Biomechanics

Besides model deformation, finite element modeling allows for the calculation of mechanical stresses and strains. Stresses inside corneal tissue are computed as force over area, and are given in the unit kilo-pascal (kPa). Strain is the deformation relative to the initial dimension, and thus unit-less. Biomechanical simulation results showed an average stress increase in the tissue underneath the pterygium of 5% (from 13.7 kPa to 14.4 kPa). Strains in the area increased from 0.0110 to 0.0120 (4.8%). As Figure 7 shows, on the anterior corneal surface area of the pterygium, stresses increased by 16%, from 9.97 kPa to 11.60 kPa (on the same area on the posterior surface, stress change was negligible with -0.3%). Strains on the anterior corneal surface under the pterygium increased from 0.0083 to 0.0097, but did not change on the posterior surface under the same area (from 0.0147 to 0.0146).

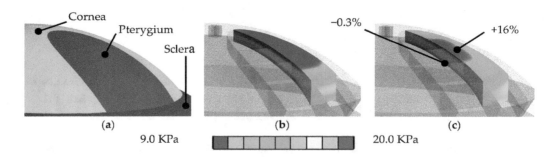

Figure 7. (a) Geometry of a cornea with pterygium. (b) Stress state before and (c) after applying the pulling force of the retracting pterygium. The color scale goes from blue (9 kPa) up to red (20 kPa). Therefore, blueish and greenish colors indicate low stress states, and orange and reddish colors indicate states of high stress. The simulation predicted an overall stress increase in corneal tissue under the pterygium of 2.4%.

4. Discussion and Conclusions

This work focused on numerical simulations of an earlier published beta-irradiation method for corneal pterygium treatment. The goal of the study was to better understand the relationship between Sr-90/Ytt-90 irradiation and clinically observed induction of corneal astigmatism, and to investigate the question of whether the retracting forces of a shrinking pterygium can be the cause of astigmatic changes. Furthermore, the model was intended to reveal the underlying biomechanical processes taking place during the treatment.

It has been shown in literature [6,7,10] that treatment with Sr-90/Ytt-90 irradiation only leads to the devascularization and reduction of the pterygium, without a single case of recurrence. Nevertheless, while corneal pachymetry remained stable after the treatment for all cases, changes in corneal astigmatism cylinder and axis were observed. It was hypothesized that the irradiation-induced retraction of the pterygium places pulling forces onto the anterior corneal surface, which as a consequence causes flattening along the central meridian of the pterygium, and ultimately leads to the induction of corneal astigmatism. Furthermore, clinical findings suggest that the amount of induced astigmatism depends on the preoperative extent of the pterygium. To the best of our knowledge, this is the first time that the mechanisms behind irradiation-induced astigmatic changes in the cornea are investigated with biomechanical simulations.

The results of biomechanical surgery simulation suggest that the clinically observed induction of corneal astigmatism after irradiation treatment might well be caused by pulling forces, exerted onto the anterior corneal surface by the retracting pterygium tissue. The simulation models, based on pre-treatment Pentacam examinations, reproduced pterygium treatment inside the computer and predicted the clinical outcome of a 25-month follow-up well, as compared to the acquired Pentacam data. Consequently, it appears likely that the biomechanical simulation model closely represents the clinical reality, and that it is biomechanical effects that cause the induction of corneal astigmatism. Since the applied pulling force of 30 Millinewton (mN) were chosen to predict postoperative astigmatism best, it remains to be proven clinically that this force corresponds to the actual forces created by pterygium retraction.

Furthermore, simulation results suggest that, in addition to astigmatic changes, the cornea would also experience flattening. Interestingly, the predicted flattening effects in the central and paracentral cornea closely corresponded to the clinical results. On the other hand, predicted wavefront aberrations only partially matched with the clinical follow-up measurements. This might have to do with the fact that the simulation model was passed on the preoperative topography measurement and that because of the pterygium, the preoperative trefoil and tetrafoil aberrations might have been imprecisely assessed prior to the surgery. Still, important aberrations such as spherical, astigmatic, and coma aberrations were well predicted with by the simulation model. The fact that our clinical findings corresponded well with a theoretical model strongly supports the hypothesis that pterygium treatment by Sr-90/Ytt-90 irradiation can induce astigmatism as well as central and paracentral corneal flattening.

Even though the employed simulation model was patient-specific with respect to corneal shape, it has the limitation of assuming non-individualized biomechanical properties. Further limitations of the modeling are the assumed amount of pulling forces, the fact that the modeling only considered the anterior section of the eye and was working with an average intraocular pressure of 15 mmHg, and, most importantly, that modeling neglected potential radiation-induced tissue modifications and multi-physical effects. Nevertheless, the model still demonstrates that forces exerted on the cornea by the contracting pterygium may well be the root cause of induced corneal astigmatism as well as corneal flattening. Finite element modeling might help in the future to further understand the biomechanical effects of pterygium surgery, define improved treatment schemes, and reduce induced corneal shape changes.

Author Contributions: Bojan Pajic provided the treatment indication, developed the study design, acquired clinical data, and contributed to writing the paper. Daniel M Aebersold performed the irradiations/treatments and substantially contributed the study design. Andreas Eggspuehler supplied surgical advice and substantially contributed to the design of the study. Frederik Theler performed finite element simulations and mathematical modeling. Harald Studer performed data analysis and contributed to writing the paper.

References

1. Taylor, H.R. Etiology of climatic droplet keratopathy and pterygium. *Br. J. Ophthalmol.* **1980**, *64*, 154–163. [CrossRef] [PubMed]
2. Cooper, J.S. Postoperative irradiation of pterygia: Ten more years of experience. *Radiology* **1978**, *128*, 753–756. [CrossRef] [PubMed]
3. Coronea, M.T.; Di Girolamo, N.; Wakefield, D. The pathogenesis of pterygia. *Curr. Opin. Ophthalmol.* **1999**, *10*, 282–288. [CrossRef]
4. Moran, D.J.; Hollows, F.C. Pterygium and ultraviolet radiation: A positive correlation. *Br. J. Ophthalmol.* **1984**, *68*, 343–346. [CrossRef] [PubMed]
5. Pajic, B.; Pugnale-Verillotte, N.; Greiner, R.H.; Pajic, D.; Eggspühler, A. Résultat de la thérapie au strontium-yttrium-90 des ptérygions. *J. Fr. Ophthalmol.* **2002**, *25*, 473–479.
6. Pajic, B.; Pallas, A.; Aebersold, D.; Gruber, G.; Greiner, R.H. Prospective Study on Exclusive, Nonsurgical Strontium-/Yttrium-90 Irradiation of Pterygia. *Strahlenther. Onkol.* **2004**, *180*, 510–516. [CrossRef] [PubMed]
7. Pajic, B.; Greiner, R.H. Long term results of non-surgical, exclusive Strontium-/Yttrium-90 Beta-irradiation of pterygia. *Radiother. Oncol.* **2005**, *74*, 25–29. [CrossRef] [PubMed]
8. Kria, L.; Ohira, A.; Amemiya, T. Immunohistochemical localization of basic fibroblast growth factor, platelet derived growth factor, transforming growth factor-β and tumor necrosis factor-α in the pterygium. *Acta Histochem.* **1996**, *98*, 195–201. [CrossRef]
9. Nakagami, T.; Watanabe, I.; Murakami, A.; Okisaka, S.; Ebihara, N. Expression of Stem Cell Factor in Pterygium. *Jpn. J. Ophthalmol.* **2000**, *44*, 193–197. [CrossRef]
10. Vastardis, I.; Pajic, B.; Greiner, R.; Pajic-Eggspuehler, B.; Aebersold, D. Prospective study of exclusive Strontium-/Yttrium-90 β- irradiation of primary and recurrent pterygia with no prior surgical excision: Clinical outcome of long-term follow-up. *Strahlenther. Onkol.* **2009**, *185*, 808–814. [CrossRef] [PubMed]
11. Wong, Y.W.; Chew, J.; Yang, H.; Tan, D.; Beuerman, R. Expression of insulin-like growth factor binding protein- 3 in pterygium tissue. *Br. J. Ophthalmol.* **2006**, *90*, 769–772. [CrossRef] [PubMed]
12. Bahrassa, F.; Datta, R. Postoperative beta radiation treatment of pterygium. *Int. J. Radiat Oncol. Biol. Phys.* **1983**, *9*, 679–684. [CrossRef]
13. Bernstein, M.; Unger, S.M. Experiences with surgery and strontium 90 in the treatment of pterygium. *Am. J. Ophthalmol.* **1960**, *49*, 1024–1029. [CrossRef]
14. De Keizer, R.J.W. Pterygium excision with or without postoperative irradiation, a double blind study. *Doc. Ophthalmol.* **1982**, *52*, 309–315. [CrossRef] [PubMed]
15. Frucht-Perry, J.; Siganos, C.S.; Ilsar, M. Intraoperative application of topical mitomycin C for pterygium surgery. *Ophthalmology* **1996**, *103*, 674–677. [CrossRef]
16. Hayasaka, S.; Noda, S.; Yukari, Y.; Setogawa, T. Postoperative installation of Mitomycin C in the treatment of recurrent pterygium. *Ophthalmic Surg.* **1989**, *20*, 580–583. [PubMed]
17. Paryani, S.B.; Scott, W.P.; Wells, J.W., Jr.; Johnson, D.W.; Chobe, R.J.; Kuruvilla, A.; Schoeppel, S.; Deshmukh, A. Management of pterygium with surgery and radiation therapy. *Int. J. Radiat. Oncol. Biol. Phys.* **1994**, *28*, 101–103. [CrossRef]
18. Rachmiel, R.; Leiba, H.; Levartovsky, S. Results of treatment with topical mitomycin C 0.02% following excision of primary pterygium. *Br. J. Ophthalmol.* **1995**, *79*, 233–236. [CrossRef] [PubMed]
19. Shusko, A.; Hovanesian, J.A. Pterygium excision with conjunctival autograft and subconjunctival amniotic membrane as antirecurrence agents. *Can. J. Ophthalmol.* **2016**, *51*, 412–416. [CrossRef] [PubMed]
20. Pajic, B.; Vastardis, I.; Rajkovic, P.; Pajic-Eggspuehler, B.; Aebersold, DM.; Cvejic, Z. A mathematical approach to human pterygium shape. *Clin. Ophthalmol.* **2016**, *10*, 1343–1349. [CrossRef] [PubMed]

21. Studer, H.P.; Larrea, X.; Riedwyl, H.; Büchler, P. Biomechanical Model of Human Cornea Based on Stromal Microstructure. *J. Biomech.* **2010**, *43*, 836–842. [CrossRef] [PubMed]
22. Studer, H.P.; Büchler, P.; Ridewly, H. Importance of Multiple Loading Scenarios for the Identification of Material Coefficients of the Human Cornea. *CMBBE* **2012**, *15*, 93–99. [CrossRef] [PubMed]
23. Studer, H.P.; Riedwyl, H.; Amstutz, C.A.; Hanson, J.V.; Büchler, P. Patient-specific finite-element simulation of the human cornea: A clinical validation study on cataract surgery. *J. Biomech.* **2013**, *46*, 751–758. [CrossRef] [PubMed]
24. Studer, H.P.; Pradhan, K.R.; Reinstein, D.Z.; Businaro, E.; Archer, T.J.; Gobbe, M.; Roberts, C.J. Biomechanical Modeling of Femtosecond Laser Keyhole Endokeratophakia Surgery. *J. Refract. Surg.* **2015**, *31*, 480–486. [CrossRef] [PubMed]
25. Whitford, C.; Studer, H.; Boote, C.; Meek, K.M.; Elsheikh, A. Biomechanical Model of the Human Cornea: Considering Shear Stiffness and Regional Variation of Collagen Anisotropy and Density. *JMBBM* **2015**, *42*, 76–87. [CrossRef] [PubMed]
26. Markert, B.; Ehlers, W.; Karajan, N. A general polyconvex strain-energy function for fiber-reinforced materials. *Proc. Appl. Math. Mech.* **2005**, *5*, 245–246. [CrossRef]
27. Aghamohammadzadeh, H.; Newton, R.; Meek, K. X-ray scattering used to map the preferred collagen orientation in the human cornea and limbus. *Structure* **2004**, *12*, 249–256. [CrossRef] [PubMed]
28. Elsheikh, A.; Wang, D.; Pye, D. Determination of the modulus of elasticity of the human cornea. *J. Refract. Surg.* **2007**, *23*, 808–818. [PubMed]
29. Elsheikh, A.; Anderson, K. Comparative study of corneal strip extensometry and inflation tests. *J. R. Soc. Interface* **2008**, *2*, 177–185. [CrossRef] [PubMed]
30. Pinsky, P.M.; van der Heide, D.; Chernyak, D. Computational modeling of mechanical anisotropy in the cornea and sclera. *J. Cataract Refract. Surg.* **2005**, *31*, 136–145. [CrossRef] [PubMed]
31. Pandolfi, A.; Manganiello, F. A model for the human cornea: Constitutive formulation and numerical analysis. *Biomech. Model. Mechanobiol.* **2006**, *5*, 237–246. [CrossRef] [PubMed]

17

Evaluation of Laser-Assisted Trans-Nail Drug Delivery with Optical Coherence Tomography

Meng-Tsan Tsai [1,2,3], Ting-Yen Tsai [1], Su-Chin Shen [4,5], Chau Yee Ng [3,5], Ya-Ju Lee [6], Jiann-Der Lee [1,7] and Chih-Hsun Yang [3,5,*]

[1]   Department of Electrical Engineering, Chang Gung University, Taoyuan 33302, Taiwan;
      mengtsan@gmail.com (M.-T.T.); trendy1991818@gmail.com (T.-Y.T.); jdlee@mail.cgu.edu.tw (J.-D.L.)
[2]   Medical Imaging Research Center, Institute for Radiological Research, Chang Gung University and Chang
      Gung Memorial Hospital at Linkou, Taoyuan 33302, Taiwan
[3]   Department of Dermatology, Chang Gung Memorial Hospital, Linkou 33305, Taiwan;
      charlene870811@gmail.com
[4]   Department of Ophthalmology, Chang Gung Memorial Hospital, Linkou 33305, Taiwan;
      suchin@adm.cgmh.org.tw
[5]   College of Medicine, Chang Gung University, Taoyuan 33302, Taiwan
[6]   Institute of Electro-Optical Science and Technology, National Taiwan Normal University,
      Taipei 11677, Taiwan; yajulee@ntnu.edu.tw
[7]   Department of Neurosurgery, Chang Gung Memorial Hospital, LinKou 33305, Taiwan
*   Correspondence: dermadr@hotmail.com

Academic Editor: Dragan Indjin

Abstract: The nail provides a functional protection to the fingertips and surrounding tissue from external injuries. The nail plate consists of three layers including dorsal, intermediate, and ventral layers. The dorsal layer consists of compact, hard keratins, limiting topical drug delivery through the nail. In this study, we investigate the application of fractional CO_2 laser that produces arrays of microthermal ablation zones (MAZs) to facilitate drug delivery in the nails. We utilized optical coherence tomography (OCT) for real-time monitoring of the laser–skin tissue interaction, sparing the patient from an invasive surgical sampling procedure. The time-dependent OCT intensity variance was used to observe drug diffusion through an induced MAZ array. Subsequently, nails were treated with cream and liquid topical drugs to investigate the feasibility and diffusion efficacy of laser-assisted drug delivery. Our results show that fractional CO_2 laser improves the effectiveness of topical drug delivery in the nail plate and that OCT could potentially be used for in vivo monitoring of the depth of laser penetration as well as real-time observations of drug delivery.

Keywords: drug delivery; nail; optical coherence tomography; fractional laser; laser ablation

---

1. Introduction

The nail is a modified form of stratum corneum, with a thick laminated keratinized structure overlying the nail bed and matrix. However, the thick structure limits drug delivery to the nail bed, which is problematic when it comes to treating nail diseases such as onychomycosis. The nail plate is composed of 25 sheets of keratinized cells that can be divided into dorsal, intermediate, and ventral layers. Compared with the intermediate layer, the dorsal and ventral layers are thinner. The dorsal and ventral layers consist of harder skin-type keratin with lipids. In contrast, the intermediate layer is composed of hair-type keratin with few lipids, making the intermediate layer more flexible. Therefore, the dorsal layer forms a barrier for drug delivery [1–4]. To improve the efficiency of drug delivery through the nail, a new strategy is to produce micropores on the nail to remove the dorsal layer [5,6]. Therefore, the development of permeation-enhanced techniques for skin has become an important area of study to improve drug delivery. Recently, transdermal drug delivery became a new route of drug and vaccine administration, providing the advantages of avoiding the first-pass metabolism, sustained therapeutic action, and better patient compliance [7,8]. Strategies to bypass the tightly packed stratum corneum, the rate-limiting step in transdermal drug penetration, will facilitate topical medication delivery deep into the skin. Several methods have been developed to improve transdermal drug delivery, including chemical enhancers [9,10], nanocarriers [11,12], microneedles [13,14], sonophoresis [15,16], and iontophoresis [17,18]. The biocompatibility and biotoxicity of chemical enhancers and nanocarriers are important issues. For microneedles, although new biodegradable polymers reduce the risk of microneedles retained in skin tissue, these materials are not able to produce sufficient mechanical strength to penetrate the skin barrier. On the contrary, metallic microneedles can easily penetrate the skin barrier but may cause allergic reactions. Both ultrasound and iontophoresis to facilitate drug delivery have been proposed in previous studies, but accurate control of the treatment depth remains a challenging issue.

The development of laser techniques has promoted various applications, in particular for therapies and biomedical imaging. In therapeutic applications, lasers offer an excellent solution in clinical medicine because they result in less bleeding, reduced infections, and minimized incision areas [19]. With a pulsed high-energy laser, the biological tissue can be coagulated, and even ablated, which enables skin tightening, hemangioma treatment, and the removal of unwanted hair and blood vessels [20–24]. Ablative fractional lasers are primarily used to treat photodamaged skin, deep rhytides and scarring. Current fractional laser systems for dermatology include carbon dioxide (CO_2, 10,600 nm) and erbium-doped yttrium aluminum garnet (Er:YAG, 2940 nm) lasers. The fractional CO_2 laser produces deep vertical holes down to the dermis to assist the delivery of topically applied drugs into the skin. Recently, this approach was used in the treatment of fungal nail diseases [25]. The micro-channel array created by a fractional CO_2 laser creates tiny pores on the skin surface that enhance the penetration of topically applied drugs. Penetration-enhanced techniques for skin and nails are rapidly developing, enabling significant increases in the efficiency of disease treatment.

Currently, various optical imaging approaches to monitor transdermal drug delivery have been proposed, such as confocal laser scanning microscopy (CLSM) [26], two-photon microscopy (TPM) [27], infrared microscopic imaging (IMI) [28], and Raman microscopy (RM) [28]. Although both CLSM and TPM can provide cellular-level resolution, their imaging depth is limited to hundreds of micrometers, which is not deep enough to observe drug diffusion beneath the skin surface. Moreover, CLSM or TPM need extra fluorescent labeling. Compared to CLSM and TPM, IMI provides a wider imaging field, but skin specimens must be carefully prepared before imaging, and IMI cannot be used for in vivo imaging. The imaging depth of RM is limited when used for studies on drug delivery. The thickness of nails ranges from hundreds of micrometers to several millimeters, making the approaches mentioned earlier unsuitable for investigating drug delivery via nails. Moreover, these methods do not acquire depth and time-resolved information of the dynamics of drug diffusion from the nail surface to the nail bed. Therefore, in this paper, we propose the use of optical coherence tomography (OCT) to investigate the dynamics of transdermal drug delivery.

OCT uses backscattered tissue signals to reconstruct the 2D/3D morphology of biological tissue [29–31]. Compared to ultrasound imaging, OCT provides higher resolutions in both the transverse and depth directions (up to 1–10 μm). Moreover, OCT can probe deeper tissue structures than of microscopic techniques such as confocal microscopy, TPM, and harmonic generation microscopy [32–34]. Besides this deeper imaging depth, OCT imaging is noninvasive, has a high imaging speed, and can be used for internal hollow organ scanning with concomitant use of an endoscope. Various functional OCT with different purposes have been developed including optical coherence angiography [35,36], polarization-sensitive OCT for the measurement of tissue birefringence [37,38], and optical coherence elastography [39,40]. In previous studies, we have demonstrated that the photothermolysis of human skin induced by an ablative laser can be monitored with OCT [41]. Furthermore, preliminary OCT results have proven the feasibility of laser-assisted therapy [42]. In this study, we investigate the time-dependent variation of OCT intensity during the diffusion process of drug particles. Additionally, we also estimate the time-dependent speckle variance (SV) [43–46] of OCT intensity, observe in vivo laser-assisted drug delivery, and evaluate the diffusion ability of different drug preparations (liquid and cream drugs) in nails treated with fractional CO_2 laser. Finally, we evaluate the relative diffusion velocities of cream and liquid drugs in the nail by estimating the center-of-mass locations of time-dependent SV.

2. Experiment Method and Setup

The experiments in this study were approved by the Chang Gung Medical Foundation Institutional Review Board (No. 101-2921A3) and were conducted in the outpatient clinic of the Department of Dermatology of Chang Gung Memorial Hospital, Taipei, Taiwan. The volunteers were subjected to irradiance by a fractional CO_2 laser (UltraPulse Encore Active FXTM; Lumenis, Santa Clara, CA, USA) under various exposure energies of 20, 30, 40, and 50 mJ. The average power and the pulse width of the used CO_2 laser are 330 W and 0.15 ms, respectively. Single laser pulse induced each MAZ on the nail plate. The maximum output energy was up to 50 mJ. The fingernails of the volunteers were exposed to laser energies of 20, 30, 40, and 50 mJ. Fingernails were scanned by the OCT system after laser exposure to discern induced photothermolysis. Liquid or cream topical drugs (Sulconazole Nitrate) were then applied to the exposed region of the fingernail, and we scanned the nail continuously with OCT. The liquid drug we used was an Exelderm solution consisting of Sulconazole nitrate with a concentration of 1%, and the cream drug we used was Exelderm cream composed of Sulconazole nitrate with a concentration of 1%. The Exelderm solution is a solution of propylene glycol, poloxamer 407, polysorbate 20, butylated hydroxyanisole, and purified water, with sodium hydroxide. Exelderm cream is in an emollient cream base, which consists of propylene glycol, stearyl alcohol, isopropyl myristate, cetyl alcohol, polysorbate 60, sorbitan monostearate, glyceryl stearate and PEG-100 stearate, ascorbyl palmitate, and purified water with sodium hydroxide. Additionally, previous reports have demonstrated that propylene glycol is a drug load enhancer and that sodium hydroxide is an uptake rate enhancer [47]. Before OCT measurement, the finger was immersed into the ultrasonic cleaner to remove the dust in microthermal ablation zones (MAZs) for 5 min and then dried in air for 30 min.

In this study, a swept-source OCT (SS-OCT) system was set up for in vivo fingernail scanning. The setup of the SS-OCT system is similar to that of a previous study [42]. A swept source (HSL-20, Santec Corp., Aichi, Japan) at 1.3 μm was used as the light source of the OCT system with a scanning spectrum of 110 nm. The longitudinal and transverse resolutions are approximately 7 and 5 μm, respectively. The physical scanning range is $3 \times 3 \times 3$ mm^3. The maximum imaging depth of this OCT system is approximately 3 mm. Because the light source can provide a scan rate of 100 kHz, the corresponding frame rate of the OCT system was set to 100 frames/s. Unconscious motion by the volunteer during the OCT measurement was reduced using a specially designed mount fabricated by a 3D printer to fix the finger stably. Moreover, to investigate the feasibility of laser-assisted drug diffusion, the drug was rubbed on the nails and scanned with OCT. We record sequential 2D OCT images before and after the drug application.

3. Results and Discussion

Fractional laser ablation causes tissue vaporization, producing a microthermal ablation zone (MAZ) array. However, the induced MAZ penetration depth is hard to predict because of differences in the optical properties of biological tissues. To investigate the induced photothermolysis on the nail, four fingernails of a 26-year-old volunteer were sequentially exposed to fractional CO_2 laser with exposure energies of 50, 40, 30, and 20 mJ. The four treated nails were then scanned in vivo by the OCT system to acquire 3D microstructural images. Figure 1 shows the OCT results of four fingernails after exposure to these laser energies. Figure 1a–h represent the top view of the 3D OCT images and the representative cross-sectional images of four nails, respectively, which were obtained after laser exposures to energies of 50, 40, 30, and 20 mJ. Laser exposure induced MAZs as indicated by white arrows in Figure 1. Figure 1a–d demonstrate the increased size and penetration depth of MAZs corresponding to the increasing exposure energy. Based on the OCT results, the penetration depth and the diameter of the induced MAZ corresponding to exposure energy can be estimated. The average penetration depths of Figure 1a–d are 372, 321, 290, and 255 μm, respectively. Additionally, the average diameters of Figure 1a–d are 203, 183, 171, and 137 μm, respectively. The results show that an exposure energy of 50 mJ provides a deeper penetration depth while sparing the nail bed. Therefore, we chose 50 mJ as the optimal exposure energy to induce MAZ on the nails in the following experiments.

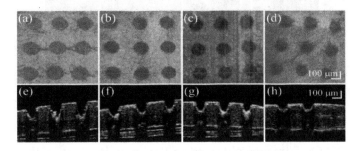

Figure 1. In vivo (**a–d**) top-view and (**e–h**) representative cross-sectional OCT images of four fingernails after fractional laser exposures to (from left to right) energies of 50, 40, 30, and 20 mJ. The red-dash lines in (**a–d**) indicate the corresponding locations of (**e–h**).

To understand the influence on the OCT intensity of the unexposed and exposed nail regions after the drug application, a fingernail of one 22-year-old male volunteer was exposed to a fractional CO_2 laser with an exposure energy of 50 mJ. In this case, only one-half of the fingernail was exposed, while the other half was spared. The finger was later fixed on the specially designed mount for motion reduction and scanned with OCT. We compare the difference of drug delivery between untreated nail and the laser-treated nail by treating both sides with liquid drug preparation and scanned with OCT. The scanning range covered both regions of the nail, and the changes before and after drug application were recorded. We analyze the intensity variation of OCT signal beneath the nail surface. A segmentation algorithm proposed in our previous study was used to explore the OCT signal beneath the nail surface [48,49]. Figure 2 shows the time-series 2D OCT images obtained at the same location of the fingernail. Figure 2a is the OCT image obtained before liquid drug application, where the left part is the untreated nail structure and the right part represents the laser-treated nail with MAZs. Figure 2b–l were obtained at various times after the liquid drug application. In Figure 2b, the strongly scattered spots, which are indicated by the white arrows, are a result of the aggregation of drug particles.

Figure 3 shows the averaged A-scan profiles of the unexposed and treated regions, as marked by the yellow and white lines in Figure 2a. Here, the A-scan represents a one-dimensional scan along the depth direction, representing the relationship between the backscattered intensity and the depth. For both lines, 11 adjacent A-scans, corresponding to a transverse range of 50 μm, were chosen for the acquisition of an averaged A-scan profile. Thus, Figure 3a represents the averaged A-scan profiles of the yellow line in Figure 2 obtained at 0, 2.0, 4.0, 6.0, 8.0, and 10.0 s after the drug application. In contrast, Figure 3b plots the averaged A-scan profiles of the white line in Figure 2 obtained at 0, 2.0, 4.0, 6.0, 8.0, and 10.0 s after the drug application. The yellowish region in Figure 3 represents the nail layer, and the greenish region indicates the tissue beneath the nail bed. In Figure 3a, the time-series of averaged A-scan profiles illustrate that there is no significant change in the backscattered intensity, especially in the yellowish region. In comparison to the results of Figure 3a, after the drug application, changes in the backscattered intensity of the yellowish region in Figure 3b was observed, marked by the black arrows. Our results show that the changes in OCT backscattered intensity can be used to identify the drug's diffusion. However, because the vessels exist in the soft tissue of skin beneath the nail bed (the greenish region), which also result in OCT intensity variation, it is hard to tell whether these changes are due to the diffusion of drug particles or the motion of red blood cells in the soft tissue layer. Therefore, in this study, we focus on investigating the intensity variation of the nail plate.

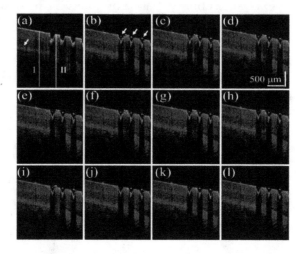

Figure 2. Time-series 2D OCT images obtained at the same location of the fingernail after 50 mJ fractional laser exposure. OCT images obtained (**a**) before the liquid drug application and at (**b**) 0 s; (**c**) 0.2 s; (**d**) 0.4 s; (**e**) 0.6 s; (**f**) 0.8 s; (**g**) 1.0 s; (**h**) 2.0 s; (**i**) 4.0 s; (**j**) 6.0 s; (**k**) 8.0 s; and (**l**) 10.0 s after the liquid drug application. The white arrows indicate that the stronger OCT backscattered signal resulted from the aggregation of drug particles. The yellow arrow indicates the nail bed. The yellow and white lines indicate the locations for estimation of the averaged A-scan profiles of the unexposed and treated regions.

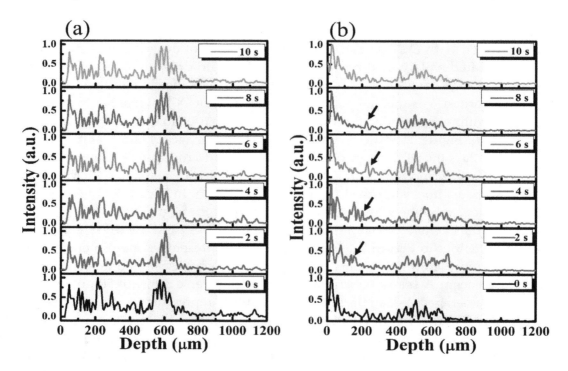

Figure 3. (**a**) Averaged A-scan profiles of the yellow line (the unexposed region) in Figure 2 and (**b**) the averaged A-scan profiles of the white line (the exposed region) in Figure 2 obtained at time points of 0, 2.0, 4.0, 6.0, 8.0, and 10.0 s after the drug application. The black arrows indicate the variation in OCT backscattered intensity after the drug application.

According to the results in Figure 3, the diffusion of drug particles results in the variation of OCT backscattered intensity. Therefore, to quantitatively evaluate the intensity variation, the SV between the time-series OCT images was estimated. First, the OCT image obtained at the point of the drug application was used as a reference, and the OCT images obtained at various time points after the drug application were then individually compared with the reference image to acquire a corresponding SV image. Therefore, an SV image at time t after the drug application can be estimated as

$$SV_{t_n}(x,z) = \frac{\left\{I_{t_0}(x,z) - \frac{1}{2}[I_{t_0}(x,z) + I_{t_n}(x,z)]\right\}^2 + \left\{I_{t_n}(x,z) - \frac{1}{2}[I_{t_0}(x,z) + I_{t_n}(x,z)]\right\}^2}{2} \tag{1}$$

where x, z are the pixel locations in the transverse and longitudinal directions, respectively [43,44], and t_0 and t_n represent the start of the drug application and the nth time point after the drug application, respectively. In our previous study, although SV can be used to observe the diffusion of water through fingernails after fractional laser exposure, it was found to be difficult to further investigate the depth-resolved drug diffusion because of the shadowing effect resulting from particle diffusion [46]. Thus, to reduce the shadowing effect, Equation (1) can be revised as

$$SVR_{t_n}(x,z) = SV_{t_n}(x,z) \times e^{\frac{1}{\gamma}\sum_{i=1}^{z} SV_{t_n}(x,i)} \tag{2}$$

where γ is an attenuation coefficient. To reject the contribution of speckle noise, we set the threshold SV value to 0.05, using the time-series 2D images to estimate the SV values before the drug application.

Subsequently, liquid and cream drugs were tested to study the feasibility of drug diffusion through MAZs. We repeat the same experiment protocol of Figure 2. First, the fingernails of one 24-year-old male volunteer were exposed to a fractional CO_2 laser with an exposure energy of 50 mJ. During OCT scanning, the finger was fixed on the specially designed mount to reduce motion artifacts, and the same location of fingernail was continuously scanned by the OCT system to obtain a time series of 2D OCT images. The liquid drug preparation was then applied to the nail surface and the nail was continuously scanned for 60 s. To compare the intensity variance before and after the drug application, a 2D OCT image was obtained at the beginning of the drug application as the reference image, and time-series OCT images were recorded after the drug application to estimate the SV images. Finally, the OCT image and corresponding SV image at each time point were merged into an SV-OCT image.

Figure 4a shows a 2D OCT image of the nail after fractional laser exposure with an exposure energy of 50 mJ, and Figure 4b–l represent time-series SV-OCT images obtained after the liquid drug application. To indicate the corresponding location of the SV signal in the nail, the OCT structural image and SV image were merged. The OCT structural intensity is shown in the gray scale, and the SV signal is shown in the red scale. Here, the occurrence of the SV signal indicates the location of intensity variance due to the moving particles, but the SV value is not proportional to the particle concentration. Strong backscattered spots, which are indicated by the white arrows in Figure 4b, moved with time, as shown in Figure 4b–l. These strong backscattered spots are a result of the aggregation of drug particles. The thickness of the liquid drug on the nail surface gives a redundant optical path difference, which will probably cause SV estimation errors. Therefore, a segmentation algorithm proposed in our previous study was performed before SV estimation [46]. Based on this segmentation algorithm, the nail surface can be detected, allowing the nail surfaces of the time-series OCT images to be realigned with the nail surface of the reference image. Since the blood flow in the soft tissue beneath the nail layer also causes time-dependent variations in OCT backscattered intensity, it is difficult to differentiate the SV contributions of the drug diffusion and the vessels in the soft tissue layer. Therefore, only SV signals in the nail structure are presented in this study; nevertheless, observations of the drug diffusion in the nail layer enable us to identify whether the drug particles have reached the nail bed. In Figure 4c, the SV signal began to occur around the boundaries of the induced MAZs, and the area of SV distribution then increased with time. After 10 s, the SV signal could be observed in the whole nail region.

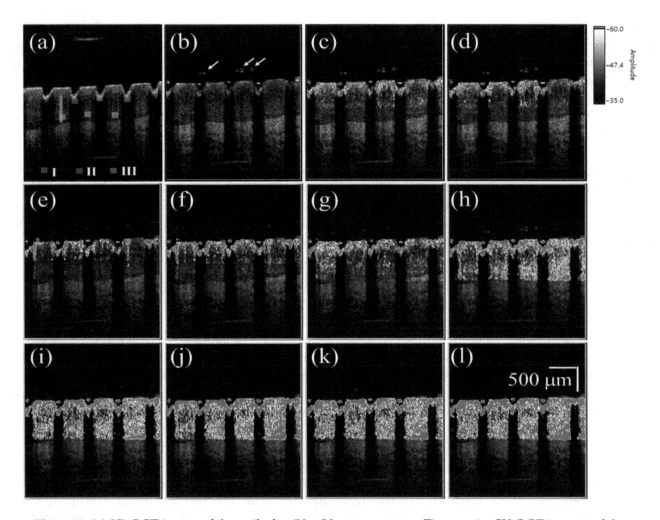

Figure 4. (a) 2D OCT image of the nail after 50 mJ laser exposure. Time-series SV-OCT images of the treated nail obtained after the liquid drug application at (**b**) 0 s; (**c**) 0.2 s; (**d**) 0.4 s; (**e**) 0.6 s; (**f**) 0.8 s; (**g**) 1.0 s; (**h**) 2.0 s; (**i**) 4.0 s; (**j**) 6.0 s; (**k**) 8.0 s; and (**l**) 10.0 s. The white arrows indicate the stronger backscattered signal, resulting from the drug particles. The scalar bar in (**l**) represents a length of 500 μm in length.

To investigate the diffusion of the cream drug in the fingernail, the same finger in the experiment of Figure 4 was utilized again and the same experimental procedure was repeated on the next day of the liquid drug experiment. To avoid the accumulation of drug particles in the nail, the nails were immersed into the ultrasound cleaner to remove the unwanted depositions in the MAZs before each experiment. Additionally, in our method, we used the B-scan obtained in the beginning of the drug application as the reference image to estimate the SV. Therefore, the effect induced by the residual drug can be greatly reduced. The cream drug preparation was then rubbed onto the nail surface and simultaneously scanned by the OCT system for 60 s. Figure 5a shows a 2D OCT image of the treated nail obtained before the cream drug application, where the induced MAZ forms an inverted pyramid shape. Figure 5b–l are the time-series SV-OCT images obtained at various time points after the cream drug application. White color represents the tissue structure, and the red color indicates the existence of an SV signal. After the drug application, the cream drug preparation occupied the MAZs, causing a stronger backscattered intensity in the MAZ region. From Figure 5b–d, we can see that the SV signal only existed on the nail surface, and gradually occurred in the nail structure as time increased. After 10 s, SV was observed in the entire nail structure. This SV is a result of the time-dependent variation of OCT intensity due to the diffusion of drug particles. Again, only SV signals in the nail layer are presented. Additionally, a comparison of Figures 4 and 5 suggests that the SV signals found in the MAZ of Figure 5 were absent in the MAZ of Figure 4. This is because the MAZs in Figure 5 were occupied by the cream drug particles. After applying the segmentation algorithm, an intact nail surface was found in Figure 5, and the MAZs in Figure 5 were included in the SV estimation. However, in the OCT images obtained from the experiment with the liquid drug after processing the segmentation algorithm, the MAZs were not included in the SV estimation.

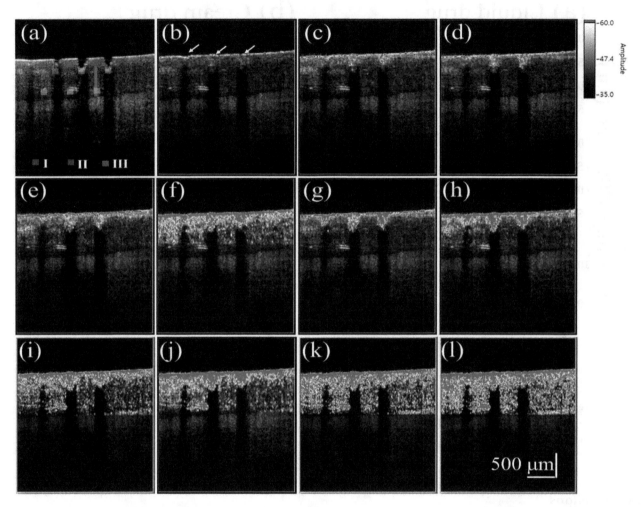

Figure 5. (a) 2D OCT image of the nail after fractional laser exposure with an exposure energy of 50 mJ. Time-series SV-OCT images of the nail obtained at (b) 0 s; (c) 0.2 s; (d) 0.4 s; (e) 0.6 s; (f) 0.8 s; (g) 1.0 s; (h) 2.0 s; (i) 4.0 s; (j) 6.0 s; (k) 8.0 s; and (l) 10.0 s after the cream drug application. The white arrows indicate that the MAZs were filled with the cream drug. The scalar bar in (l) represents a length of 500 μm in length.

For the study of drug particles diffusion behavior in nail layers, three regions (Regions I, II, and III in Figures 4 and 5) were selected for analysis. Three orange squares located at the tip regions of the MAZs in Figures 4 and 5 (Region I) were averaged, as were the three red squares located at the upper nail regions in Region II and the three white squares located in the middle of the two MAZs (Region III). For each region, the summation of the SV values of three colored square was averaged to acquire an averaged summation result at various time points. Figure 6a,b show the averaged summations of SV values of Regions I, II, and III in Figures 4 and 5, respectively. From Figure 6a, we see that the averaged summation of the SV values in Region I increased after the drug application, reaching a saturation level after approximately 15 s. The results for Regions II and III in Figure 6a indicate that the averaged SV summation started to increase after 1 s. In comparison, Figure 6b shows the same trend for region I, but the summations only start to increase after 2 s in Regions II and III. Figure 6 show that MAZs effectively improve the drug diffusion through the nail layer. Three regions in each depth range (indicated by red, orange and white squares in Figures 4a and 5a) are selected to estimate the average summation of SV values. The standard deviation of the three regions at the same depth range is shown in Figure 6.

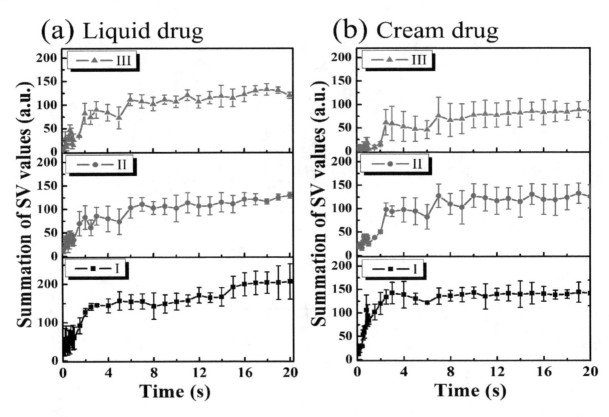

Figure 6. (**a**) Averaged summation of SV values of Regions I, II, and III indicated by the squares in Figure 4 as a function of time; (**b**) Averaged summation of SV values of Regions I, II, and III indicated by the squares in Figure 5 as a function of time.

4. Conclusions

In this study, we demonstrated that using a fractional ablative laser produces MAZ arrays on fingernails that facilitate drug delivery. However, the induced depth of photothermolysis is difficult to predict. Therefore, we used OCT for in vivo evaluation of photothermolysis on nail induced by the fractional CO_2 laser. In addition, we propose a method here for in vivo observations of drug diffusion through the induced MAZs based on the evaluation of the time-dependent OCT intensity. In this study, the exposure energy for producing microthermal ablation zones in nails was set to be 50 mJ, which is the maximum output energy of the CO_2 laser. From OCT scanning results, 50 mJ laser energy can induce an averaged penetration depth of more than 370 μm in nails, making drug particles easily penetrate the nail barrier and reach the skin tissue beneath the nail. These results suggest that OCT could serve as a potential tool for in vivo observations of drug diffusion.

Acknowledgments: This research was supported in part by the Ministry of Science and Technology (MOST) and Chang Gung Memorial Hospital, Taiwan, Republic of China, under grants MOST104-2221-E-182A-004-MY2, MOST104-2221-E-182-027-MY2, MOST105-2221-E-182-016-MY3, CMRPD2F0131, and CMRPD2B0033.

Author Contributions: Meng-Tsan Tsai and Chih-Hsun Yang designed the experiments; Ting-Yen Tsai and Ya-Ju Lee performed the experiments; Meng-Tsan Tsai, Su-Chin Shen, Chau Yee Ng, Chih-Hsun Yang, and Jiann-Der Lee analyzed the data; Meng-Tsan Tsai, Chau Yee Ng and Chih-Hsun Yang wrote the paper.

References

1. Gupchup, G.V.; Zatz, J.L. Structural characteristics and permeability properties of the human nail: A review. *J. Cosmet. Sci.* **1999**, *50*, 363–385.
2. Repka, M.A.; O'Haver, J.; See, C.H.; Gutta, K.; Munjal, M. Nail morphology studies as assessments for onychomycosis treatment modalities. *Int. J. Pharm.* **2002**, *245*, 25–36. [CrossRef]
3. Shivakumar, H.; Juluri, A.; Desai, B.; Murthy, S.N. Ungual and transungual drug delivery. *Drug Dev. Ind. Pharm.* **2012**, *38*, 901–911. [CrossRef] [PubMed]
4. Gupta, A.K.; Paquet, M. Improved efficacy in onychomycosis therapy. *Clin. Dermatol.* **2013**, *31*, 555–563. [CrossRef] [PubMed]
5. Elkeeb, R.; AliKhan, A.; Elkeeb, L.; Hui, X.; Maibach, H.I. Transungual drug delivery: Current status. *Int. J. Pharm.* **2010**, *384*, 1–8. [CrossRef] [PubMed]
6. Chiu, W.S.; Belsey, N.A.; Garrett, N.L.; Moger, J.; Price, G.J.; Delgado-Charro, M.B.; Guy, R.H. Drug delivery into microneedle-porated nails from nanoparticle reservoirs. *J. Control. Release* **2015**, *220*, 98–106. [CrossRef] [PubMed]
7. Prausnitz, M.R.; Langer, R. Transdermal drug delivery. *Nat. Biotechnol.* **2008**, *26*, 1261–1268. [CrossRef] [PubMed]
8. Wong, T.W. Electrical, magnetic, photomechanical and cavitational waves to overcome skin barrier for transdermal drug delivery. *J. Control. Release* **2014**, *193*, 257–269. [CrossRef] [PubMed]
9. Man, G.; Elias, P.M.; Man, M.-Q. Therapeutic benefits of enhancing permeability barrier for atopic eczema. *Dermatol. Sin.* **2015**, *33*, 84–89. [CrossRef]
10. Hu, L.; Man, H.; Elias, P.M.; Man, M.-Q. Herbal medicines that benefit epidermal permeability barrier function. *Dermatol. Sin.* **2015**, *33*, 90–95. [CrossRef]
11. Merino, V.; Escobar-Chávez, J.J. *Current Technologies to Increase the Transdermal Delivery of Drugs*; Bentham Science Publishers: Sharjah, United Arab Emirates, 2010.
12. Goswami, S.; Bajpai, J.; Bajpai, A. Designing gelatin nanocarriers as a swellable system for controlled release of insulin: An in vitro kinetic study. *J. Macromol. Sci. A* **2009**, *47*, 119–130. [CrossRef]
13. Van der Maaden, K.; Jiskoot, W.; Bouwstra, J. Microneedle technologies for (trans) dermal drug and vaccine delivery. *J. Control. Release* **2012**, *161*, 645–655. [CrossRef] [PubMed]
14. Tsioris, K.; Raja, W.K.; Pritchard, E.M.; Panilaitis, B.; Kaplan, D.L.; Omenetto, F.G. Fabrication of silk microneedles for controlled-release drug delivery. *Adv. Funct. Mater.* **2012**, *22*, 330–335. [CrossRef]
15. Smith, N.B. Perspectives on transdermal ultrasound mediated drug delivery. *Int. J. Nanomed.* **2007**, *2*, 585–594.
16. Azagury, A.; Khoury, L.; Enden, G.; Kost, J. Ultrasound mediated transdermal drug delivery. *Adv. Drug Del. Rev.* **2014**, *72*, 127–143. [CrossRef] [PubMed]
17. Bounoure, F.; Skiba, M.L.; Besnard, M.; Arnaud, P.; Mallet, E.; Skiba, M. Effect of iontophoresis and penetration enhancers on transdermal absorption of metopimazine. *J. Dermatol. Sci.* **2008**, *52*, 170–177. [CrossRef] [PubMed]
18. Escobar-Chavez, J.J.; Merino, V.; López-Cervantes, M.; Rodriguez-Cruz, I.M.; Quintanar-Guerrero, D.; Ganem-Quintanar, A. The use of iontophoresis in the administration of nicotine and new non-nicotine drugs through the skin for smoking cessation. *Curr. Drug Disc. Technol.* **2009**, *6*, 171–185. [CrossRef]
19. Jelínková, H. *Lasers for Medical Applications: Diagnostics, Therapy and Surgery*; Elsevier: Amsterdam, The Netherlands, 2013.
20. Stafford, R.J.; Fuentes, D.; Elliott, A.A.; Weinberg, J.S.; Ahrar, K. Laser-induced thermal therapy for tumor ablation. *Crit. Rev. Biomed. Eng.* **2010**, *38*, 79–100. [CrossRef] [PubMed]
21. Longo, C.; Galimberti, M.; De Pace, B.; Pellacani, G.; Bencini, P.L. Laser skin rejuvenation: Epidermal changes and collagen remodeling evaluated by in vivo confocal microscopy. *Laser Med. Sci.* **2013**, *28*, 769–776. [CrossRef] [PubMed]
22. Chung, S.H.; Mazur, E. Surgical Applications of femtosecond lasers. *J. Biophotonics* **2009**, *2*, 557–572. [CrossRef] [PubMed]
23. Garvie-Cook, H.; Stone, J.M.; Yu, F.; Guy, R.H.; Gordeev, S.N. Femtosecond pulsed laser ablation to enhance drug delivery across the skin. *J. Biophotonics* **2016**, *9*, 144–154. [CrossRef] [PubMed]

24. Lee, W.-R.; Shen, S.-C.; Al-Suwayeh, S.A.; Yang, H.-H.; Yuan, C.-Y.; Fang, J.-Y. Laser-assisted topical drug delivery by using a low-fluence fractional laser: Imiquimod and macromolecules. *J. Control. Release* **2011**, *153*, 240–248. [CrossRef] [PubMed]

25. Lim, E.-H.; Kim, H.-R.; Park, Y.-O.; Lee, Y.; Seo, Y.-J.; Kim, C.-D.; Lee, J.-H.; Im, M. Toenail onychomycosis treated with a fractional carbon-dioxide laser and topical antifungal cream. *J. Am. Acad. Dermatol.* **2014**, *70*, 918–923. [CrossRef] [PubMed]

26. Stumpp, O.F.; Bedi, V.P.; Wyatt, D.; Lac, D.; Rahman, Z.; Chan, K.F. In vivo confocal imaging of epidermal cell migration and dermal changes post nonablative fractional resurfacing: Study of the wound healing process with corroborated histopathologic evidence. *J. Biomed. Opt.* **2009**, *14*, 024018. [CrossRef] [PubMed]

27. Hanson, K.M.; Behne, M.J.; Barry, N.P.; Mauro, T.M.; Gratton, E.; Clegg, R.M. Two-photon fluorescence lifetime imaging of the skin stratum corneum pH Gradient. *Biophys. J.* **2002**, *83*, 1682–1690. [CrossRef]

28. Xiao, C.; Moore, D.J.; Rerek, M.E.; Flach, C.R.; Mendelsohn, R. Feasibility of tracking phospholipid permeation into skin using infrared and Raman microscopic imaging. *J. Investig. Dermatol.* **2005**, *124*, 622–632. [CrossRef] [PubMed]

29. Huang, D.; Swanson, E.A.; Lin, C.P.; Schuman, J.S.; Stinson, W.G.; Chang, W.; Hee, M.R.; Flotte, T.; Gregory, K.; Puliafito, C.A. Optical coherence tomography. *Science* **1991**, *254*, 1178–1181. [CrossRef] [PubMed]

30. Ahmad, A.; Shemonski, N.D.; Adie, S.G.; Kim, H.-S.; Hwu, W.-M.W.; Carney, P.S.; Boppart, S.A. Real-time in vivo computed optical interferometric tomography. *Nat. Photonics* **2013**, *7*, 444–448. [CrossRef] [PubMed]

31. Wu, C.T.; Tsai, M.T.; Lee, C.K. Two-level optical coherence tomography scheme for suppressing spectral saturation artifacts. *Sensors* **2014**, *14*, 13548–13555. [CrossRef] [PubMed]

32. Deka, G.; Wu, W.-W.; Kao, F.-J. In vivo wound healing diagnosis with second harmonic and fluorescence lifetime imaging. *J. Biomed. Opt.* **2013**, *18*, 061222. [CrossRef] [PubMed]

33. Yeh, A.T.; Kao, B.; Jung, W.G.; Chen, Z.P.; Nelson, J.S.; Tromberg, B.J. Imaging wound healing using optical coherence tomography and multiphoton microscopy in an in vitro skin-equivalent tissue model. *J. Biomed. Opt.* **2006**, *9*, 248–253. [CrossRef] [PubMed]

34. Cobb, M.J.; Chen, Y.; Underwood, R.A.; Usui, M.L.; Olerud, J.; Li, X.D. Noninvasive assessment of cutaneous wound healing using ultrahigh-resolution optical coherence tomography. *J. Biomed. Opt.* **2006**, *11*, 064002. [CrossRef] [PubMed]

35. Wang, H.; Baran, U.; Wang, R.K. In vivo blood flow imaging of inflammatory human skin induced by tape stripping using optical microangiography. *J. Biophotonics* **2015**, *8*, 265–272. [CrossRef] [PubMed]

36. Liu, G.; Jia, W.; Sun, V.; Choi, B.; Chen, Z. High-resolution imaging of microvasculature in human skin in vivo with optical coherence tomography. *Opt. Express* **2012**, *20*, 7694–7705. [CrossRef] [PubMed]

37. Sakai, S.; Yamanari, M.; Miyazawa, A.; Matsumoto, M.; Nakagawa, N.; Sugawara, T.; Kawabata, K.; Yatagai, T.; Yasuno, Y. In vivo three-dimensional birefringence analysis shows collagen differences between young and old photo-aged human skin. *J. Investig. Dermatol.* **2008**, *128*, 1641–1647. [CrossRef] [PubMed]

38. Sakai, S.; Yamanari, M.; Lim, Y.; Nakagawa, N.; Yasuno, Y. In vivo evaluation of human skin anisotropy by polarization-sensitive optical coherence tomography. *Biomed. Opt. Express* **2011**, *2*, 2623–2631. [CrossRef] [PubMed]

39. Nguyen, T.-M.; Song, S.; Arnal, B.; Huang, Z.; O'Donnell, M.; Wang, R.K. Visualizing ultrasonically induced shear wave propagation using phase-sensitive optical coherence tomography for dynamic elastography. *Opt. Lett.* **2014**, *39*, 838–841. [CrossRef] [PubMed]

40. Wang, S.; Larin, K.V. Optical Coherence Elastography for Tissue Characterization: A Review. *J. Biophotonics* **2015**, *8*, 279–302. [CrossRef] [PubMed]

41. Tsai, M.-T.; Yang, C.-H.; Shen, S.-C.; Lee, Y.-J.; Chang, F.-Y.; Feng, C.-S. Monitoring of wound healing process of human skin after fractional laser treatments with optical coherence tomography. *Biomed. Opt. Express* **2013**, *4*, 2362–2375. [CrossRef] [PubMed]

42. Yang, C.-H.; Tsai, M.-T.; Shen, S.-C.; Ng, C.Y.; Jung, S.-M. Feasibility of ablative fractional laser-assisted drug delivery with optical coherence tomography. *Biomed. Opt. Express* **2014**, *5*, 3949–3959. [CrossRef] [PubMed]

43. Mariampillai, A.; Standish, B.A.; Moriyama, E.H.; Khurana, M.; Munce, N.R.; Leung, M.K.; Jiang, J.; Cable, A.; Wilson, B.C.; Vitkin, I.A. Speckle variance detection of microvasculature using swept-source optical coherence tomography. *Opt. Lett.* **2008**, *33*, 1530–1532. [CrossRef] [PubMed]

44. Cadotte, D.W.; Mariampillai, A.; Cadotte, A.; Lee, K.K.; Kiehl, T.-R.; Wilson, B.C.; Fehlings, M.G.; Yang, V.X. Speckle variance optical coherence tomography of the rodent spinal cord: In vivo feasibility. *Biomed. Opt. Express* **2012**, *3*, 911–919. [CrossRef] [PubMed]

45. Lee, C.-K.; Tseng, H.-Y.; Lee, C.-Y.; Wu, S.-Y.; Chi, T.-T.; Yang, K.-M.; Chou, H.-Y.E.; Tsai, M.-T.; Wang, J.-Y.; Kiang, Y.-W. Characterizing the localized surface plasmon resonance behaviors of Au nanorings and tracking their diffusion in bio-tissue with optical coherence tomography. *Biomed. Opt. Express* **2010**, *1*, 1060–1074. [CrossRef] [PubMed]

46. Mahmud, M.S.; Cadotte, D.W.; Vuong, B.; Sun, C.; Luk, T.W.; Mariampillai, A.; Yang, V.X. Review of speckle and phase variance optical coherence tomography to visualize microvascular networks. *J. Biomed. Opt.* **2013**, *18*, 050901. [CrossRef] [PubMed]

47. Murthy, S.N.; Vaka, S.R.K.; Sammeta, S.M.; Nair, A.B. Transcreen-N™: Method for rapid screening of trans-ungual drug delivery enhancers. *J. Pharm. Sci.* **2009**, *98*, 4264–4271. [CrossRef] [PubMed]

48. Tsai, M.-T.; Yang, C.-H.; Shen, S.-C.; Chang, F.-Y.; Yi, J.-Y.; Fan, C.-H. Noninvasive characterization of fractional photothermolysis induced by ablative and non-ablative lasers with optical coherence tomography. *Laser Phys.* **2013**, *23*, 075604. [CrossRef]

49. Wijesinghe, R.E.; Lee, S.-Y.; Kim, P.; Jung, H.-Y.; Jeon, M.; Kim, J. Optical Inspection and Morphological Analysis of Diospyros kaki Plant Leaves for the Detection of Circular Leaf Spot Disease. *Sensors* **2016**, *16*, 1282. [CrossRef] [PubMed]

Permissions

List of Contributors

Prince Manta and Deepak N. Kapoor
School of Pharmaceutical Sciences, Shoolini University of Biotechnology and Management Sciences, Solan 173212, India

Rupak Nagraik and Avinash Sharma
School of Bioengineering and Food Technology, Shoolini University of Biotechnology and Management Sciences, Solan 173212, India

Akshay Kumar
Department of Surgery, Medanta Hospital, Gurugram 122001, India

Pritt Verma and Shravan Kumar Paswan
Departments of Pharmacology, CSIR-National Botanical Research Institute, Lucknow 226001, India

Dmitry O. Bokov
Institute of Pharmacy, Sechenov First Moscow State Medical University, 8 Trubetskaya St., Moscow 119991, Russia

Juber Dastagir Shaikh
Department of Neurology, MGM Newbombay Hospital, Vashi, Navi Mumbai 400703, India

Roopvir Kaur
Department of Anesthesiology, Government Medical College, Amritsar 143001, India

Ana Francesca Vommaro Leite and Silas Jose Braz Filho
Department of Medicine, University of Minas Gerais, Passos 37902-313, Brazil

Nimisha Shiwalkar
Department of Anesthesiology, MGM Hospital, Navi Mumbai 410209, India

Purnadeo Persaud
Department of Medicine, Kansas City University, Kansas City, MO 64106, USA

Marius Albrecht and Julia Walther
Department of Medical Physics and Biomedical Engineering, Technische Universitaet Dresden, Carl Gustav Carus Faculty of Medicine, Fetscherstraße 74, 01307 Dresden, Germany

Maksim Zibin
«DIAMANT» Dental Clinic, 443090 Samara, Russia

Christian Schnabel
Department of Medical Physics and Biomedical Engineering, Technische Universitaet Dresden, Carl Gustav Carus Faculty of Medicine, Fetscherstraße 74, 01307 Dresden, Germany
Department of Anesthesiology and Intensive Care Medicine, Technische Universität Dresden, Clinical Sensing and Monitoring, Carl Gustav Carus Faculty of Medicine, Fetscherstraße 74, 01307 Dresden, Germany

Juliane Mueller, Jonas Golde and Edmund Koch
Department of Anesthesiology and Intensive Care Medicine, Technische Universität Dresden, Clinical Sensing and Monitoring, Carl Gustav Carus Faculty of Medicine, Fetscherstraße 74, 01307 Dresden, Germany

Masayuki Tanabe and Makiko Kobayashi
Faculty of Advanced Science and Technology, Kumamoto University, Kumamoto 8608555, Japan

Tai Chieh Wu and Che Hua Yang
College of Mechanical and Electrical Engineering, National Taipei University of Technology, Taipei 10608, Taiwan

Elena Timchenko and Pavel Timchenko
Department of Laser and Biotechnical Systems, Samara National Research University, 443086 Samara, Russia

Larisa Volova
Research and Production Center "Samara Tissue Bank", Samara State Medical University, 443079 Samara, Russia

Oleg Frolov
Department of Physics, Samara National Research University, 443086 Samara, Russia

Irina Bazhutova
Department of Dentistry, Samara State Medical University, 443079 Samara, Russia

Harald Studer
Eye Clinic Orasis, Swiss Eye Research Foundation, CH-5734 Reinach, Switzerland
OCTlab, Department of Ophthalmology, University of Basel, CH-4001 Basel, Switzerland

Rufeng Li, Yibei Wang, Hong Xu and Binjie Qin
School of Biomedical Engineering, Shanghai Jiao Tong University, Shanghai 200240, China

Baowei Fei
Emory University School of Medicine, Georgia Institute of Technology, Atlanta, GA 30329 USA

Chih-Ling Huang
Center for Fundamental Science, Kaohsiung Medical University, Kaohsiung 807, Taiwan

Meng-Jia Lian and Wei-Ming Chen
School of Dentistry, College of Dental Medicine, Kaohsiung Medical University, Kaohsiung 807, Taiwan

Yi-Hsuan Wu
Department of Medicinal and Applied Chemistry, College of Life Science, Kaohsiung Medical University, Kaohsiung 807, Taiwan

Wen-Tai Chiu
Department of Biomedical Engineering, National Cheng Kung University, Tainan 701, Taiwan

Brigitte Pajic-Eggspuehler and Joerg Mueller
Eye Clinic Orasis, Swiss Eye Research Foundation, CH-5734 Reinach, Switzerland

Zeljka Cvejic
Department of Physics, Faculty of Sciences, University of Novi Sad, Trg Dositeja Obradovica 4, 21000 Novi Sad, Serbia

Bojan Pajic
Eye Clinic Orasis, Swiss Eye Research Foundation, CH-5734 Reinach, Switzerland
Department of Physics, Faculty of Sciences, University of Novi Sad, Trg Dositeja Obradovica 4, 21000 Novi Sad, Serbia
Division of Ophthalmology, Department of Clinical Neurosciences, Geneva University Hospitals, CH-1205 Geneva, Switzerland
Faculty of Medicine of the Military Medical academy, University of Defence, 11000 Belgrade, Serbia

Su-Chin Shen
Department of Ophthalmology, Chang Gung Memorial Hospital, Linkou 33305, Taiwan
College of Medicine, Chang Gung University, Taoyuan 33302, Taiwan

Olga Streltsova, Anton Kuyarov and Muhhamad Shuaib Abdul Malik Molvi
E.V. Shakhov Department of Urology, Privolzhsky Research Medical University, 10/1 Minin and Pozharsky Sq., 603950 Nizhny Novgorod, Russia

Svetlana Zubova
N.A. Semashko Nizhny Novgorod Regional Clinical Hospital, 190 Rodionova St., 603126 Nizhny Novgorod, Russia

Valery Lazukin
Department of Medical Physics and Informatics, Privolzhsky Research Medical University, 10/1 Minin and Pozharsky Sq., 603950 Nizhny Novgorod, Russia

Ekaterina Tararova
Nizhny Novgorod Regional Oncology Dispensary, 190 Rodionova St., 603126 Nizhny Novgorod, Russia

Elena Kiseleva
Institute of Experimental Oncology and Biomedical Technologies, Privolzhsky Research Medical University, 10/1 Minin and Pozharsky Sq., 603950 Nizhny Novgorod, Russia

Byung Jun Park, Seung Rag Lee, Hyun Jin Bang, Byung Yeon Kim, Jeong Hun Park, Dong Guk Kim and Young Jae Won
Medical Device Development Center, Osong Medical Innovation Foundation, Cheongju, Chungbuk 361-951, Korea

Sung Soo Park
Department of Surgery, Korea University College of Medicine, Seoul 02841, Korea

Mitra Almasian, Leah S. Wilk, Daniel M. de Bruin, Paul R. Bloemen and Ton G. van Leeuwen
Department of Biomedical Engineering & Physics, Academic Medical Center, University of Amsterdam, 1105 AZ Amsterdam, The Netherlands

Sanne M. Jansen
Department of Biomedical Engineering & Physics, Academic Medical Center, University of Amsterdam, 1105 AZ Amsterdam, The Netherlands
Department of Plastic, Reconstructive & Hand Surgery, Academic Medical Center, University of Amsterdam, 1105 AZ Amsterdam, The Netherlands

Simon D. Strackee
Department of Plastic, Reconstructive & Hand Surgery, Academic Medical Center, University of Amsterdam, 1105 AZ Amsterdam, The Netherlands

Mark I. van Berge Henegouwen and Suzanne S. Gisbertz
Department of Surgery, Academic Medical Center, University of Amsterdam, 1105 AZ Amsterdam, The Netherlands

Sybren L. Meijer
Department of Pathology, Academic Medical Center, University of Amsterdam, 1105 AZ Amsterdam, The Netherlands

Udaya Wijenayake and Soon-Yong Park
School of Computer Science and Engineering, Kyungpook National University, 80 Daehakro, Bukgu, Daegu 41566, Korea

Jiří Přibil and Ivan Frollo
Institute of Measurement Science, Slovak Academy of Sciences, 841 04 Bratislava, Slovak Republic

Anna Přibilová
Faculty of Electrical Engineering and Information Technology, Slovak University of Technology in Bratislava, 812 19 Bratislava, Slovak Republic

Tatsuto Iida, Shunsuke Kiya and Kosuke Kubota
Department of Systems Life Engineering, Maebashi Institute of Technology, Maebashi 371-0816, Japan

Yasutomo Nomura
Department of Systems Life Engineering, Maebashi Institute of Technology, Maebashi 371-0816, Japan
Laboratory for Nano-Bio Probes, RIKEN Center for Biosystems Dynamics Research, Suita 565-0874, Japan

Takashi Jin
Laboratory for Nano-Bio Probes, RIKEN Center for Biosystems Dynamics Research, Suita 565-0874, Japan

Akitoshi Seiyama
Human Health Sciences, Graduate School of Medicine, Kyoto University, Kyoto 606-8507, Japan

Robert Bogdanowicz and Michał Sobaszek
Faculty of Electronics, Telecommunications and Informatics, Gdansk University of Technology, Narutowicza 11/12, 80-233 Gdansk, Poland

Paweł Niedziałkowski, Wioleta Białobrzeska, Zofia Cebula and Tadeusz Ossowski
Department of Analytical Chemistry, Faculty of Chemistry, University of Gdansk, Wita Stwosza 63, 80-308 Gdansk, Poland

Dariusz Burnat and Mateusz Śmietana
Institute of Microelectronics and Optoelectronics, Warsaw University of Technology, Koszykowa 75, 00-662 Warszawa, Poland

Petr Sezemsky and Vitezslav Stranak
Institute of Physics and Biophysics, Faculty of Science, University of South Bohemia, Branisovska 1760, 370 05 Ceske Budejovice, Czech Republic

Marcin Koba
Institute of Microelectronics and Optoelectronics, Warsaw University of Technology, Koszykowa 75, 00-662 Warszawa, Poland
National Institute of Telecommunications, Szachowa 1, 04-894 Warszawa, Poland

Mengqi Zhu, Zhonghua Huang, Chao Ma and Yinlin Li
School of Mechatronical Engineering, Beijing Institute of Technology, Beijing 100081, China

Daniel M. Aebersold
Department of Radiation Oncology, Inselspital, Bern University Hospital, University of Bern, CH-3010 Bern, Switzerland

Andreas Eggspuehler
Department of Neurology, Schulthess Klinik, CH-8008 Zuerich, Switzerland

Frederik R. Theler
Optimo Medical, CH-2503 Biel, Switzerland

Harald P. Studer
Eye Clinic Orasis, Swiss Eye Research Foundation, CH-5734 Reinach, Switzerland
OCTlab, Department of Ophthalmology, University of Basel, CH-4001 Basel, Switzerland

Ting-Yen Tsai
Department of Electrical Engineering, Chang Gung University, Taoyuan 33302, Taiwan

Meng-Tsan Tsai
Department of Electrical Engineering, Chang Gung University, Taoyuan 33302, Taiwan
Medical Imaging Research Center, Institute for Radiological Research, Chang Gung University and Chang Gung Memorial Hospital at Linkou, Taoyuan 33302, Taiwan
Department of Dermatology, Chang Gung Memorial Hospital, Linkou 33305, Taiwan

Chau Yee Ng and Chih-Hsun Yang
Department of Dermatology, Chang Gung Memorial Hospital, Linkou 33305, Taiwan
College of Medicine, Chang Gung University, Taoyuan 33302, Taiwan

Ya-Ju Lee
Institute of Electro-Optical Science and Technology, National Taiwan Normal University, Taipei 11677, Taiwan

Jiann-Der Lee
Department of Electrical Engineering, Chang Gung University, Taoyuan 33302, Taiwan
Department of Neurosurgery, Chang Gung Memorial Hospital, LinKou 33305, Taiwan

Index